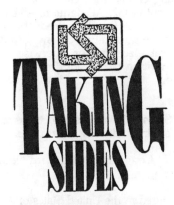

TAKING SIDES

Clashing Views on Controversial Bioethical Issues

4th edition

Edited, Selected, and with Introductions by

Carol Levine

The Dushkin Publishing Group, Inc.

Taking Sides ® is a registered trademark of
The Dushkin Publishing Group, Inc.

Library of Congress Catalog Card Number:
90-84858

Manufactured in the United States of America

Fourth Edition, Third Printing
ISBN: 0-87967-936-0

Printed on Recycled Paper

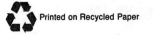

The Dushkin Publishing Group, Inc.
Sluice Dock, Guilford, CT 06437

PREFACE

This is a book about choices—hard and tragic choices. The choices are hard not only because they often involve life and death but also because there are convincing arguments on both sides of the issues. An ethical dilemma, by definition, is one that poses a conflict not between good and evil but between one good principle and another that is equally good. The choices are hard because the decisions that are made—by individuals, groups, and public policy makers—will influence the kind of society we have today and the one we will have in the future.

Although the views expressed in the selections in this volume are strong—even passionate—ones, they are also subtle ones, concerned with the nuances of the particular debate. *How* one argues matters in bioethics; you will see and have to weigh the significance of varying rhetorical styles and appeals throughout this volume.

Although there are no easy answers to any of the issues in the book, the questions will be answered in some fashion—partly by individual choices and partly by decisions that are made by professionals and government. We must make them the best answers possible, and that can only be done by informed and thoughtful consideration. This book, then, can serve as a beginning for what ideally will become an ongoing process of examination and reflection.

Changes to this edition Although I have retained the basic structure of the third edition, I have made some significant internal changes. There are eight entirely new issues: *Should Thawing Unused Frozen Embryos Be Permitted?* (Issue 2); *The Maternal-Fetal Relationship: Can Compelled Medical Treatment of Pregnant Women Be Justified?* (Issue 4); *Is Physician-Assisted Suicide Ethical?* (Issue 6); *Should Surgical Patients Be Screened for HIV?* (Issue 10); *Do Physicians Have an Ethical Duty to Treat AIDS Patients?* (Issue 11); *Should Ethical Standards of International Research Be "Culturally Relevant"?* (Issue 13); *Should Dying Patients Have Greater Access to Experimental Drugs?* (Issue 20); and *Should the United States Follow the Canadian Model of a National Health Program?* (Issue 21). Two of these new issues (Issue 13 and Issue 21) reflect the trend toward considering international dimensions of biomedical ethics.

For four issues, I have retained the issue from the previous edition but have replaced one of the selections in order to more sharply focus the debate or to bring the debate up to date. The more straightforward of these substitutions are found in *Are There Limits to Confidentiality?* (Issue 8) and *Should Animal Experimentation Be Permitted?* (Issue 15). For the remaining two substitutions, a word of explanation may avoid confusion among users familiar with the third edition. For *Is There a Moral Right to Abortion?* (Issue 1) and *Is It Ever Morally Right to Withhold Food and Water from Dying Patients?* (Issue 7), I have only substituted one selection but have also rephrased the questions to make the readings more

i

compatible. The authors whose writings remain from the third edition have not changed their minds; I have changed the question and the order in which the readings appear. For Issue 7, a reading from a previous edition has been brought back by popular demand.

In all, 20 new readings are included in this edition. Part introductions, issue introductions, and postscripts have been revised as necessary.

Supplements An *Instructor's Manual with Test Questions* (multiple-choice and essay) is available through the publisher, and a general guidebook, *Using Taking Sides in the Classroom*, which discusses methods and techniques for using the pro-contra approach in any classroom setting, is also available.

Acknowledgments I received helpful comments and suggestions from the many users of *Taking Sides* across the United States and Canada. Their suggestions have enhanced the quality of this edition of the book and are reflected in the new selections and issues.

Special thanks go to those who responded with specific suggestions for the fourth edition:

Keith Boone
Denison University

Thomas E. Brown
Atlantic Community College

John Engelhard
Hope College

Marc D. Hiller
University of New Hampshire

David James
Old Dominion University

Lawrence R. Krupka
Michigan State University

Joe Mosca
Monmouth College

Connie Veldink
Everett Community College

Allen D. Verhey
Hope College

For this edition, Lauri Posner was an invaluable researcher, commentator, critic, and one-person support system. She also prepared the *Instructor's Manual*. Marna Howarth and Julie Rothstein of The Hastings Center staff responded to inquiries efficiently, promptly, and with great good humor. For their assistance in previous editions, which gave me a solid base from which to proceed, I want to thank Paul Homer, Eric Feldman, and Arthur Caplan. I would particularly like to thank Daniel Callahan, director of The Hastings Center, and William Gaylin, its president, for their early encouragement in this project. Although I am no longer on the staff of the Center, I continue to benefit from that experience. Finally, I dedicate this edition to the memory of my father, King Solomon, who died in January 1989; and to my granddaughter, Hannah Levine Pickar, who was born in October 1990.

Carol Levine
New York City

CONTENTS IN BRIEF

CONTENTS

Professor of Christian ethics Beverly Wildung Harrison argues that women ought to decide whether or not to bear children on the basis of their own moral preparedness to become mothers. Psychologist Sidney Callahan asserts that a woman's moral obligation to continue a pregnancy arises from both her status as a member of the human community and her unique life-giving female reproductive power.

The American Medical Association's Board of Trustees concludes that the man and woman who provided the sperm and egg should decide about the disposition of an unused frozen embryo and that they may legally and ethically decide to thaw and dispose of it. Philosopher David T. Ozar argues that the responsible parties have a moral obligation to preserve frozen embryos until they are implanted in a woman's womb or can no longer survive implantation.

Professor of law John A. Robertson believes that infertile couples have a right
to arrange for a surrogate mother to bear the husband's child and that the
ethical and legal problems that might result are not very different from those
that already exist in adoption and artificial insemination by a donor. Professor of law Herbert T. Krimmel takes the position that it is immoral to bear a
child for the purpose of giving it up and that surrogate mother arrangements
will put additional strain on our society's shared moral values.

Physician Frank A. Chervenak and philosopher Laurence B. McCullough
argue that respect for maternal autonomy is not an absolute ethical principle
and that a physician's obligation to honor the autonomy of the mother must
be weighed against the obligation to promote the best interests of the fetus.
Philosopher Lawrence J. Nelson and physician Nancy Milliken believe that
the decision of a competent woman to forgo medical treatment likely to
benefit her fetus should not be overridden, even if others disagree with her
choice.

Physician Bernard C. Meyer argues that physicians must use discretion in
communicating bad news to patients. Adherence to a rigid formula of truth
telling fails to appreciate the differences among patients in their readiness to
hear and understand the information. Philosopher Sissela Bok challenges the
traditional physicians' view by arguing that the harm resulting from dis-

closure is less than they think and is outweighed by the benefits, including the important one of giving the patient the right to choose among treatments.

Physician Sidney H. Wanzer and a group of nine other physicians believe that it is not immoral for a physician to assist in the rational suicide of a terminally ill person. Physician and lawyer David Orentlicher argues that treatment designed to bring on death, by definition, does not heal and is therefore fundamentally inconsistent with the physician's role.

Physician Joanne Lynn and professor of religious studies James F. Childress claim that nutrition and hydration are not morally different from other life-sustaining medical treatments that may on occasion be withheld or withdrawn, according to the patient's best interest. Professor of religion Gilbert Meilaender asserts that removing the ordinary human care of feeding aims to kill and is morally wrong.

Physician Mark Siegler declares that medical confidentiality, as it has traditionally been understood by patients and doctors, has been eradicated by third-party interests and modern medical practice. Physician Michael H. Kottow argues that any breach of patient confidentiality causes harms that are more serious than hypothetical benefits.

Psychiatrist Thomas S. Szasz maintains that the detention of persons in mental institutions against their will is a crime against humanity. People are committed not because they are "mentally ill" or "dangerous" but because society wants to control their behavior. Psychiatrist Paul Chodoff believes that the rights of the mentally ill to be treated are being set aside in the rush to give them their freedom. He favors a return to the use of medical criteria by psychiatrists, albeit with legal safeguards.

Surgeon Robert W. M. Frater and physician assistant Douglas Condit argue that preoperative HIV screening is in the best interests of patients, health care workers, and employers as long as it is performed in an atmosphere of confidentiality and mandatory, supportive counseling. Surgeon Lynn Peterson believes that from both a practical and ethical point of view, physicians should not rely on preoperative HIV screening for their own protection but should instead follow universal infection control procedures.

Philosopher Albert R. Jonsen asserts that refusing treatment in specific cases, because it is inconvenient, risky, or burdensome, casts a shadow on the most precious value of medicine, its commitment to service. Attorney James W. Tegtmeier argues that it is improper to assert that physicians have an ethical duty to treat individuals with AIDS because the grounds for imposing such a duty are too weak to support that conclusion.

The late psychologist Stanley Milgram believed that the central moral justification for allowing deceptive experiments is that the vast majority of subjects who take part in them find them acceptable after the rationale is explained. Social psychologist Diana Baumrind argues that the costs of using deception in research to subjects, the profession, and society outweigh any benefits.

Physician and researcher Michele Barry believes that basic ethical principles that guide human investigation must be interpreted in ways that are appropriate to different cultural settings, many of which were unfamiliar to the international bodies that originally formulated these principles. Physician and journal editor Marcia Angell argues that just as *scientific* standards cannot be compromised because of local traditions, so too with ethical standards.

system of routine removal, in which physicians would retrieve organs from newly-dead persons unless the next of kin refuses.

Pediatric surgeon Michael R. Harrison believes that if anencephalic newborns were treated as brain-dead rather than as brain-absent, their organs could be transplanted and their families could be offered the consolation that their loss provided life for another child. Philosopher John D. Arras and pediatric neurologist Shlomo Shinnar argue that the current principles of the strict definition of brain death are sound public policy and good ethics.

Attorney Lori B. Andrews believes that donors, recipients, and society will benefit from a market in body parts so long as owners—and no one else—retain control over their bodies. Ethicist Thomas H. Murray argues that the gift relationship should govern transfer of body parts because it honors important human values, which are diminished by market relationships.

Philosopher Daniel Callahan believes that government has an obligation to provide those health care resources that help people live out a natural life span. Beyond that point, only the means necessary for the relief of suffering, not those for life-extending technology, should be provided. Sociologist Amitai Etzioni argues that rationing health care for the elderly would encourage conflict between generations and would invite restrictions on health care for other groups.

Physician Nathaniel Pier argues that the current, cautious system of drug approval consigns large numbers of people with AIDS to death, without giving them the dignity of a chance to fight back by taking experimental medications. Physician Douglas D. Richman believes that unproven therapies are unlikely to prolong life or improve its quality and instead have significant potential for harm.

Physicians Steffie Woolhandler and David U. Himmelstein propose a sweeping reform of health care financing, following the Canadian model of a single-source system of payment, to ensure equity of access and efficiency. Physician Ronald Bronow, on behalf of an organization entitled Physicians Who Care, believes that problems of underfinancing and rationing in the Canadian system would be magnified in the American setting.

INTRODUCTION

Medicine and Moral Arguments
Carol Levine

In the fall of 1975, a twenty-one-year-old woman lay in a New Jersey hospital—as she had for months—in a coma, the victim of a toxic combination of barbiturates and alcohol. Doctors agreed that her brain was irreversibly damaged and that she would never recover. Her parents, after anguished consultation with their priest, asked the doctors and hospital to disconnect the respirator that was artificially maintaining their daughter's life. When the doctors and hospital refused, the parents petitioned the court to be made her legal guardian so that they could authorize the withdrawal of treatment. After hearing all the arguments, the court sided with the parents, and the respirator was removed. Contrary to everyone's expectations, however, the young woman did not die but began to breathe on her own (perhaps because, in anticipation of the court order, the nursing staff had gradually weaned her from total dependence on the respirator). She lived for ten years until her death in June 1985—comatose, lying in a fetal position and fed with tubes—in a New Jersey nursing home.

The young woman's name was Karen Ann Quinlan, and her case brought national attention to the thorny ethical questions raised by modern medical technology: When, if ever, should life-sustaining technology be withdrawn? Is the sanctity of life an absolute value? What kinds of treatment are really beneficial to a patient in a "chronic vegetative state" like Karen's? And, perhaps the most troubling question, who shall decide? These and similar questions are at the heart of the growing field of biomedical ethics or (as it is usually called) *bioethics*.

Ethical dilemmas in medicine are, of course, nothing new. They have been recognized and discussed in Western medicine since a small group of physicians—led by Hippocrates—on the Isle of Cos in Greece, around the fourth century B.C., subscribed to a code of practice that newly graduated physicians still swear to uphold today. But unlike earlier times, when physicians and scientists had only limited abilities to change the course of disease, today they can intervene in profound ways in the most fundamental processes of life and death. Moreover, ethical dilemmas in medicine are no longer considered the sole province of professionals. Professional codes of ethics, to be sure, offer some guidance, but they are usually unclear and ambiguous about what to do in specific situations. More important, these codes assume that whatever decision is to be made is up to the professional, not the patient. Today, to an ever-greater degree, lay people—patients, families, lawyers, clergy, and others—want to and have become involved in ethical decision-making not only in individual cases, such as the Quinlan case, but also in large societal decisions, such as how to allocate scarce medical resources, including high-technology machinery, newborn intensive care units, and the expertise of physicians. While questions about the physician-patient relationship and individual cases are still prominent in bioethics (see, for example, Issue 5 on truth-telling and Issue 6 on assisting dying patients in suicide), today the field covers a broad range of other decisions as well, such as the harvesting of organs (Issues 16 and 17), containing the costs of health care (Issues 19 and 21), and the future of animal experimentation (Issue 15).

This involvement is part of broader social trends: a general disenchantment with the authority of all professionals and, hence, a greater readiness to challenge the traditional belief that "doctor knows best"; the growth of various civil rights movements among women, the aged, and minorities—of which the patients' rights movement is a spin-off; the enormous size and complexity of the health care delivery system, in which patients and families often feel alienated from the professional; the increasing cost of medical care, much of it at public expense; and the growth of the "medical model" in which conditions that used to be considered outside the scope of physicians' control, such as alcoholism and behavioral problems, have come to be considered diseases.

Bioethics began in the 1950s as an intellectual movement among a small group of physicians and theologians who started to examine the questions raised by the new medical technologies that were starting to emerge as the result of the heavy expenditure of public funds in medical research after World War II. They were soon joined by a number of philosophers who had become disillusioned with what they saw as the arid abstractions of much analytic philosophy at the time, and by lawyers who sought to find principles in the law that would guide ethical decision-making or, if such principles were not there, to develop them by case law and legislation or regulation. Although these four disciplines—medicine, theology, philosophy, and law—still dominate the field, today bioethics is an interdisciplinary effort, with political scientists, economists, sociologists, anthropologists, nurses, allied health professionals, policymakers, psychologists, and others contributing their special perspectives to the ongoing debates.

The issues discussed in this volume attest to the wide range of bioethical dilemmas, their complexity, and the passion they arouse. But if bioethics today is at the frontiers of scientific knowledge, it is also a field with ancient roots. It goes back to the most basic questions of human life: What is right? What is wrong? How should people act toward others? And why?

While the *bio* part of *bioethics* gives the field its urgency and immediacy, we should not forget that the root word is *ethics.*

APPLYING ETHICS TO MEDICAL DILEMMAS

To see where bioethics fits into the larger framework of academic inquiry, some definitions are in order. First, *morality* is the general term for an individual's or a society's standards of conduct, both actual and ideal, and of the character traits that determine whether people are considered "good" or "bad." The scientific study of morality is called *descriptive ethics*; a scientist— generally an anthropologist, sociologist, or historian—can describe in empirical terms what the moral beliefs, judgments, or actions of individuals or societies are and what reasons are given for the way they act or what they believe. The philosophical study of morality, on the other hand, approaches the subject of morality in one of two different ways: either as an analysis of the concepts, terms, and methods of reasoning (*metaethics*) or as an analysis of what those standards or moral judgments ought to be (*normative ethics*). Metaethics deals with meanings of moral terms and logic; normative ethics, with which the issues in this volume are concerned, reflects on the kinds of actions and principles that will promote moral behavior.

Because normative ethics accepts the idea that some acts and character traits are more moral than others (and that some are immoral), it rejects the rather popular idea that ethics is relative. Because different societies have different moral codes and values, ethical relativists have argued that there can be no universal moral judgments: What is right or wrong depends on who does it and where, and whether society approves. Although it is certainly true that moral values are embedded in a social, cultural, and political context, it is also true that certain moral judgments are universal. We think it is wrong, for example, to sell people into slavery—whether or not a certain society approved or even whether or not the person wanted to be a slave. People may not agree about what these universal moral values are or ought to be, but it is hard to deny that some such values exist. This issue is tackled directly in Issue 13, which discusses the conflict between cultural relevancy and universal standards in the context of clinical research.

The other relativistic view rejected by normative ethics is the notion that whatever feels good *is* good. In this view, ethics is a matter of personal preference, weightier than one's choice of which automobile to buy, but not much different in kind. Different people, having different feelings, can arrive at equally valid moral judgments, according to the relativistic view. Just as we should not disregard cultural factors, we should not overlook the role of emotion and personal experience in arriving at moral judgments. But to give emotion ultimate authority would be to consign reason and rationality—the bases of moral argument—to the ethical trash heap. At the very least, it would be impossible to develop a just policy concerning the care of vulnerable persons, like the mentally retarded or newborns, who depend solely on the vagaries of individual caretakers.

Thus, if normative ethics is one branch of philosophy, bioethics is one branch of normative ethics; it is normative ethics applied to the practice of medicine and science. There are other branches—business ethics, legal ethics, journalism ethics, and military ethics, for example. One common term for the entire grouping is *applied and professional ethics*, because these ethics deal with the ethical standards of the members of a particular profession and how they are applied in the professionals' dealings with each other and the rest of society. Bioethics is based on the belief that some solutions to the dilemmas that arise in medicine and science are more moral than others and that these solutions can be determined by moral reasoning and reflection.

ETHICAL THEORIES

If the practitioners of bioethics do not rely solely on cultural norms and emotions, what are their sources of determining what is right or wrong? The most comprehensive source is a theory of ethics—a broad set of moral principles (or perhaps just one overriding principle) that is used in measuring human conduct. Divine law is one such source, of course, but even in the Western religious traditions of bioethics (both the Jewish and Catholic religions have rich and comprehensive commentaries on ethical issues, and the Protestant religion a less cohesive but still important tradition) the law of God is interpreted in terms of human moral principles. A theory of ethics must be acceptable to many groups, not just the followers of one religious tradition. Most writers outside the religious traditions (and some within them) have looked to one of three major traditions in ethics: teleological theories, deontological theories, and natural law theories.

Teleological Theories
Teleological theories are based on the idea that the end or purpose (from the Greek *telos* or end) of the action determines its rightness or wrongness. The most prominent teleological theory is *utilitarianism*. In its simplest formulation, an act is moral if it brings more good consequences than bad ones. Utilitarian theories are derived from the works of two English philosophers: Jeremy Bentham (1748–1832) and John Stuart Mill (1806–1873). Rejecting the absolutist religious morality of his time, Bentham proposed that "utility"— the greatest good for the greatest number—should guide the actions of human beings. Invoking the hedonistic philosophy of Epicurean Greeks, Bentham said that pleasure (*hedon* in Greek) is good and pain is bad. Therefore, actions are right if they promote more pleasure than pain and wrong if they promote more pain than pleasure. Mill found the highest utility in "happiness," rather than pleasure. (Mill's philosophy is echoed, you will recall, in the Declaration of Independence's espousal of "life, liberty, and the pursuit of happiness.") Other utilitarians have looked to a range of

utilities, or goods (including friendship, love, devotion, and the like) that they believe ought to be weighed in the balance—the utilitarian calculus.

Utilitarianism has a pragmatic appeal. It is flexible, and it seems impartial. However, its critics point out that utilitarianism can be used to justify suppression of individual rights for the good of society ("the ends justify the means") and that it is difficult to quantify and compare "utilities," however they are defined.

Utilitarianism, in its many forms, has had a powerful influence on bioethical discussion, partly because it is the closest to the case-by-case risk/benefit ratio that physicians use in clinical decision-making. Joseph Fletcher, a Protestant theologian who was one of the pioneers in bioethics in the 1950s, developed a utilitarian theory that he called *situation ethics*. He argued that a true Christian morality does not blindly follow moral rules but acts from love and sensitivity to the particular situation and the needs of those involved. He has enthusiastically supported most modern technologies on the grounds that they lead to good ends.

Other writers in this volume who use a utilitarian theory to arrive at their moral judgments are Bernard C. Meyer (Issue 5), who defends the withholding of the truth from dying patients on the grounds that it leads to better consequences than truth-telling; Lori B. Andrews (Issue 18), who supports a market in body parts; and Jerod M. Loeb and his colleagues (Issue 15), who defend animal research.

Deontological Theories

The second major type of ethical theory is *deontological* (from the Greek *deon* or duty). The rightness or wrongness of an act, these theories hold, should be judged on whether it conforms to a moral principle or rule, not on whether it leads to good or bad consequences. The primary exponent of a deontological theory was Immanuel Kant (1724–1804), a German philosopher. Kant declared that there is an ultimate norm, or supreme duty, which he called the "Moral Law." He held that an act is moral only if it springs from a "good will," the only thing that is good without qualification.

We must do good things, said Kant, because we have a duty to do them, not because they result in good consequences or because they give us pleasure (although that can happen as well). Kant constructed a formal "Categorical Imperative," the ultimate test of morality: "I ought never to act except in such a way that I can also will that my maxim should become universal law." Recognizing that this formulation was far from clear, Kant said the same thing in three other ways. He explained that a moral rule must be one that can serve as a guide for everyone's conduct; it must be one that permits people to treat each other as ends in themselves, not solely as means to another's ends; and it must be one that each person can impose on himself by his own will, not one that is solely imposed by the state, one's parents, or God. Kant's Categorical Imperative, in the simplest terms, says that all persons have equal moral worth and no rule can be moral unless all people can apply it autonomously to all other human beings. Although on its own, Kant's Categorical Imperative is merely a formal statement with no moral content at all, he gave some examples of what he meant: "Do not commit suicide," and "Help others in distress."

Kantian ethics is criticized by many who note that Kant gives little guidance on what to do when ethical principles conflict, as they often do. Moreover, they say, his emphasis on autonomous decision-making and individual will neglects the social and communal context in which people live and make decisions. It leads to isolation and unreality. These criticisms notwithstanding, Kantian ethics has stimulated much current thinking in bioethics. The idea that certain actions are in and of themselves right or wrong underlies, for example, Sissela Bok's appeal to truth-telling (Issue 5); Diana Baumrind's attack on deception in research (Issue 12); and Albert R. Jonsen's affirmation of a physician's duty to treat AIDS patients (Issue 11).

Two modern deontological theorists are the philosophers John Rawls and Robert M. Veatch. In *A Theory of Justice* (1971), Rawls places the highest value on equitable distribution of society's resources. He believes that society has a fundamental obligation to correct the inequalities of historical circumstance and natural endowment of its least well-off members. According to this theory, some action is good only if it benefits the least well-off. (It can also benefit others, but that is secondary.) His social justice theory has influenced bioethical writings concerning the allocation of scarce resources.

Robert M. Veatch has applied Rawlsian principles to medical ethics. In his book *A Theory of Medical Ethics* (1981), he offers a model of social contract among professionals, patients, and society that emphasizes mutual respect and responsibilities. This contract model will, he hopes, avoid the narrowness of professional codes of ethics and the generalities and ambiguities of more broadly based ethical theories.

Natural Law Theory

The third strain of ethical theory that is prominent in bioethics is *natural law theory*, first developed by St. Thomas Aquinas (1223–1274). According to this theory, actions are morally right if they accord with our nature as human beings. The attribute that is distinctively human is the ability to reason and to exercise intelligence. Thus, argues this theory, we can know the good, which is objective and can be learned through reason. References to natural law theory are prominent in the works of Catholic theologians and writers; they see natural law as ultimately derived from God, but knowable through the efforts of human beings. The influence of natural law theory can be seen in this volume in Sidney Callahan's pro-life feminist opposition to abortion (Issue 1) and Gilbert Meilaender's arguments against removing food and water from dying patients (Issue 7).

Theory of Virtue

The *theory of virtue*, another ethical theory with deep roots in the Aristotelian tradition, has recently been revived in bioethics. This theory stresses not the morality of any particular actions or rules but the disposition of individuals to act morally, to be virtuous. In its modern version, its primary exponent is Alasdair MacIntyre, whose book *After Virtue* (1980) urges a return to the Aristotelian model. Gregory Pence has applied the theory of virtue directly to medicine in *Ethical Options in Medicine* (1980); he lists temperance in personal life, compassion for the suffering patient, professional competence, justice, honesty, courage, and practical judgment as the virtues most desirable in physicians. Although this theory has not yet been as fully developed in bioethics as the utilitarian or deontological theories, it is likely to have particular appeal for physicians—many of which have resisted formal ethics education on the grounds that moral character is the critical factor and that one can best learn to be a moral physician by emulating one's mentors.

Although various authors, in this volume and elsewhere, appeal in rather direct ways to either utilitarian or deontological theories, often the various types are combined. One may argue both that a particular action is immoral in and of itself and that it will have bad consequences (some commentators say even Kant used this argument). In fact, probably no single ethical theory is adequate to deal with all the ramifications of the issues. In that case we can turn to a middle level of ethical discussion. Between the abstractions of ethical theories (Kant's Categorical Imperative) and the specifics of moral judgments (always obtain informed consent from a patient) is a range of concepts—ethical principles—that can be applied to particular cases.

ETHICAL PRINCIPLES

In its four years of deliberation, the National Commission for the Protection of Human Subjects of Biomedical and Behavioral Research grappled with some of the most difficult issues facing researchers and society: When, if ever, is it ethical to do research on the fetus, on children, or on people in mental institutions? This commission—which was composed of people from various religious backgrounds, professions, and social strata—was finally able to agree on specific recommendations on these questions, but only after they had finished their work did the commissioners try to determine what ethical principles they had used in reaching a consensus. In their Belmont Report (1978), named after the conference center where they met to discuss this question, the commissioners outlined what they considered to be the three most important ethical principles (respect for persons, beneficence, and justice) that should govern the conduct of research with human beings. These three principles, they believed, are generally accepted in our cultural tradition and can serve as basic justifications for the many particular ethical prescriptions and evaluations of human action. Because of the principles' general acceptance and widespread applicability, they are at the basis of most bioethical discussion. Although philosophers argue about whether other principles—preventing harm to others or loyalty, for example—ought to be accorded equal weight with these three or should be included under another umbrella, they agree that these principles are fundamental.

Respect for Persons
Respect for persons incorporates at least two basic ethical convictions, according to the Belmont Report. Individuals should be treated as autonomous agents, and persons with diminished autonomy are entitled to protection. The derivation from Kant is clear. Because human beings have the capacity for rational action and moral choice, they have a value independent of anything that they can do or provide to others. Therefore, they should be treated in a way that respects their independent choices and judgments. Respecting autonomy means giving weight to autonomous persons' considered opinions and choices, and refraining from interfering with their choices unless those choices are clearly detrimental to others. However, since the capacity for autonomy varies by age, mental disability, or other circumstances, those people whose autonomy is diminished must be protected—but only in ways that serve their interests and do not interfere with the level of autonomy that they do possess.

Two important moral rules are derived from the ethical principle of respect for persons: informed consent and truth-telling. Persons can exercise autonomy only when they have been fully informed about the range of options open to them, and the process of informed consent is generally considered to include the elements of information, comprehension, and voluntariness. Thus, a person can give informed consent to some medical procedure only if he or she has full information about the risks and benefits, understands them, and agrees voluntarily—that is, without being coerced or pressured into agreement. Although the principle of informed consent has become an accepted moral rule (and a legal one as well), it is difficult—some say impossible—to achieve in a real-world setting. It can easily be turned into a legalistic parody or avoided altogether. But as a moral ideal it serves to balance the unequal power of the physician and patient.

Another important moral ideal derived from the principle of respect for persons is truth-telling. It held a high place in Kant's theory. In his essay "The Supposed Right to Tell Lies from Benevolent Motives," he wrote: "If, then, we define a lie merely as an intentionally false declaration towards another man, we need not add that it must injure another . . . ; for it always injures another; if not another individual, yet mankind generally. . . . To be truthful in all declarations is therefore a sacred and conditional command of reasons, and not to be limited by any other expediency." (See Issue 5.)

Other important moral rules that are derived from the principle of respect for persons are confidentiality and privacy. (See Issue 8.)

Beneficence
Most physicians would probably consider beneficence (from the Latin *bene* or good) the most basic ethical principle. In the Hippocratic Oath it is used this

way: "I will apply dietetic measures for the benefit of the sick according to my ability and judgment; I will keep them from harm and injustice." And further on, "Whatever houses I may visit, I will comfort and benefit the sick, remaining free of all intentional injustice." The phrase *Primum non nocere* (First, do no harm) is another well-known version of this idea, but it appears to be a much later, Latinized version—not from the Hippocratic period.

The philosopher William Frankena has outlined four elements included in the principle of beneficence: (1) one ought not to inflict evil or harm; (2) one ought to prevent evil or harm; (3) one ought to remove evil or harm; and (4) one ought to do or promote good. Frankena arranged these elements in hierarchical order, so that the first takes precedence over the second, and so on. In this scheme, it is more important to avoid doing evil or harm than to do good. But in the Belmont Report, beneficence is understood as an obligation—first to do no harm, and second, to maximize possible benefits and minimize possible harms.

The principle of beneficence is at the basis of Joanne Lynn and James F. Childress's defense of withholding fluids and nutrition from some dying patients (Issue 7), and Paul Chodoff's defense of involuntary commitment of mental patients (Issue 9).

Justice

The third ethical principle that is generally accepted is justice, which means "what is fair" or "what is deserved." An injustice occurs when some benefit to which a person is entitled is denied without good reason or when some burden is imposed unduly, according to the Belmont Report. Another way of interpreting the principle is to say that equals should be treated equally. However, some distinctions—such as age, experience, competence, physical condition, and the like—can justify unequal treatment. Those who appeal to the principle of justice are most concerned about which distinctions can be made legitimately and which ones cannot. (See Issue 19.)

One important derivative of the principle of justice is the recent emphasis on "rights" in bioethics. Given the successes in the 1960s and 1970s of civil rights movements in the courts and political arena, it is easy to understand the appeal of "rights talk." An emphasis on individual rights is part of the American tradition, in a way that emphasis on the "common good" is not. The language of rights has been prominent in the abortion debate, for instance, where the "right to life" has been pitted against the "right to privacy" or the "right to control one's body." The "right to health care" is a potent rallying cry, though it is one that is difficult to enforce legally. Although claims to rights may be effective in marshaling political support and in emphasizing moral ideals, those rights may not be the most effective way to solve ethical dilemmas. Our society, as philosopher Ruth Macklin has pointed out, has not yet agreed on a theory of justice in health care that will determine who has what kinds of rights and—the other side of the coin—who has the obligation to fulfill them.

WHEN PRINCIPLES CONFLICT

These three fundamental ethical principles—beneficence, respect for persons, and justice—all carry weight in ethical decision-making. But what happens when they conflict? That is what this book is all about.

On each side of the issues included in this volume are writers who appeal, explicitly or implicitly, to one or more of these principles. For example, in Issue 9, Thomas S. Szasz sees respect for persons as paramount: Let people decide autonomously, he argues, whether or not they would wish to be treated in a psychiatric hospital. But Paul Chodoff looks to beneficence as the overriding principle, arguing that it is sometimes necessary to ignore autonomy in order to benefit people—and living a life without psychosis is clearly a benefit. In Issue 4, Frank A. Chervenak and Laurence B. McCullough appeal to justice to argue in favor of sometimes overriding a pregnant woman's decision to forgo medical treatment that might benefit her fetus. But Lawrence J. Nelson and Nancy Milliken see the woman's autonomy as more important: Let the woman decide, even if others disagree.

Some of the issues are concerned with how to interpret a particular principle: Whether, for example, it is more beneficent to allow a market in body parts (Issue 18); or whether a totally voluntary system of obtaining organs for transplant is more just than one that involves some required interventions (see Issue 16).

Will it ever be possible to resolve such fundamental divisions—those that are not merely matters of procedure or interpretation but of fundamental differences in principle? Lest the situation seem hopeless, consider that some consensus does seem to have been reached on questions that seemed equally tangled a few decades ago. The idea that government should play a role in regulating human subjects research was hotly debated, but it is now generally accepted (at least if the research is medical, not social or behavioral in nature, and is federally funded). And the appropriateness of using the criteria of brain death for determining the death of a person (and the possibility of subsequent removal of their organs for transplantation) has largely been accepted and written into state laws. The idea that a hopelessly ill patient has the legal and moral right to refuse treatment that will only prolong dying is also well established (though it is often hard to exercise because hospitals and physicians continue to resist it). Finally, nearly everyone now agrees that health care is distributed unjustly in this country—a radical idea only a few years ago. There is, of course, sharp disagreement about whose responsibility it is to rectify the situation—the government's or the private sector's.

Although there is consensus in some areas, in others there is only controversy. This book will introduce you to some of the ongoing debates. Whether we will be able to move beyond opposing views to a realm of moral consensus will depend on society's willingness to struggle with these issues and to make the hard choices that are required.

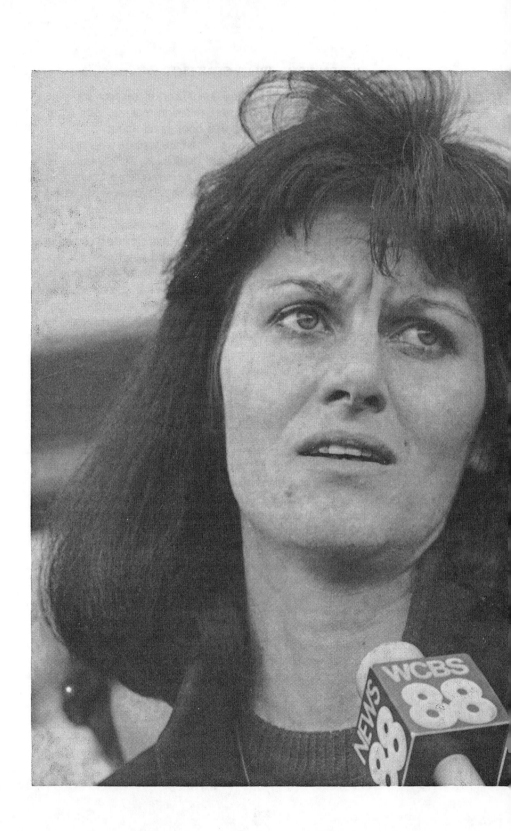

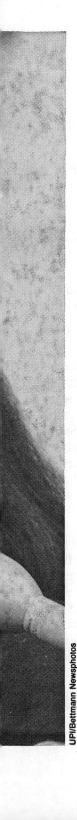

PART 1

Choices in Reproduction

Few bioethical issues could be of greater significance than questions concerning reproduction. This is an area fraught with conflicting and competing interests and precedents that have important implications for the future. Advances in medical technology, such as in vitro fertilization, frozen embryos, and changes in social mores that have made surrogate mothering more acceptable, have opened new possibilities to couples who might otherwise not have been able to have children. Our enhanced understanding of fetal development and ability to intervene on its behalf create new pressures to override the mother's wishes. The centuries-old debate about abortion takes on new significance in the modern era when abortion is safe and legal, but still highly controversial. The issues in this section come to grips with some of the most perplexing and fundamental questions that confront medical practitioners and society.

Is There a Moral Right to Abortion?

Should Thawing Unused Frozen
    Embryos Be Permitted?

Should Women Be Allowed to Bear
    Babies for a Fee?

The Maternal-Fetal Relationship: Can
    Compelled Medical Treatment of
    Pregnant Women Be Justified?

1

ISSUE 1

Is There a Moral Right to Abortion?

YES: Beverly Wildung Harrison, from *Our Right to Choose: Toward a New Ethics of Abortion* (Beacon Press, 1983)

NO: Sidney Callahan, from "Abortion and the Sexual Agenda: A Case for Prolife Feminism," *Commonweal* (April 1986)

ISSUE SUMMARY

YES: Professor of Christian ethics Beverly Wildung Harrison argues that women ought to decide whether or not to bear children on the basis of their own moral preparedness to become responsible mothers.
NO: Psychologist Sidney Callahan asserts that a woman's moral obligation to continue a pregnancy arises from both her status as a member of the human community and her unique life-giving female reproductive power.

Abortion is the most divisive bioethical issue of our time. The issue has been a persistent one in history, but in the past twenty years or so the debate has polarized. One view—known as "pro-life"—sees abortion as the wanton slaughter of innocent life. The other view—"pro-choice"—considers abortion as an option that must be available to women if they are to control their own reproductive lives. In the pro-life view, women who have access to "abortion on demand" put their own selfish whims ahead of an unborn child's right to life. In the pro-choice view, women have the right to choose to have an abortion—especially if there is some overriding reason, such as preventing the birth of a child with a severe genetic defect or one conceived as a result of rape or incest.

Behind these strongly held convictions, as political scientist Mary Segers has pointed out, are widely differing views of what determines value (that is, whether value is inherent in a thing or ascribed to it by human beings), the relation between law and morality, and the use of limits of political solutions to social problems, as well as the value of scientific progress. Those who condemn abortion as immoral generally follow a classical tradition in which abortion is a public matter because it involves our conception of how we ought to live together in an ideal society. Those who accept the idea of abortion, on the other hand, generally share the liberal, individualistic ethos of contemporary society. To them, abortion is a private choice, and public policy ought to reflect how citizens actually behave, not some unattainable ideal.

This is what we know about abortion practices in America today: It has been legal since the 1973 Supreme Court decision of *Roe v. Wade* declared that a woman has a constitutional right to privacy, which includes an abortion. It is seven times safer than childbirth, although there are some unknown risks—primarily the effect of repeated abortions on subsequent pregnancies. Abortion is common: Each year about 1.6 million abortions are performed. That is, one out of four pregnancies (and half of all unintended pregnancies) end in abortion. About 90 percent of all abortions are performed within the first 12 weeks of pregnancy by a method called suction aspiration. Eighty percent of the women who have abortions are unmarried, and nearly 63 percent are between the ages of 15 and 24. (In comparison, however, in 1965 there were between 200 thousand and 1.2 million illegal abortions, and 20 percent of all deaths from childbirth or pregnancy were caused by botched abortions.)

If abortion today is legal, safe, and common, it undeniably involves the killing of fetal life, and so the question remains: Is it ethical? At the heart of the issue are two complex questions. Does the fetus have a moral status that entitles it to life, liberty, and the pursuit of happiness as guaranteed by the Constitution? And even if it does, does a woman's rights to the same freedoms outweigh those of the fetus?

The selections that follow are written from two different feminist perspectives. Beverly Wildung Harrison asserts that the moral decision about abortion should rest with the woman herself. She believes that assigning special obligations to women to forgo abortion consigns women to an inferior status in society. Sidney Callahan seeks to broaden what she sees as Harrison's and other feminists' excessively narrow focus on "rights." She argues that women, as members of the human community with unique life-giving powers, have a moral obligation not to terminate a pregnancy and that society should provide the support that women need to enhance their lives.

YES
Beverly Wildung Harrison

OUR RIGHT TO CHOOSE

THE WIDER MORAL FRAMEWORK FOR THE ACT OF ABORTION

I argue that a society which would deny the conditions of procreative choice to women, or which treats women merely or chiefly as reproductive means to some purported end of that society's own self-perpetuation, is one that mandates women's inferior status as less than full, rational beings, denying women full claim to intrinsic value in the process. Likewise, a society that incorporates a perdurable structure of coercion, even violence, against women as morally appropriate to its functioning, but claims that it upholds the sanctity of or respect for human life is deluded. . . .

It is little wonder, then, that feminist efforts to articulate a moral argument about bodily integrity and its relevance to procreation are met with almost incredulous disbelief, derision, or trivialization in the ethical literature on abortion. To be sure, when fetal life is adjudged full, existent human life, appeals to body-right will not have automatic, overriding force because where two existent human beings are involved there will be a conflict of rights. (Such conflicts occur all the time in our social world.) But this recognition of *possible* conflict of rights is not usually what is assumed in discussions of the morality of abortion. Rather, appeals women make to their right to bodily self-control and self-direction are treated, at best, as non-moral, morally irrelevant, or ethically confused and, at worst, as selfish, whimsical, or positive evidence of the immorality of women who choose to have or to defend legal abortions.

I claim that the fact of women's biological fertility and capacity for childbearing in no way overrides our moral claim to the "right" of bodily integrity, because this moral claim is inherent to human well-being. Furthermore, if the full implications of women's history were comprehended, including the morally onerous attitudes and violent practices toward women, then reproductive self-determination would be understood to reinforce the substantive social justice claim about bodily integrity. Reproductive choice for women is requisite to any adequate notion of what constitutes a good society. Transformed social conditions of reproduction are absolutely critical to all women's well-being. No society that coerces women at the level of reproduction may lay claim to moral adequacy.

I agree strongly with those who have argued that the notion of "rights" is intrinsically social; it pertains to conditions of relationship between existent beings. I would insist one ought not to impute the existence of "rights" in a social relation unless all parties fall within some justifiable definition of "existents" vis-à-vis our human relations. In discussing the moral meaning of fetal life, we cannot afford to overlook the social character of "rights." When anyone invokes the claim that a fetus has "a right to life," we are justified in being wary, unless or until a plausible account is given of the criteria grounding the contention that a fetus is properly a full member of the class of human beings.

I have also stressed a more utilitarian or "concrete consequentialist" argument for procreative choice that correlates with but is logically discrete from the foregoing one: namely that given women's overall, continuing, disadvantaged socioeconomic situation, together with the de facto reality of childbearing, women should have procreative choice. Women most frequently must provide the life energy, physical and emotional support, and, increasingly, the economic wherewithal for infant survival, growth, and development. Under such circumstances, optimal conditions of procreative choice for women are mandatory.

I have constructed my case to put both good society or rights arguments and utilitarian teleological arguments in the forefront, not only because of my own methodological convictions but, even more important, because so much contemporary philosophical and religioethical analysis approaches the morality of abortion with such a weak sense of the relevance of these considerations. No moralist would be considered reputable if he or she argued the morality of economic life either by abdicating reflection on the meaning of a good society or by ignoring the concrete effects of economic policy and practice on people's lives. But, indeed, it *is* acceptable to discuss the morality of abortion without examining the implications of our moral judgments on what a "good society" should be and without taking into account the actual condition of women in society. Hence my ongoing contention is that, given the present climate of opinion among ethicists, it is necessary to insist that the positive principle of justice and the issue of social welfare, or social utility, are both at stake in procreative choice, or noncoercion in childbearing.

If one approaches the question of the morality of abortion without an acute sense of the viability of all these moral claims, then the question of the moral valuation of fetal life inevitably appears to be the only relevant question and the moral problematic of abortion seems to pose a fairly simple moral quandary. If, however, one recognizes the moral dubiousness of a society that treats women as less than full persons with an appropriate and serious moral claim to well-being, self-respect, self-direction and noncoercion in childbearing, and if one also recognizes the disadvantaged state of most women's lives, one's approach to the morality of abortion must shift. Even if one holds, as I do *not*, that fetal life is, from conception or at the point when the genetic code is implanted, essentially a *full, existent* human life, it is necessary to comprehend that we are dealing with a genuine moral dilemma, a conflict of "rights," not a moral chimera in which the "innocent party"—the fetal "person"—is, *by definition*, the "wronged" party in the moral equation.

To address the question "When does human life begin?" or to ask more precisely "What is the moral status of fetal life?" is something we are bound to do, given our modern scientific understanding of embryological development. Yet the questions are a far more intricate matter than they may appear at face value. Biological science itself is a complex, cultural construct, and biological scientists themselves differ over the moral implications of their paradigm. None of us nontechnical interpreters of these scientific data proceed untouched by our own operating cultural and social understandings. In fact, beneath the diverse judgments moralists make about the meaning of fetal life lie differing philosophies of nature and of science, including quite disparate views of biological theory, as well as conflicting methodological assumptions about how scientific "fact" and moral valuation interrelate. . . .

Even though there are reasonable grounds for positing the existence of a genetically developed individuated human body form from sometime after the midpoint of pregnancy onward, it does not follow that we should consider a fetus to be "a person" from this earliest possible point of species differentiation. Many have argued that the term *person* should be reserved to designate those who *actually belong* to the moral community by virtue of criteria derived from our understanding of living human beings. In a notable defense of this position, philosopher Mary Anne Warren has proposed the following criteria for "personhood":

> I suggest that the traits which are most central to the concept of personhood, or humanity in the moral sense, are, very roughly, the following:
> 1. consciousness (of objects and events external and/or internal to the being), and in particular the capacity to feel pain;
> 2. reasoning (the developed capacity to solve new and relatively complex problems);
> 3. self-motivated activity (activity which is relatively independent of either genetic or direct external control);
> 4. the capacity to communicate, by whatever means, messages of an indefinite variety of types, that is, not just with an indefinite number of possible contents, but on indefinitely many possible topics;
> 5. the presence of self-concepts, and self-awareness, either individual or social, or both.

Warren does not suppose that any of these criteria are indisputable, but what she does maintain, correctly I believe, is that a fetus possesses *none* of the criteria that come to mind when we think normatively of a "person." . . .

In the debate over the morality of abortion, those who correlate "personhood" with any level of gestational maturation seem to me to obscure, or to fail to appreciate, the integrity of arguments formulated by pro-choice supporters about the importance of "quality of life" questions regarding procreation or birth. Whether or not we wish to acknowledge it, the constitutive foundations of personality are bound up not with biological maturation of the human species life form but with the quality of our social relations. For centuries, even millennia, we human beings have permitted ourselves the luxury of imagining that our personal life follows inexorably from our existence as a natural or species life form, ignoring the now growing evidence that it is our human social relations, the quality of our interaction with each other, that conditions all that we become after birth. Ours is a world in which there is "a crisis of the personal"—that is, a loss of the very conditions that make it possible for individuals who share human species being to live, grow, and thrive as genuinely personal beings having deeply centered personal relations to others. A biologically reductionist understanding of our species, which fully conflates the biologically human and the "person," threatens to intensify this crisis in our human moral relations. Ironically, the "fetishizing of fetuses" in the abortion debate may well exacerbate our already overdeveloped tendency to consider ourselves "normatively human" quite apart from the world of social relations our moral action creates. The birth of an infant, understood from the standpoint of organic embryological development, is an event. Birth is an inexorable watershed in organic process, however, because the care and nurturance of a newborn inaugurates an infinitely complex series of actions. . . .

With respect to the abortion controversy, it is worth remembering that *any* definition of "a human life" or "person" that neglects the moral reality required to nurture and sustain life after birth is very dangerous to our self-understanding. A "pro-life" movement that invites us to "respect" fetal rights from conception or genetic implantation onward actually undermines us by tempting us to imagine that personal rights inhere in natural processes, apart from any genuine covenant of caring, including the human re-solve to create viable conditions of life for all who are born among us. Human rights are qualities that ought to inhere in our social relations. Any use of the concept that neglects this fact invites us to take with less than full seriousness the sort of claim we ought to be making when we say that human beings have "a right to life." Early fetal life does *not* yet possess even the minimal organic requirements for participation in the sphere of human rights. And like Mary Anne Warren, I do not believe that even the highly developed fetus can yet be said to have "an intrinsic right to life." Even so, I recognize that it is morally wise to extend such respect, de facto, to fetuses in late stages of gestation. But to do so is also and simultaneously to insist that rights are moral relations, born of our freedom as mature, other-regarding persons. In extending "a right to life" to fetuses in late stages of development, we are attesting that it is a good use of our freedom as agents, from a moral point of view, to do so.

To argue that *we* may appropriately predicate to fetuses, in the late stages of gestation, "a right to life" does not mean, however, that the life of the pregnant woman should be overridden in decisions about late-stage pregnancies. Rather, it means that abortions, at least in the second half of gestation, are not to be undertaken without serious justifications. My own belief is that the physical and emotional well-being of the pregnant woman, as a valuable existent person, still outweighs the incremental value of the fetus her life sustains. Of course, it is true that in the later stages of pregnancy, abortions are matters of high risk for pregnant women. But doctors, who under most existing laws have discretion as to whether an abortion is advisable at this stage, are themselves not likely to be "frivolous" about the decisions that confront them given the danger of late abortions. . . .

[A]bortions will continue to be available whether or not they are legal. Ironically, then, those persons insisting that a human life begins at conception or at an early stage of genetic human development may help to create a situation in which abortions, though they will not cease, will occur at a later stage of gestation. . . .

Persons of authentic theological sensibility must continue to insist that every child who is born among us deserves to be embraced in a covenant of life and affirmation that includes not merely the love of a mother, or a father, but the active concern and respect of the wider community. We must never imagine that the conditions for such deeply humane covenant exist. I noted at the outset that if women did not have to deliberate the questions relating to our procreative power in an atmosphere of taboo, we would be able to turn our attention to the positive moral task I have commended: what it means for us to use our procreative power responsibly. In the present condemnatory atmosphere, such moral reasoning will go largely undeveloped.

Even so, the deepest reappropriation of the theological theme of the covenant that women can make requires our perception of procreation as a moral act, one we must enter into with maximum awareness of what it means to bear a child. We are still a long way from a historical situation in which women really will have the conditions that make such a genuine covenant and choice an easy matter. Safe surgical abortion has created only the negative conditions for procreative choice. We often now live in situations where it is easier to say no than to say yes to this prospective covenant. The current circumstances in which women choose abortions are often dominated by desperation. And yet it is now possible to begin to anticipate what it would mean to incorporate this covenantal image into the total process of species reproduction. When such a covenant of life is embodied in the birth of every child, an incredible reduction in human suffering will have been accomplished.

Any of us who have experienced human joy in the knowledge of our birth at some level have heard God's call to life through the "yes" of our parents. Without that yes, life is immeasurably impoverished. In fact, it is necessary to put the point more strongly. Those who are born in the absence of such an act of human covenant by already living persons (of course, not merely by our biological parents) frequently do not really live at all. Our acknowledgment of each other in relation is not an optional addition to life, an afterthought; it is constitutive of life itself. For a vital human life to be born, a woman must say yes in a strong and active way and enter positively into a life-bearing, demanding, and, at times, extremely painful process. Freedom to say yes, which, of course, also means the freedom to say no, is constitutive of the sacred covenant of life itself. Failure to see this is also failure to see how good, how strong and real, embodied existence is in this world we are making together.

NO   Sidney Callahan

ABORTION AND THE SEXUAL AGENDA: A CASE FOR PROLIFE FEMINISM

The abortion debate continues. In the latest and perhaps most crucial development, prolife feminists are contesting prochoice feminist claims that abortion rights are prerequisites for women's full development and social equality. The outcome of this debate may be decisive for the culture as a whole. Prolife feminists, like myself, argue on good feminist principles that women can never achieve the fulfillment of feminist goals in a society permissive toward abortion.

These new arguments over abortion take place within liberal political circles. This round of intense intra-feminist conflict has spiraled beyond earlier right-versus-left abortion debates, which focused on "tragic choices," medical judgments, and legal compromises. Feminist theorists of the prochoice position now put forth the demand for unrestricted abortion rights as a *moral imperative* and insist upon women's right to complete reproductive freedom. They morally justify the present situation and current abortion practices. Thus it is all the more important that prolife feminists articulate their different feminist perspective.

These opposing arguments can best be seen when presented in turn. Perhaps the most highly developed feminist arguments for the morality and legality of abortion can be found in Beverly Wildung Harrison's *Our Right to Choose* (Beacon Press, 1983) and Rosalind Pollack Petchesky's *Abortion and Woman's Choice* (Longman, 1984). Obviously it is difficult to do justice to these complex arguments, which draw on diverse strands of philosophy and social theory and are often interwoven in prochoice feminists' own version of a "seamless garment." Yet the fundamental feminist case for the morality of abortion, encompassing the views of Harrison and Petchesky, can be analyzed in terms of four central moral claims: (1) the moral right to control one's own body; (2) the moral necessity of autonomy and choice in personal responsibility; (3) the moral claim for the contingent value of fetal life; (4) the moral right of women to true social equality.

From Sidney Callahan, "Abortion and the Sexual Agenda: A Case for Prolife Feminism," *Commonweal*, vol. 123 (April 25, 1986). Copyright © 1986 by the Commonweal Foundation. Reprinted by permission.

1. The moral right to control one's own body. Prochoice feminism argues that a woman choosing an abortion is exercising a basic right of bodily integrity granted in our common law tradition. If she does not choose to be physically involved in the demands of a pregnancy and birth, she should not be compelled to be so against her will. Just because it is *her* body which is involved, a woman should have the right to terminate any pregnancy, which at this point in medical history is tantamount to terminating fetal life. No one can be forced to donate an organ or submit to other invasive physical procedures for however good a cause. Thus no woman should be subjected to "compulsory pregnancy." And it should be noted that in pregnancy much more than a passive biological process is at stake.

From one perspective, the fetus is, as Petchesky says, a "biological parasite" taking resources from the woman's body. During pregnancy, a woman's whole life and energies will be actively involved in the nine-month process. Gestation and childbirth involve physical and psychological risks. After childbirth a woman will either be a mother who must undertake a twenty-year responsibility for child rearing, or face giving up her child for adoption or institutionalization. Since hers is the body, hers the risk, hers the burden, it is only just that she alone should be free to decide on pregnancy or abortion.

The moral claim to abortion, according to the prochoice feminists, is especially valid in an individualistic society in which women cannot count on medical care or social support in pregnancy, childbirth, or child rearing. A moral abortion decision is never made in a social vacuum, but in the real life society which exists here and now.

2. The moral necessity of autonomy and choice in personal responsibility. Beyond the claim for individual *bodily* integrity, the prochoice feminists claim that to be a full adult *morally*, a woman must be able to make responsible life commitments. To plan, choose, and exercise personal responsibility, one must have control of reproduction. A woman must be able to make yes-or-no decisions about a specific pregnancy, according to her present situation, resources, prior commitments, and life plan. Only with such reproductive freedom can a woman have the moral autonomy necessary to make mature commitments, in the area of family, work, or education.

Contraception provides a measure of personal control, but contraceptive failure or other chance events can too easily result in involuntary pregnancy. Only free access to abortion can provide the necessary guarantee. The chance biological process of an involuntary pregnancy should not be allowed to override all the other personal commitments and responsibilities a woman has: to others, to family, to work, to education, to her future development, health, or well-being. Without reproductive freedom, women's personal moral agency and human consciousness are subjected to biology and chance.

3. The moral claim for the contingent value of fetal life. Prochoice feminist exponents like Harrison and Petchesky claim that the value of fetal life is contingent upon the woman's free consent and subjective acceptance. The fetus must be invested with maternal valuing in order to become human. This process of "humanization" through personal consciousness and "sociality" can only be bestowed by the woman in whose body and psychosocial system a new life must mature. The meaning and value of fetal life are constructed by the woman; without this personal conferral there only exists a biological, physiological process. Thus fetal interests or fetal rights can never outweigh the woman's prior interest and rights. If a woman does not consent to invest her pregnancy with meaning or value, then the merely biological process can be freely terminated. Prior to her own free choice and conscious investment, a woman cannot be described as a "mother" nor can a "child" be said to exist.

Moreover, in cases of voluntary pregnancy, a woman can withdraw consent if fetal genetic defects or some other problem emerges at any time before birth. Late abortion should thus be granted without legal restrictions. Even the minimal qualifications and limitations on women embedded in *Roe v. Wade* are unacceptable—repressive remnants of patriarchal unwillingness to give power to women.

4. The moral right of women to full social equality. Women have a moral right to full social equality. They should not be restricted or subordinated because of their sex. But this morally required equality cannot be realized without abortion's certain control of reproduction. Female social equality depends upon being able to compete and participate as freely as males can in the structures of educational and economic life. If a woman cannot control when and how she will be pregnant or rear children, she is at a distinct disadvantage, especially in our male-dominated world.

Psychological equality and well-being is also at stake. Women must enjoy the basic right of a person to the free exercise of heterosexual intercourse and full sex-

ual expression, separated from procreation. No less than males, women should be able to be sexually active without the constantly inhibiting fear of pregnancy. Abortion is necessary for women's sexual fulfillment and the growth of uninhibited feminine self-confidence and ownership of their sexual powers.

But true sexual and reproductive freedom means freedom to procreate as well as to inhibit fertility. Prochoice feminists are also worried that women's freedom to reproduce will be curtailed through the abuse of sterilization and needless hysterectomies. Besides the punitive tendencies of a male-dominated health-care system, especially in response to repeated abortions or welfare pregnancies, there are other economic and social pressures inhibiting reproduction. Genuine reproductive freedom implies that day care, medical care, and financial support would be provided mothers, while fathers would take their full share in the burdens and delights of raising children.

Many prochoice feminists identify feminist ideals with communitarian, ecologically sensitive approaches to reshaping society. Following theorists like Sara Ruddick and Carol Gilligan, they link abortion rights with the growth of "maternal thinking" in our heretofore patriarchal society. Maternal thinking is loosely defined as a responsible commitment to the loving nature of specific human beings as they actually exist in socially embedded interpersonal contexts. It is a moral perspective very different from the abstract, competitive, isolated, and principled rigidity so characteristic of patriarchy.

HOW DOES A PROLIFE FEMINIST RESPOND to these arguments? Prolife feminists grant the good intentions of their prochoice counterparts but protest that the prochoice position is flawed, morally inadequate, and inconsistent with feminism's basic demands for justice. Prolife feminists champion a more encompassing moral ideal. They recognize the claims of fetal life and offer a different perspective on what is good for women. The feminist vision is expanded and refocused.

1. From the moral right to control one's own body to a more inclusive ideal of justice. The moral right to control one's own body does apply to cases of organ transplants, mastectomies, contraception, and sterilization; but it is not a conceptualization adequate for abortion. The abortion dilemma is caused by the fact that 266 days following a conception in one body, another body will emerge. One's own body no longer exists as a single unit but is engendering another organism's life. This dynamic passage from conception to birth is genetically ordered and universally found in the human species. Pregnancy is not like the growth of cancer or infestation by a biological parasite; it is the way every human being enters the world. Strained philosophical analogies fail to apply: having a baby is not like rescuing a drowning person, being hooked up to a famous violinist's artificial life-support system, donating organs for transplant—or anything else.

As embryology and fetology advance, it becomes clear that human development is a continuum. Just as astronomers are studying the first three minutes in the genesis of the universe, so the first moments, days, and weeks at the beginning of human life are the subject of increasing scientific attention. While neonatology pushes the definition of viability ever earlier, ultrasound and fetology expand the concept of the patient *in utero*. Within such a continuous growth process, it is hard to defend logically any demarcation point after conception as the point at which an immature form of human life is so different from the day before or the day after, that it can be morally or legally discounted as a nonperson. Even the moment of birth can hardly differentiate a nine-month fetus from a newborn. It is not surprising that those who countenance late abortions are logically led to endorse selective infanticide.

The same legal tradition which in our society guarantees the right to control one's own body firmly recognizes the wrongfulness of harming other bodies, however immature, dependent, different looking, or powerless. The handicapped, the retarded, and newborns are legally protected from deliberate harm. Prolife feminists reject the suppositions that would except the unborn from this protection.

After all, debates similar to those about the fetus were once conducted about feminine personhood. Just as women, or blacks, were considered too different, too underdeveloped, too "biological," to have souls or to possess legal rights, so the fetus is now seen as "merely" biological life, subsidiary to a person. A woman was once viewed as incorporated into the "one flesh" of her husband's person; she too was a form of bodily property. In all partriarchal unjust systems, lesser orders of human life are granted rights only when wanted, chosen, or invested with value by the powerful.

Fortunately, in the course of civilization there has been a gradual realization that justice demands the powerless and dependent be protected against the uses of power wielded unilaterally. No human can be treated as a means to an end without consent. The fetus is an immature, dependent form of human life which only needs time and protection to develop. Surely, immaturity and dependence are not crimes.

In an effort to think about the essential requirements of a just society, philosophers like John Rawls recommend imagining yourself in an "original position," in which your position in the society to be created is hidden by a "veil of ignorance." You will have to weigh the possibility that any inequalities inherent in that society's practices may rebound upon you in the worst, as well as in the best, conceivable way. This thought experiment helps ensure justice for all.

Beverly Harrison argues that in such an envisioning of society everyone would institute abortion rights in order to guarantee that if one turned out to be a woman one would have reproductive freedom. But surely in the original position and behind the "veil of ignorance," you would have to contemplate the possibility of being the particular fetus to be aborted. Since everyone has passed through the fetal stage of development, it is false to refuse to imagine oneself in this state when thinking about a potential world in which justice would govern. Would it be just that an embryonic life—in half the cases, of course, a female life—be sacrificed to the right of a woman's control over her own body? A woman may be pregnant without consent and experience a great many penalties, but a fetus killed without consent pays the ultimate penalty.

It does not matter . . . whether the fetus being killed is fully conscious or feels pain. We do not sanction killing the innocent if it can be done painlessly or without the victim's awareness. Consciousness becomes important to the abortion debate because it is used as a criterion for the "personhood" so often seen as the prerequisite for legal protection. Yet certain philosophers set the standard of personhood so high that half the human race could not meet the criteria during most of their waking hours (let alone their sleeping ones). Sentience, self-consciousness, rational decision-making, social participation? Surely no infant, or child under two, could qualify. Either our idea of person must be expanded or another criterion, such as human life itself, be employed to protect the weak in a just society. Prolife feminists who defend the fetus emphatically identify with an immature state of growth passed through by themselves, their children, and everyone now alive.

IT ALSO SEEMS A TRAVESTY OF JUST PROcedures that a pregnant woman now, in effect, acts as sole judge of her own case, under the most stressful conditions. Yes, one can acknowledge that the pregnant woman will be subject to the potential burdens arising from a pregnancy, but it has never been thought right to have an interested party, especially the more powerful party, decide his or her own case when there may be a conflict of interest. If one considers the matter as a case of a powerful versus a powerless, silenced claimant, the prochoice feminist argument can rightly be inverted: since hers is the body, hers the risk, and hers the greater burden, then how in fairness can a woman be the sole judge of the fetal right to life?

Human ambivalence, a bias toward self-interest, and emotional stress have always been recognized as endangering judgment. Freud declared that love and hate are so entwined that if instant thoughts could kill, we would all be dead in the bosom of our families. In the case of a woman's involuntary pregnancy, a complex, long-term solution requiring effort and energy has to compete with the immediate solution offered by a morning's visit to an abortion clinic. On the simple, perceptual plane, with imagination and thinking curtailed, the speed, ease, and privacy of abortion, combined with the small size of the embryo, tend to make early abortions seem less morally serious—even though speed, size, technical ease, and the private nature of an act have no moral standing.

As the most recent immigrants from nonpersonhood, feminists have traditionally fought for justice for themselves and the world. Women rally to feminism as a new and better way to live. Rejecting male aggression and destruction, feminists seek alternative, peaceful, ecologically sensitive means to resolve conflicts while respecting human potentiality. It is a chilling inconsistency to see prochoice feminists demanding continued access to assembly-line, technological methods of fetal killing—the vacuum aspirator, prostaglandins, and dilation and evacuation. It is a betrayal of feminism, which has built the struggle for justice on the bedrock of women's empathy. After all, "maternal thinking" receives its name from a mother's unconditional acceptance and nurture of dependent, immature life. It is difficult to develop concern for women, children, the poor and the dispossessed—and to care about peace—and at the same time ignore fetal life.

2. From the necessity of autonomy and choice in personal responsibility to an expanded sense of responsibility. A distorted idea of morality overemphas-

izes individual autonomy and active choice. Morality has often been viewed too exclusively as a matter of human agency and decisive action. In moral behavior persons must explicitly choose and aggressively exert their wills to intervene in the natural and social environments. The human will dominates the body, overcomes the given, breaks out of the material limits of nature. Thus if one does not choose to be pregnant or cannot rear a child, who must be given up for adoption, then better to abort the pregnancy. Willing, planning, choosing one's moral commitments through the contracting of one's individual resources becomes the premier model of moral responsibility.

But morality also consists of the good and worthy acceptance of the unexpected events that life presents. Responsivenss and response-ability to things unchosen are also instances of the highest human moral capacity. Morality is not confined to contracted agreements of isolated individuals. Yes, one is obligated by explicit contracts freely initiated, but human beings are also obligated by implicit compacts and involuntary relationships in which persons simply find themselves. To be embedded in a family, a neighborhood, a social system, brings moral obligations which were never entered into with informed consent.

Parent-child relationships are one instance of implicit moral obligations arising by virtue of our being part of the interdependent human community. A woman, involuntarily pregnant, has a moral obligation to the now-existing dependent fetus whether she explicitly consented to its existence or not. No prolife feminist would dispute the forceful observations of prochoice feminists about the extreme difficulties that bearing an unwanted child in our society can entail. But the stronger force of the fetal claim presses a woman to accept these burdens; the fetus possesses rights arising from its extreme need and the interdependency and unity of humankind. The woman's moral obligation arises both from her status as a human being embedded in the interdependent human community and her unique lifegiving female reproductive power. To follow the prochoice feminist ideology of insistent individualistic autonomy and control is to betray a fundamental basis of the moral life.

3. From the moral claim of the contingent value of fetal life to the moral claim for the intrinsic value of human life. The feminist prochoice position which claims that the value of the fetus is contingent upon the pregnant woman's bestowal—or willed, conscious "construction"—of humanhood is seriously flawed. The inadequacies of this position flow from the erroneous premises (1) that human value and rights can be granted by individual will; (2) that the individual woman's consciousness can exist and operate in an *a priori* isolated fashion; and (3) that "mere" biological, genetic human life has little meaning. Prolife feminism takes a very different stance toward life and nature.

Human life from the beginning to the end of development *has* intrinsic value, which does not depend on meeting the selective criteria or tests set up by powerful others. A fundamental humanist assumption is at stake here. Either we are going to value embodied human life and humanity as a good thing, or take some variant of the nihilist position that assumes human life is just one more random occurrence in the universe such that each instance of human life must explicitly be justified to prove itself worthy to continue. When faced with a new life, or an involuntary pregnancy, there is a world of difference in whether one first asks, "Why continue?" or "Why not?" Where is the burden of proof going to rest? The concept of "compulsory pregnancy" is as distorted as labeling life "compulsory aging."

In a sound moral tradition, human rights arise from human needs, and it is the very nature of a right, or valid claim upon another, that it cannot be denied, conditionally delayed, or rescinded by more powerful others at their behest. It seems fallacious to hold that in the case of the fetus it is the pregnant woman alone who gives or removes its right to life and human status solely through her subjective conscious investment or "humanization." Surely no pregnant woman (or any other individual member of the species) has created her own human nature by an individually willed act of consciousness, nor for that matter been able to guarantee her own human rights. An individual woman and the unique individual embryonic life within her can only exist because of their participation in the genetic inheritance of the human species as a whole. Biological life should never be discounted. Membership in the species, or collective human family, is the basis for human solidarity, equality, and natural human rights.

4. The moral right of women to full social equality from a prolife feminist perspective. Prolife feminists and prochoice feminists are totally agreed on the moral right of women to the full social equality so far denied them. The disagreement between them concerns the definition of the desired goal and the best means to get there. Permissive abortion laws do not bring women reproductive freedom, social equality, sexual fulfillment, or full personal development.

Pragmatic failures of a prochoice feminist position combined with a lack of moral vision are, in fact, causing disaffection among young women. Middle-aged prochoice feminists blamed the "big chill" on the general conservative backlash. But they should look rather to their own elitist acceptance of male models of sex and to the sad picture they present of women's lives. Pitting women against their own offspring is not only morally offensive, it is psychologically and politically destructive. Women will never climb to equality and social empowerment over mounds of dead fetuses, numbering now in the millions. As long as most women choose to bear children, they stand to gain from the same constellation of attitudes and institutions that will also protect the fetus in the woman's womb— and they stand to lose from the cultural assumptions that support permissive abortion. Despite temporary conflicts of interest, feminine and fetal liberation are ultimately one and the same cause.

Women's rights and liberation are pragmatically linked to fetal rights because to obtain true equality, women need (1) more social support and changes in the structure of society, and (2) increased self-confidence, self-expectations, and self-esteem. Society in general, and men in particular, have to provide women more support in rearing the next generation, or our devastating feminization of poverty will continue. But if a woman claims the right to decide by herself whether the fetus becomes a child or not, what does this do to paternal and communal responsibility? Why should men share responsibility for child support or child rearing if they cannot share in what is asserted to be the woman's sole decision? Furthermore, if explicit intentions and consciously accepted contracts are necessary for moral obligations, why should men be held responsible for what *they* do not voluntarily choose to happen? By prochoice reasoning, a man who does not want to have a child, or whose contraceptive fails, can be exempted from the responsibilities of fatherhood and child support. Traditionally, many men have been laggards in assuming parental responsibility and support for their children; ironically, ready abortion, often advocated as a response to male dereliction, legitimizes male irresponsibility and paves the way for even more male detachment and lack of commitment.

For that matter, why should the state provide a system of day care or child support, or require workplaces to accommodate women's maternity and the needs of child rearing? Permissive abortion, granted in the name of women's privacy and reproductive freedom, ratifies the view that pregnancies and children are a woman's private individual responsibility. More and more frequently, we hear some version of this old rationalization: if she refuses to get rid of it, it's her problem. A child becomes a product of the individual woman's freely chosen investment, a form of private property resulting from her own cost-benefit calculation. The larger community is relieved of moral responsibility.

With legal abortion freely available, a clear cultural message is given: conception and pregnancy are no longer serious moral matters. With abortion as an acceptable alternative, contraception is not as responsibly used; women take risks, often at the urging of male sexual partners. Repeat abortions increase, with all their psychological and medical repercussions. With more abortion there is more abortion. Behavior shapes thought as well as the other way round. One tends to justify morally what one has done; what becomes commonplace and institutionalized seems harmless. Habituation is a powerful psychological force. Psychologically it is also true that whatever is avoided becomes more threatening; in phobias it is the retreat from anxiety-producing events which reinforces future avoidance. Women begin to see themselves as too weak to cope with involuntary pregnancies. Finally, through the potency of social pressure and the force of inertia, it becomes more and more difficult, in fact almost unthinkable, *not* to use abortion to solve problem pregnancies. Abortion becomes no longer a choice but a "necessity." . . .

New feminist efforts to rethink the meaning of sexuality, femininity, and reproduction are all the more vital as new techniques for artificial reproduction, surrogate motherhood, and the like present a whole new set of dilemmas. In the long run, the very long run, the abortion debate may be merely the opening round in a series of far-reaching struggles over the role of human sexuality and the ethics of reproduction. Significant changes in the culture, both positive and negative in outcome, may begin as local storms of controversy. We may be at one of those vaguely realized thresholds when we had best come to full attention. What kind of people are we going to be? Prolife feminists pursue a vision for their sisters, daughters, and granddaughters. Will their great-granddaughters be grateful?

POSTSCRIPT

Is There a Moral Right to Abortion?

Although the Supreme Court consistently upheld the legality of abortion in a series of cases in the early and mid–1980s, its July 1989 ruling in the case of *Webster v. Reproductive Health Services* was widely seen as a harbinger of change. The changing composition of the Court, pro-life activism, and the Reagan administration's stance against abortion has led to a social and legal climate that might ultimately overturn *Roe v. Wade*. The *Webster* decision, however, was not a clear-cut victory for either pro-life or pro-choice advocates. By upholding the constitutionality of Missouri's restrictive abortion statutes, the Court gave more power to state legislatures and courts in regulating abortion. It did not, however, directly revoke the right to an abortion.

Much of the debate and activism following *Webster* has focused on state election campaigns; the results have been mixed, with pro-life candidates winning in some races and losing in others. Legislatures seeking to restrict abortions have most commonly required unmarried women under 18 to obtain consent or to inform one or both parents; in some cases a judicial appeal is permitted. Such laws in Minnesota and Ohio were upheld by the Supreme Court in June 1990. However, sweeping antiabortion legislation failed to be enacted in Louisiana, Florida, and Idaho. The most restrictive legislation was passed in Guam; its enactment has been stayed pending a court challenge.

For generally supportive analyses of *Webster,* see Charles H. Baron, "Abortion and Legal Process in the United States: An Overview of the Post-*Webster* Legal Landscape," and Lynn D. Wardle, "The Road to Moderation: The Significance of *Webster* for Legislation Restricting Abortion," two of a series of four articles in *Law, Medicine & Health Care* (Winter 1989). In "The Right of Privacy Protects the Doctor-Patient Relationship," *Journal of the American Medical Association* (February 9, 1990), George J. Annas, Leonard H. Glantz, and Wendy K. Mariner criticize the Court's decision.

The literature on abortion is large and often impassioned. John Noonan's views against abortion are found in *A Private Choice: Abortion in America in the Seventies* (The Free Press, 1979). Paul Ramsey's *Ethics at the Edges of Life* (Yale, 1978) is another eloquent statement of the pro-life stance.

Judith Jarvis Thomson's article "A Defense of Abortion," *Philosophy and Public Affairs* (Fall, 1971), is a classic philosophical defense of the feminist argument that a woman has the right to control her body. In her article, "On the Moral and Legal Status of Abortion," *The Monist* (January, 1973), Mary Anne Warren goes even further, asserting that the fetus is not a person and that abortion is always permissible. In *Abortion and Woman's Choice* (Longman, 1984), Rosalind Pollack Petchesky presents a communitarian view of abortion, stressing the social context in which women must make reproductive choices.

Abortion: Understanding Differences (Plenum, 1984), edited by Sidney Callahan and Daniel Callahan, is a collection of articles by pro-choice and pro-life women on the relationship of views about abortion to other values. Other volumes that present a range of viewpoints on abortion are Kristin Luker, *Abortion and the Politics of Motherhood* (University of California Press, 1984); Jay L. Garfield and Patricia Hennessey, eds., *Abortion: Moral and Legal Perspectives* (University of Massachusetts Press, 1984); and Hyman Rodman, Betty Sarvis, and Joy Walker Bonar, *The Abortion Question* (Columbia University Press, 1987). Laurence H. Tribe has written a thoughtful analysis in *Abortion: The Clash of Absolutes* (Norton, 1990).

ISSUE 2

Should Thawing Unused Frozen Embryos Be Permitted?

YES: American Medical Association, from "Board of Trustees Report: Frozen Pre-Embryos," *Journal of the American Medical Association* (May 9, 1990)

NO: David T. Ozar, from "The Case Against Thawing Unused Frozen Embryos," *Hastings Center Report* (August 1985)

ISSUE SUMMARY

YES: The American Medical Association's Board of Trustees concludes that the man and woman who provided the sperm and egg should decide about the disposition of an unused frozen embryo, and that they may legally and ethically decide to thaw and dispose of it.

NO: Philosopher David T. Ozar argues that the responsible parties have a moral obligation to preserve frozen embryos until they are implanted in a woman's womb or can no longer survive implantation.

Since the birth of Louise Joy Brown—the world's first documented test-tube baby—in July 1978, in vitro fertilization (IVF) has become relatively common-place. Thousands of babies have been born to previously infertile couples. With this technique, more properly called external fertilization, a ripe egg is removed through surgery from the mother's ovary and then mixed in a special solution with the male sperm (egg cells and sperm cells are some-times referred to as "gametes"). After two or three days, if fertilization occurs, the resulting embryo is implanted in the mother's uterine wall. (The technical term for this early stage of embryonic development is "pre-embryo," but "embryo" is the most commonly used term.) The process is painful, expensive ($3,000 to $6,000 per try, with three to four tries not uncommon), and successful only some of the time. Success rates vary from institution to institution, depending on experience, but fewer than 10 percent of women who begin the process of egg retrieval ultimately give birth to a baby.

In an effort to decrease the risks and costs of surgery, women in IVF programs are given drugs that stimulate ovulation. More than one egg is then produced for retrieval and fertilization. As a result, more embryos are available than can be implanted at a single time. The extra embryos are often frozen and saved for later implantation, which may be necessary because of the timing of the reproductive cycle, a failure on the first attempt to achieve implantation, or the wishes of the couple to have another IVF child. Freezing significantly reduces the capacity of the embryos to be implanted. Nevertheless, in 1988 alone, more than 70 infants were born after having started life in a test tube and then a freezer, and nearly 10,000 embryos were stored in laboratory freezers.

As IVF centers have proliferated and as the demand of infertile couples for this service has increased, the debate about the morality of producing test-tube babies has waned. Nevertheless, some theologians, feminists, and others remain opposed to artificially assisted reproduction on moral or policy grounds. Some oppose it on the grounds that it violates the natural order of things; others claim that it places undue emphasis on women as breeders and on the importance of bearing a genetically related child. Still others point out that it is unfair that this procedure is available only to the wealthy. Even those who accept IVF as an ethical procedure are concerned about informed consent, quality control, and inequities in access.

The main ethical debate has moved to the subsequent and related question of what to do with unused frozen embryos. Are they property to be disposed of at will? Human life with all its rights? Or something in-between? Three cases illustrate the kinds of real-life problems that can arise. In 1983 a wealthy couple named Rios died in a plane crash, leaving behind frozen embryos in an Australian lab and a legal tangle about who would control their estate. In 1989 Junior and Mary Sue Davis, about to be divorced, went to court over the disposition of the seven frozen embryos that resulted from their participation in a Tennessee fertility clinic. Mrs. Davis wanted to have them implanted so that she might have a chance to be a mother; Mr. Davis wanted to remain childless. In another 1989 case the Yorks, a New York couple who had entered an IVF program in Virginia, moved to California and asked to have their frozen embryos moved to a Los Angeles fertility clinic. The Virginia clinic refused, claiming that the embryos should be implanted only at their facility.

In the following selections, the Board of Trustees of the American Medical Association recommends that the two persons who provided the egg and the sperm have the primary authority to decide what to do with any frozen embryos they do not intend to use themselves. They may donate them to others for implantation or for research, or they may allow them to thaw and deteriorate. David T. Ozar argues that whether one believes that the embryo has rights from the instant of conception or that the embryo has no moral rights at all, frozen embryos ought to be preserved until they are implanted in a woman's womb or are no longer viable.

YES   American Medical Association

FROZEN PRE-EMBRYOS

While in vitro fertilization (IVF) has enabled many previously infertile couples to have children, it has also posed troubling legal and ethical dilemmas. This report, which was prepared by the Committee on Medico-legal Problems and the Council on Ethical and Judicial Affairs, will discuss the legal and ethical issues created by the freezing of human pre-embryos and will indicate how rights, if any, should be allocated among the two gamete providers, the frozen pre-embryos, and third parties. (Because fertilized eggs are frozen before the embryonic stage of development, they are referred to as pre-embryos.) . . .

For the reasons described in the remainder of this report, the Board of Trustees recommends as follows:

1. Primary authority for frozen pre-embryos rests with the two gamete providers, and they must agree to any disposition of the pre-embryos.

2. Agreements by the gamete providers for the future disposition of their pre-embryos should generally be enforceable. However, either gamete provider should be able to show that changed circumstances make enforcement of the agreement unreasonable. The gamete providers should not be required to enter into an agreement that will govern the future disposition of their pre-embryos.

3. Frozen pre-embryos may be used by the gamete providers, donated for use by other parties, or donated for research. The frozen pre-embryos also may be allowed to thaw and deteriorate. . . .

DECISION-MAKING AUTHORITY

Whether frozen pre-embryos are considered to be persons, body parts, or something in between, this country's cultural and legal traditions indicate that the logical persons to exercise control over a frozen pre-embryo are the man and woman who provided the sperm and ovum.

First, the gamete providers have a fundamental interest at stake, their potential for procreation.[1] Indeed, the federal constitution, many state

From American Medical Association, "Board of Trustees Report: Frozen Pre-Embryos," *Journal of the American Medical Association*, vol. 263, no. 18 (May 9, 1990), pp. 2484-2487. Copyright © 1990 by the American Medical Association. Reprinted by permission.

constitutions, and society in general recognize that individuals must be allowed to control the exercise of their reproductive capacities.[2] Consequently, individuals should be able to protect that interest in the absence of compelling reasons to override their choice. Even though the government may limit the individual's freedom of reproductive choice,[3] the government does not grant decision-making authority to private third parties but rather restricts the individual's ability to choose among potential courses of action.

From the perspective of the pre-embryo's interests, the gamete providers are also the logical decision makers. By way of analogy, parents have long been recognized as the proper decision makers for their children. It is they who are most concerned with their children's welfare and most willing to undergo sacrifices on behalf of their children. Accordingly, the law has deferred to parental choices on all aspects of their children's lives[4] as long as the child is not neglected or abused.[5] Similarly, the gamete providers are the persons who are most concerned with the interests of the pre-embryo and most likely to protect those interests.

The gamete providers are the logical decision makers also from the perspective of pre-embryos as body parts. Individuals have traditionally been accorded primary control over their body parts. While people may donate their organs, semen, or blood to others, they cannot be compelled to give them up.[6]

The conclusion that the providers of the sperm and ovum should exercise primary control over a frozen pre-embryo means that couples [in in vitro fertilization programs] have priority over the physicians who perform the IVF. Hence, the gamete providers would have the authority to decide when a frozen pre-embryo should be thawed for transfer and which woman would receive the pre-embryo. In addition, they would be able to change physicians and move their pre-embryos to other facilities for implantation.

On showing a sufficiently compelling interest, governments might impose certain limitations on the ability of individuals to move their pre-embryos from one facility to another. For example, the state may regulate the procedures for IVF and pre-embryo transfer. The state may require, if a frozen pre-embryo is to be thawed for transfer to the woman, that the thawing and transfer be performed by a licensed facility. Other potential limitations on the authority of the gamete providers will be discussed below in the section "Extent of Decision-Making Authority."

In some cases, a couple may cede part of their control to their physician when they sign an agreement to undergo IVF. For example, they may decide that, if they become divorced, the physician should choose another couple to use their frozen pre-embryos. The advisability of such transfers of control and the extent to which they should be enforced are discussed in the section of this report on "Advance Agreements."

If one of the gamete providers dies while the pre-embryos are still frozen, the other provider should assume full decision-making authority. While the provider who has died may have wanted to designate a surrogate decision maker, no surrogate would have the same degree of interest as the surviving gamete provider. Family law provides a useful analogy here. When a parent dies, the surviving parent becomes the child's sole guardian.[7] In some cases, the surviving provider will die or both providers will die simultaneously. Just as parents may designate a guardian for their minor children in the event that both die,[8] gamete providers should be able to designate a recipient or guardian of their pre-embryos.

In the event that the gamete providers do not indicate their intent in advance, an appropriate presumption would be to assume that the couple would want the pre-embryos used by someone else. According to data at one clinic, more than 75% of gamete providers choose to have their pre-embryos donated to other couples in the event that the gamete providers cannot use them.[9] Consequently, the fertility clinic should be able to make the pre-embryos available for use, with preference given to relatives of the couple, as long as the gamete providers are given notice of the policy by the clinic. With notice, the policy need not cause any unfairness to the gamete providers, since they could override the policy by an advance directive.

EXTENT OF DECISION-MAKING AUTHORITY

The second important issue to be resolved with frozen pre-embryos is what decisions regarding their use are permissible. In addition to being used by the gamete providers or donated to others for use, the pre-embryos could be used for research or be allowed to thaw and deteriorate (in such a manner as to prevent their survival).

A consensus has developed that the gamete providers should be able to use the pre-embryos themselves or donate them to others. Some commentators question, however, whether the pre-embryos may be used by single people.

Such a situation would arise, for example, if the gamete providers wished to donate their pre-embryos to a particular single woman or to make their pre-embryos available to an infertile woman, regardless of her marital status. Alternatively, the male gamete provider might die and the woman might still want to use the pre-embryos.

Some people have argued that it is not fair to the potential child to be raised by a single parent. There has been some evidence that children from single-parent households do not do as well academically as children from two-parent households.[10,11] However, this finding may reflect differences in income, education, and other socioeconomic factors between the single parents and the parental couples. Indeed, other studies do not find disparities in aptitude among children depending on the number of parents, and some research suggests that girls who have a single mother are more independent and more achievement oriented.[10]

Even if children generally benefit from being raised by two parents, it does not follow that single individuals should be denied parenthood. This country's constitutional tradition recognizes as fundamental the right to procreate and to raise children according to individual preferences.[2,12-14] This tradition rejects the view that government should try to produce "perfect" children by engaging in social engineering. In addition, a denial of parenthood to single individuals raises serious equal-protection concerns and would therefore not be appropriate.

Whether a couple may choose to allow their frozen pre-embryos to thaw and deteriorate (in such a manner as to prevent their survival) is a question that turns on moral, religious, and philosophical views about personhood. This report takes no position on the question of when personhood status begins. Instead, the report will work within the existing body of law on abortion and will reach conclusions about the treatment of frozen pre-embryos based on that law.

If a woman may choose to abort her fetus, it arguably follows that she should be able to allow a frozen pre-embryo to thaw and deteriorate (in such a manner as to prevent its survival). The pre-embryo has a much smaller chance of being a child than a fetus. In addition, the "natural" course of a frozen pre-embryo is to deteriorate. Unlike a fetus, it will not become a child if left alone. On the other hand, a frozen pre-embryo does not intrude on the woman's bodily integrity.

As long as a woman can lawfully abort her fetus, however, it would be inconsistent and ineffectual to have a rule against the thawing and deterioration of a frozen pre-embryo. A couple that wanted to dispose of its pre-embryo could have it transferred to the woman's uterus. The woman could then immediately abort the pre-embryo.

In addition, it would be difficult to draft a rule aimed at preventing the deterioration of frozen pre-embryos. A couple intent on not having the pre-embryo develop into a child could donate the pre-embryo to a woman whom they knew to be incapable of becoming pregnant, or the couple could ask that the pre-embryo be transferred to the female partner's uterus during the time of her cycle when her uterus is not receptive to pregnancy.

It has been suggested that, if a couple does not use a frozen pre-embryo by a certain time, they be required to donate the pre-embryo to another couple. There are several problems with this proposal. Such a rule would treat couples who use

IVF differently from couples who conceive naturally. The latter are not subject to the dictates of society in deciding when to have their children. In addition, an arbitrary time limit would prevent some couples from acting on a subsequent desire to use their pre-embryos to have a child. Finally, even if there would be no parental obligations after donation, the couple should have a right to decide not to have a genetically related child.

The Council on Ethical and Judicial Affairs has previously addressed the question of whether pre-embryos produced by IVF may be used for research. The Council observed that research on pre-embryos in vitro plays an important role in providing society with a better understanding of how genetic defects arise and are transmitted and how they might be prevented or treated.[15] Consequently, the Council concluded that research on pre-embryos is permissible as long as the pre-embryos are not destined for transfer to a woman's uterus and as long as the research is conducted in accordance with the Council's guidelines on fetal research.[15]

DISPUTES BETWEEN THE GAMETE PROVIDERS

In some cases, the providers of the gametes will be unable to agree on the use of their pre-embryos. For example, after a divorce, one may want to have a child with the pre-embryos while the other may want the pre-embryos thawed and discarded. Several considerations suggest that the man and woman should presumptively have an equal say in the use of their pre-embryos and that, therefore, the pre-embryos could not be used by either party without the consent of the other party. First, the man and woman both have contributed half of the pre-embryo's most important component, its genetic code. In addition, whether a person chooses to become a parent and assume all of the accompanying obligations is a particularly personal and fundamental decision. Even if the individual could be absolved of any parental responsibilities, he or she may feel strongly about not having offspring. The absence of a legal duty does not eliminate the moral duty many would feel toward any genetic offspring. Moreover, the far-reaching social implications of requiring individuals to have unwanted children counsels caution. In addition to concerns about the child's economic needs, psychological needs of these children are often left unsatisfied.

Accordingly, the choice not to have children should not be overridden by another person's desire to have offspring. A woman could not insist, for example, that she have access to the sperm of a man that had been frozen for his later use, without the man's permission. In addition, the gamete provider who wants to use the frozen pre-embryos can fulfill his or her desire to have children without frustrating the other gamete provider's desire not to have children. For example, the gamete provider could try IVF with a new partner or turn to adoption. While the gamete provider may not be willing to adopt one of the many children available for adoption (and the preference for genetically related children is understandable), the desire for a genetically related child (or a particular kind of child) should not justify imposing parenthood on the other gamete provider. . . .

In some disputes, the issue will be whether the frozen pre-embryos should be donated to others, used for research, or allowed to thaw and deteriorate (in such a manner as to prevent their survival). In these cases as well, the pre-embryos should not be changed from their frozen state unless both gamete providers agree to the change.

Some commentators have suggested bases for giving one of the gamete providers priority in a dispute. It has been argued that the woman should have priority because she has undergone greater medical risks than the man during the IVF process. In effect, then, she has assumed certain burdens in reliance on the man's willingness to help her have a child. However, we generally do not force one person to waive his or her rights because of another person's reliance. A couple who relies on a pregnant woman's promise to let them adopt her child or a candidate who relies on a citizen's promise to vote for the candidate has no resources if the promisor changes his or her mind.

Priority for the woman might be deduced by analogy to abortion law. Under current law, a woman's right to choose between abortion and childbirth cannot be overridden by the man who would be the child's father.[16] However, in that case the woman's bodily integrity is at stake, a concern not present when pre-embryos are stored in a freezer. Thus, it does not follow from principles of abortion law that the woman's desire to procreate with the pre-embryos should override the man's desire not to procreate.

There is a legitimate concern that neutral rules for the resolution of disputes between gamete providers would, as a practical matter, systematically disadvantage women. Since men have longer reproductive lives than women, for example, their ability to have genetically related offspring is not as likely to be stymied by a lack of access to their frozen pre-embryos. Legal and policy decision makers, therefore, must monitor the impact of the rules governing frozen pre-embryos and, where appropriate, modify the rules to prevent gender-based inequalities.

Another basis proposed for giving one of the gamete providers priority in a dispute is a theory of implied consent. It has been argued that, by virtue of their participation in IVF, the providers of the sperm and ovum have consented to have a child. Consequently, if one wants to use a frozen pre-embryo to have a child and the other does not want to use the pre-embryo, the pre-embryo should be available to the person who wants the child. There are several problems with this theory of implied consent. First, it is not clear that the gamete providers consented to anything more than the creation of a pre-embryo that would become a child whose parenting they would share as a married couple. Specific consent to use the pre-embryo for any other purpose would therefore be required before such a use could be made of the pre-embryo. In addition, society has recognized that an individual's feelings about reproductive decisions may reasonably change with the passage of time. Thus, for example, under current law a woman cannot be bound by an agreement not to abort her fetus, nor can a surrogate mother be bound by her decision to turn her child over to the father of the child.[17] Similarly, a pregnant woman's agreement to give her child up for adoption can be revoked, at least until she actually delivers the child to the adoptive parents.[18] Consequently, until the time for pre-embryo transfer, it would be inappropriate to assume that there is binding consent by either party to have the pre-embryo transferred to a woman's uterus.

ADVANCE AGREEMENTS

The inappropriateness of assuming binding consent suggests that disputes over the use of frozen pre-embryos cannot always be appropriately resolved by a prior general agreement, even a written one, between the gamete providers. The IVF guidelines of professional societies often recommend that the gamete providers specifically decide at the time of IVF about the disposition of their frozen pre-embryos in the event of divorce or other changes in circumstances.[18] The gamete providers might decide that, in the event of divorce, the woman should be able to use the pre-embryos or that the physician should choose another couple to use the pre-embryos. Advance agreements can help ensure that the gamete providers undergo IVF after a full contemplation of the consequences. In drafting their agreement, the gamete providers can be given careful and complete counseling regarding the implications of their endeavors, the potential uses of the pre-embryos, and the possibility that the passage of time will alter their circumstances and their feelings about their initial decision to become a parent through IVF. In general, therefore, these agreements should be enforced. However, decisions about the disposition of pre-embryos can have such profound consequences that the law should include provisions for either gamete provider to be able to show that changed circumstances make enforcement of the agreement unreasonable. (A challenge to an agreement might arise in a dispute between the two gamete providers or between the gamete providers and the clinic.)

Although advance agreements can be useful, gamete providers should not be *required* to enter into advance agreements providing for the disposition of their future pre-embryos, because of the potential problems with advance agreements. Gamete providers may not be able to predict how they will feel about becoming parents at some later time. Advance agreements are also problematic because of the way they are usually developed. Ideally, advance agreements would be drafted by the gamete providers to reflect their particular concerns and preferences. However, the terms of advance agreements are generally decided by the operators of IVF programs on a standardized basis for all of their patients. Consequently, the agreements may reflect the values of the program operators rather than those of the gamete providers. The standard contract of a clinic in Cleveland, Ohio, for example, stipulates that, in the event of a divorce, the couple will permit the clinic either to destroy the pre-embryos or to donate the pre-embryos to an anonymous infertile couple (*Chicago Tribune.* September 28, 1989:1A25). Under the standard contract of a clinic in Detroit, Mich, on the other hand, the pre-embryos would go to the woman or, if she does not want them, to an infertile couple (*Chicago Tribune.* September 28, 1989:1A25). Couples undergoing IVF may try to revise their clinic's standard contract, but the clinic may have sufficient monopoly power that it can effectively offer its terms on a take-it-or-leave-it basis.[19] In addition, standard contracts are not designed to encourage individual approaches.

Advance agreements have been advocated on the ground that they would preclude the need for judicial intervention to resolve disputes that might arise regarding the use of frozen pre-embryos. However, a gamete provider who did not want to be bound by his or her prior agreement could challenge the agreement in court. Indeed, in a recent case, a woman asked the court to void her agreement to have her frozen pre-embryos destroyed in the event of divorce (*Chicago Tribune.* September 28, 1989: 1A25). Similarly, written contracts in surrogate mother arrangements have not prevented litigation, nor have they been upheld routinely by the courts.[18]

There are ways to avoid costly and time-consuming lawsuits without requiring advance agreements. . . . Consequently, the adoption of clear legal rules regarding the disposition of frozen pre-embryos in the event of a dispute is an alternative approach that would eliminate the need for courts to resolve disagreements between gamete providers or between clinics and gamete providers. For example, if courts or legislatures adopted the proposal in this report that frozen pre-embryos not be used, donated, or discarded unless both gamete providers agree to the same disposition, gamete providers would have to resolve their disputes by themselves.

REFERENCES

1. *Skinner v Oklahoma,* 316 US 635 (1942).
2. *Griswold v Connecticut,* 381 US 479 (1965).
3. *Webster v Reproductive Health Services,* 109 S CT 3040 (1989).
4. *Parham v JR,* 442 US 584 (1979).
5. *Bowen v American Hospital Association,* 476 US 610 (1986).
6. Robertson JA. Ethical and legal issues in cryopreservation of human embryos. *Fertil Steril.* 1987; 47:371–381.
7. *See, eg,* Ill Ann Stat ch 110 1/2 ¶ 11-7.
8. *See, eg,* Ill Ann Stat ch 110 1/2, ¶ 11-5(b).
9. Trounson A. Preservation of human eggs and embryos. *Fertil Steril.* 1986; 46:1–12.

10. McGuire M, Alexander NJ. Artificial insemination of single women. *Fertil Steril.* 1985; 43:182–184.

11. Orentlicher D. Does mother know best? *Hastings L. J.* 1989; 40:1111–1122.

12. *Meyer v Nebraska,* 262 US 390 (1923).

13. *Prince v Massachusetts,* 321 US 158 (1944).

14. *Carey v Population Services International,* 431 US 678 (1977).

15. *Current Opinions of the Council on Ethical and Judicial Affairs of the American Medical Association—1989: In Vitro Fertilization.* Chicago, Ill: American Medical Association; 1989.

16. *Planned Parenthood of Central Missouri v Danforth,* 428 US 52 (1976).

17. *In re Baby M,* 109 NJ 396, 537 A2d 1227 (1988).

18. Committee on Ethics, American College of Obstetricians and Gynecologists. *Ethical Issues in Human in Vitro Fertilization and Embryo Placement.* Washington, DC: American College of Obstetricians and Gynecologists; 1986.

19. Robertson JA. Resolving disputes over frozen embryos. *Hastings Cent Rep.* November/December 1989; 19(6):7–12.

NO

David T. Ozar

THE CASE AGAINST THAWING UNUSED FROZEN EMBRYOS

Whether one believes that the embryo has rights from the instant of conception, or that the embryo has no moral rights at all, the conclusion about the fate of unused frozen embryos is the same: they ought to be preserved in their frozen state until they are implanted in a woman's womb or are no longer able to survive implantation. . . .

How ought people to act, what ought people to do, in regard to unused frozen embryos?

Some might argue that this question misses the point, that the real issue concerns the morality of artificial reproductive techniques themselves, of which freezing live embryos is simply one example. From this perspective all forms of fertilization other than intercourse are profoundly unnatural and immoral.[1] The real point would be that these embryos should not have been fertilized and frozen in the first place. We are uncertain about how to proceed rightly from this point because the parties acted immorally at the outset. . . .

But this response is of little help to those who must now determine what to do about existing frozen embryos. Even if the acts that brought us to this pass were profoundly immoral, what we do next is still not a morally indifferent matter. . . .

THE "INSTANT OF CONCEPTION" VIEW

There are two approaches to our obligations toward fetuses that are informative regarding frozen embryos as well. First is the most inclusive moral position regarding obligations toward the unborn—the position that holds that the conceptus has a moral right not to be killed, and the rest of us have a moral obligation not to kill the conceptus or to intend to kill it, from the first instant of its conception.[2] (This right, stated more completely, is a right not to be *directly* killed, and the obligation is an obligation not to *directly* kill or to intend to *directly* kill the conceptus. The added term, "directly," is very important in other contexts; but it is not important in the present discussion, and therefore I shall use the more simplified statement.)

This position is commonly called the "right to life" position; but I shall call it the "instant of conception" position. Many other positions on these matters affirm life-related rights, including rights not to be killed under various sets of circumstances. In calling it the "instant of conception" position, I am focusing on what is truly distinctive about it and on its substantive claims in the present discussion.

According to this position, a frozen embryo, as the fruit of human conception, has a moral right not to be killed. Therefore the doctors and researchers responsible for the care of such an embryo could not morally place it in an environment known to be lethal to it. This would preclude deliberately permitting a frozen embryo to be thawed without placing it in the only environment in which it could survive thawing, namely, a woman's womb. Nor could the parents (by any definition) or anyone else morally choose that a frozen embryo be dealt with in this way.

At the same time, the "instant of conception" position provides no basis for saying that an embryo has a moral right to be implanted in a womb. The moral right not to be killed does not automatically imply a right to the use of a womb. For an embryo may be implanted in a womb only by the free choice of the woman whose womb it is. Thus the obligation not to kill an embryo does not necessarily imply an obligation on anyone's part to offer her womb for its survival.

One possible exception is the genetic mother, the donor of the ovum whence the embryo has grown. It may be that, in bringing the embryo into being, she has undertaken an obligation to assist it in realizing its full potential for human life.

But this obligation, if it exists, does not derive from a moral right of the embryo as the kind of being that it is, but rather from the mother's freely undertaking to bring it into being. (The genetic father might have a similar obligation, but since he cannot provide the womb that the embryo needs, I shall not consider his obligations further.)

I shall not attempt to resolve here the complicated questions about the degree of responsibility of genetic parents for their offspring.[3] The point is that, if the genetic mother does have such an obligation to the embryo, then she may be obligated to accept the unused embryo into her womb. If the genetic mother refuses to do so, however, or if she dies . . . so that responsibility for the frozen embryos now falls upon the hospital-laboratory team, no one would have an *obligation* to accept the embryo into her womb. If anyone did accept it, this would be an act of charity toward the embryo, not an act of obligation or an act to which the embryo had a right.

There are then two possibilities. If no one volunteers her womb for the implantation of the unused frozen embryo, those responsible for its care will fulfill their obligations simply by not killing it, that is, by keeping it frozen. If, on the other hand, someone does volunteer for its implantation, the responsible parties would need to determine whether implantation in the womb of this particular volunteer would give the embryo a reasonable chance of survival and further development, as compared with continued freezing and the possibility of implantation in a future volunteer with more likelihood of success. It would be appropriate, also, for the responsible parties to seek out women who might desire to volunteer for implantation of unused embryos.

Since frozen embryos may deteriorate over time, let us assume that there is a point at which the hospital-laboratory team can accurately say that a particular embryo is no longer able to survive implantation. Such an embryo no longer has any potential for continued life. Because it is still frozen, it is not yet dead; yet death is its only conceivable prospect. I believe that the "instant of conception" position would conclude that such an embryo no longer has any moral right that would require its continued maintenance in the frozen state. Its condition is now analogous to that of someone who is irreversibly in the process of dying. The embryo may morally be thawed at this point, and the irreversible process of its death permitted to proceed to its conclusion.

THE VIEW THAT THE EMBRYO HAS NO MORAL RIGHTS

The obligations that I have just outlined, based as they are on the most inclusive position regarding our obligations to the unborn, constitute the most extensive set of obligations toward unused frozen embryos that can reasonably be defended. Next we must ask: Is any lesser set of obligations toward unused frozen embryos more reasonable? In order to respond, I shall look at a position that accords no moral rights at all to the unborn.

If a frozen embryo has no moral rights of its own, if it is more like a piece of property (or is just like a piece of property) rather than a bearer of rights, still those who are responsible for it will have obligations regarding its use and the consequences of its use. If certain ways of

dealing with it would lead to significantly more good than other ways, at relatively little cost in human effort, in monetary resources, and so on, then the responsible parties would be obligated to choose those ways of acting. If certain ways of acting would involve risk of significant harm, which could be avoided at relatively little cost in human effort, in monetary resources, and so on, then the responsible parties would be obligated to avoid them.

These straightforward moral principles point to the same conclusion as is defended by the "instant of conception" position, even if the embryo has no moral rights at all. My argument follows a pattern developed by Mary Anne Warren in a famous postscript to "On the Moral and Legal Status of Abortion." In response to criticisms that her criteria for having moral rights were so strict as to deny moral rights to infants, Warren argued that even when no moral rights are relevant, morality may require that human life be preserved and protected because of the negative consequences of doing otherwise.

Once the original outlay of expense and effort for freezing embryos has been made, embryos can be maintained in their frozen state at very little cost, in dollars or in human effort. Therefore if there are women who desire to bear a child and who might be successfully implanted with embryos unused by others, the moral principles just articulated argue strongly for maintaining unused embryos in their frozen state until they can be implanted. The costs of doing this are very small and the benefits to the mothers concerned (as well as to their spouses and other affected parties) are very great. In fact, if the good of enabling women to bear children can justify the sizable expense of developing or purchasing this technology in the first place, then it surely can justify the far smaller expense of maintaining unused embryos until other women who desire to bear a child have volunteered. It would also be reasonable for the doctors and researchers to seek out such women, especially if the frozen embryo does deteriorate over time, in the interests of maximizing the benefits and minimizing the costs of the process.

This same conclusion—that unused frozen embryos ought to be maintained in their frozen state for as long as they are able to survive implantation—can be reached in another way, which takes account of other consequences of the process. For even if frozen embryos do not have moral rights, they are still members of the human species with a potential for a full human life. Indeed it is precisely because of that potential that they were frozen in the first place. Consequently if hospital-laboratory teams, parents, or other responsible parties routinely followed a policy of simply disposing of unused frozen embryos, such a policy, if widely known, could have a negative impact on the ways in which we as individuals and as a community value and deal with human life generally, especially in other members of our species whose lives are in some way compromised.

Two questions need to be addressed here. One is a subtle question of social psychology. It asks how various policies concerning human life that are accepted within a community have an impact on individuals' values and future actions and on future policies within the community. The second is a normative question: What values, actions, and future policies regarding human life should we

support and reinforce in our present policy making?

We are woefully short on answers to the first question. Some have argued that a community that values many other things over the life of a fetus will experience a gradual but significant lessening in the value of human life generally, so that previously unacceptable trade-offs between human life and other values will come to be accepted. Others have claimed that there is no such linkage in human feelings or in other parts of the human psyche between our valuation of human life in the unborn and the born.

I have no expert opinion to offer on the first question, but I believe that we do have some sense of the proper answer to the second, for it is clear that a great deal is at stake here. The value that we, as individuals and as a community, attach to human life is the most fundamental element of the social morality that makes it possible for us to live together in some measure of security. Such valuing of human life is nurtured in many subtle ways in our habits and mores, and in our institutions. Such valuing is probably vulnerable as well, at least over the long run; it may even be subject to significant changes as habits, mores, and institutions change.

Thus it is not beyond the realm of possibility that widespread public acceptance of a practice in which human embryos are made when it is efficient and economical to make them and disposed of when it is efficient and economical to dispose of them would have an impact on the community's valuing of human life in other contexts, an impact that would put the lives of those already born at risk when trade-offs of efficiency and economics did not favor them. We know far too little to predict that something like this will certainly occur. But we also know far too little to predict that it certainly will not. Certainly enough is at stake that we would be foolish not to acknowledge the risk.

Only reasons of economy and efficiency support a policy of disposal. But a policy of maintaining the lives of frozen embryos for as long as they could survive implantation and of actively seeking out women who might desire to bear them would be far less expensive than the setup costs of the technology that enabled us to freeze embryos in the first place. Thus, given the possible negative impact of disposing of human embryos for reasons of efficiency and economics, clearly the far better course of action is to maintain the frozen embryos until they can no longer survive implantation and to actively support their implantation when women desiring to bear them volunteer. This course of action avoids risk of significant harm at relatively little cost.

From this it is clear that those who would accord to frozen embryos no moral rights whatsoever, but who would still be guided in their obligations by consideration of the outcomes of their actions, would reach the same conclusion regarding unused frozen embryos as those who affirm the embryos' moral rights from the instant of conception. From both perspectives, as well as each of the intermediate moral positions, the responsible parties have an obligation to preserve the frozen embryos in their frozen state until such time as they can no longer survive implantation. In addition, they should support implantation of unused embryos in women who volunteer to bear them and should make reasonable efforts to locate such women when there are implantable embryos.

FREEZING MULTIPLE EMBRYOS

The issues discussed so far presuppose the value of fertilizing multiple ova and freezing the resulting embryos on the chance that an implanted embryo will subsequently abort. Since the risk of spontaneous abortion of implanted embryos is considerable, the fertilization and freezing of multiple embryos seem a reasonable efficiency. But the previous arguments suggest that the production of embryos is not something to be undertaken lightly. So we need to reflect on the ethical appropriateness of the multiple frozen embryo procedure itself.

Some authors have argued that in vitro fertilization and the implantation of the resulting embryo are, without exception, profoundly unnatural and immoral. Obviously if this view is correct, nearly every aspect of the procedure of freezing multiple embryos is immoral; but I do not find the arguments offered in support of this view to be persuasive. Putting considerations of the just allocation of health care resources aside for the moment, I consider it a reasonable and therapeutic intervention to assist a woman who desires to bear a child by fertilizing her ovum in vitro and implanting the resulting embryo in her womb. If freezing the embryo at some point in its development will give it a better chance of surviving implantation, without harming its development in other ways, this too seems reasonable to me.

The ethical issue that has not been adequately addressed is precisely the procedure of fertilizing and freezing *multiple* embryos. The most obvious reason for this procedure is that it is easier and cheaper to fertilize several ova at the same time and to have the resulting embryos available for a second or third implantation whenever they are needed, rather than go back to fertilizing an ovum from the beginning if the first (second, third) implantation fails.

The problem is, as before, that the organisms being used to make the procedure cheaper and easier are genetically complete human organisms. It is, again, their very potential for full human life that prompts the hospital-laboratory team to fertilize and preserve them in the first place. Therefore the same considerations that argue for thoughtful caution in our dealings with unused embryos argue for a similar caution in our making and freezing of embryos at all.

If it becomes common knowledge that human embryos are fertilized and frozen in quantity in order to make a particular medical procedure easier and less expensive, could this not have a significant negative impact on individuals' and communities' values and future actions, at least over the long run? Are the benefits of such a procedure valuable enough to run the risks that the procedure involves?

In response, it could be argued that it is precisely in the interests of human life that human life is being used in this way. Everyone involved in this technology is striving to enable children to be born who otherwise could not have been born. The chances of a particular child's being born are multiplied by two or three or whatever the number, it would be argued, if we are able to fertilize and freeze two or three or more embryos at the start. Does not this goal of extending human life to those who would otherwise not have it justify the multiple frozen embryo procedure?

When we are dealing with those already born, we do not permit anyone's life to be used to improve another person's chances unless the helper undertakes the task voluntarily. If we are dealing with children or others who cannot choose on their own, we would permit one's life to be used in the interests of another in only the rarest of circumstances, if ever. Still, "using a life" usually does not mean giving a new life, as it does when multiple embryos are fertilized and frozen. On the other hand, the frozen embryo procedure is not the only way to obtain a second, third, or fourth living embryo if the first implantation should fail. So we are left with a question: If it was certain that every embryo fertilized and frozen in this procedure would have a chance for implantation, as in the policy argued for in the preceding section, then would the way in which the embryos' lives are "used" in this technology be morally acceptable? Or would manipulating the lives of human embryos in this way still pose a risk of negatively affecting the ways in which individuals and communities value and deal with human life? Considerations of efficiency and laboratory economy alone would not seem worth this risk.

But what about the value to the mothers involved, the value of bearing a child? To be sure, the good of childbearing is a great good; and the future of our species, itself a considerable good, depends on it. But a particular woman's ability to bear a child is not an absolute good; it can be outweighed by a variety of other considerations, singly or in combination. Nor is childbearing the only possible basis of parenting, which is the good that at least some candidates for this procedure seek. We must at least inquire whether adoption would not fulfill the most important needs of many who seek the assistance of reproductive technologies without the risks and costs of such technologies.

A single-minded commitment on the part of the physicians and researchers involved in reproductive technologies to enable women to bear children who would otherwise be unable to do so is understandable and perhaps even commendable. But in making policy the larger community must take more into account than the ability of patients to bear children and the ability of doctors and researchers to develop efficient procedures to this end.

The issue can be posed in a different way. Ought every woman who has healthy ova but who cannot bear children without such a procedure receive the benefits of multiple frozen embryo technology? As soon as we ask the question in this way, recognizing that many thousands of women might be candidates for the procedure (by some current estimates, 15 percent of all married couples are infertile),[4] we realize that we must consider the costs. Making the procedure available to every woman who might benefit would almost certainly draw significant resources away from other pressing health care needs or from other uses of resources within the larger community.

Is this procedure so valuable that we would be willing to close immunization programs or blood banks or a significant number of medical schools, or reduce the resources devoted to arthritis research or the like, in order to make it available to all who might benefit? Is it more valuable than efforts to provide better education to our disadvantaged young or decent survival to our elderly poor or basic foodstuffs and fresh water to the millions in the world community who cannot obtain them without assistance? We recognize immediately that the good that this technology pursues is a relative good; it must be weighed against other goods before we can know if pursuing it is worth the cost in resources, in human effort, and, as I have argued, in the risk of future harm.

At present the benefits of the multiple frozen embryo procedure are available only to the wealthy and to those who have been selected as research subjects. The latter pattern of allocating this therapy may be justified as long as the therapy is still experimental. But there is a clear injustice in giving the wealthy privileged access to an accepted therapeutic procedure. Admittedly some instances of "pure" research justify themselves only long afterwards by leading to benefits for many that could not have been foreseen. But we must ask who will benefit and how much, and how these benefits compare not only with the cost in resources and human effort, but also with the risk of future harm within the larger community.

AN UNUSUAL OPPORTUNITY

In the case of freezing multiple embryos we have an unusual opportunity for agreement on a question of reproductive morality. Richard McCormick, David Thomasma, and many others, have stressed that we cannot resolve by law and public policy a set of issues on which there is not, within the community at large, a consensus on the underlying values.[5] On the issue of the legality of abortion, and of the constitutionality of laws prohibiting or regulating it, our community appears to be profoundly divided; and this division has been deepened and entrenched by strident rhetoric on both sides.

But if I am correct in claiming that the two most frequently opposed moral positions about reproductive morality must reach the same conclusion regarding our obligations toward unused frozen embryos, then here is a possible starting point from which respectful conversation and the search for a broader consensus can begin. To be sure, different patterns of reasoning are involved in the two positions. But on this issue at least, the two sides need not begin their conversation at odds, committed to showing first of all that the other's position is without substance. On this issue there is a basis for agreement, and therefore for respect and for further conversation.

REFERENCES

1. A classic statement of this position appears in Pope Pius XXI's 1956 address to the Second World Congress on Fertility and Sterility. *Proceedings of the Second World Congress on Fertility and Sterility,* 2 vols. (Naples, Italy: University of Naples, 1957–1958), vol. I p. 40. See also Leon Kass, "Making Babies—The New Biology and the 'Old' Morality," *Public Interest,* Winter 1972, pp. 23–49, and " 'Making Babies' Revisited," *Public Interest,* Winger 1979, pp. 44–60. But also see Anthony Kosnik, *et. al., Human Sexuality: New Directions in American Catholic Thought* (New York: Paulist Press, 1977), pp. 137–40, and Margot Joan Fromer, *Ethical Issues in Sexuality and Reproduction* (St. Louis: Mosby, 1983), pp. 271–77. For a broad survey of ethical literature on in vitro fertilization, see LeRoy Walters, "Human In Vitro Fertilization: A Review of the Ethical Literature," *Hastings Center Report,* August 1979, pp. 23–43; and *Bioethics Reporter,* "Rights of Fetuses: Issues, Commentary, Literature, Court Cases, Legislation, and Bibliography," 1984.

2. For examples of this position, see John T. Noonan, Jr., "An Almost Absolute Value in History," in his *The Morality of Abortion: Legal and Historical Perspectives* (Cambridge: Harvard University Press, 1970) and Teresa Iglesias, "*In Vitro* Fertilization: The Major Issues," *Journal of Medical Ethics* vol. 10 (1984).

3. This topic has not been carefully discussed in the literature. For a thoughtful discussion of voluntariness and responsibility in regard to a fetus conceived through intercourse, see Joel Feinberg, "Abortion," in Tom Regan, ed., *Matters of Life and Death,* (New York: Random House, 1980), pp. 209–14.

4. Lori Andrews, *New Conceptions: A Consumer's Guide to the Newest Infertility Treatments, Including In Vitro Fertilization, Artificial Insemination, and Surrogate Motherhood* (New York: St. Martins Press, 1984).

5. See Richard A. McCormick, S.J., "The Abortion Dossier," "Rules for Abortion Debate," and "Public Policy on Abortion," in his *How Brave a New World?* (Garden City, N.Y.; Doubleday, 1981), and David Thomasma, *An Apology for the Value of Human Life* (St. Louis: Catholic Health Association, 1983).

POSTSCRIPT

Should Thawing Unused Frozen Embryos Be Permitted?

A committee, convened to decide what to do with the frozen embryos left by the deceased Rios couple, recommended that the embryos be destroyed. However, the legislature of the Australian state of Victoria rejected this advice and called for the embryos to be implanted in surrogate mothers and then placed for adoption if pregnancies resulted and came to term. Since so much time has passed without any further announcement, it is unlikely that any implantation took place. In the Davis case, in a controversial decision, the court found that "human life begins at conception" and awarded custody of the embryos to Mrs. Davis. In May 1990 Mrs. Davis, who has remarried, announced that she no longer intends to implant the embryos and will donate them to a fertility clinic for use by a childless couple. Her former husband is continuing to appeal the original ruling. The York case was settled out of court with the Virginia clinic agreeing to release the embryos to the couple in California.

Much of the discussion about IVF and embryo freezing has taken place abroad. Clinical in vitro fertilization has been accepted as ethical in 15 countries that established commissions to review new reproductive technologies. However, there is no consensus on embryo freezing. The most often-cited committee report is the British "Warnock Report," published in 1985 by Basil Blackwell as *A Question of Life*. LeRoy Walters analyzed the international committee statements in a Special Supplement of the *Hastings Center Report* (June 1987). An American overview can be found in a report by the Institute of Medicine and the National Research Council, "Medically Assisted Conception: An Agenda for Research" (1989).

John A. Robertson urges that couples in IVF programs stipulate binding instructions in advance regarding the disposition of frozen embryos in "Resolving Disputes Over Frozen Embryos," *Hastings Center Report* (November/December 1989). Also see Robertson's "Ethical and Legal Issues in Cryopreservation of Human Embryos," *Fertility and Sterility* (March 1987), as well as Andrea Bonnicksen's "Embryo Freezing: Ethical Issues in the Clinical Setting," *Hastings Center Report* (December 1988).

ISSUE 3

Should Women Be Allowed to Bear Babies for a Fee?

YES: John A. Robertson, from "Surrogate Mothers: Not So Novel After All," *Hastings Center Report* (October 1983)

NO: Herbert T. Krimmel, from "The Case Against Surrogate Parenting," *Hastings Center Report* (October 1983)

ISSUE SUMMARY

YES: Professor of law John A. Robertson maintains that infertile couples have a right to arrange for a surrogate mother to bear the husband's child and that the ethical and legal problems that might result are not very different from those that already exist for adoption and artificial insemination by donor.
NO: Professor of law Herbert T. Krimmel takes the position that it is immoral to bear a child for the purpose of giving it up and that surrogate mother arrangements will put additional stress on our society's shared moral values.

The desire to bear a child is a deep and natural one, and for the 2.4 million infertile married American couples, their inability to reproduce is often a source of sorrow and pain. But adoption is not an easy alternative today. Because of the availability of legal abortion and because an increasing number of unwed teenage mothers are choosing to keep their babies, there are fewer babies available through adoption agencies—particularly the healthy, white newborns that are in greatest demand. The new reproductive technologies of external fertilization and embryo transfer are available only to a few women who meet rigid medical criteria.

Under these circumstances, it is not surprising that, when the wife is infertile, some couples are turning to surrogate mothers—women who will bear the husband's baby for a fee and then give it up for legal adoption. This is the way it works: A broker (usually a lawyer) puts an infertile couple in contact with potential surrogates who have been recruited (usually through newspaper advertisements) and screened for medical and psychological characteristics. If the couple and the surrogate agree, they sign a contract specifying in detail the fee (usually $10,000), the surrogate's responsibilities to care for her health during pregnancy, the conditions under which she would have an abortion, the transfer of legal custody, and the like. The price

40

tag is high. In addition to the surrogate's fee, the couple will have to pay the broker ($5,000 to $10,000), the doctor who performs the insemination, the doctor who delivers the baby, and other medical costs. The total costs can run to $30,000 or more.

In the past such arrangements were almost certainly carried out in secret, and probably without any money changing hands, between friends and relatives. But in 1980 Elizabeth Kane (a pseudonym), a married woman with three children, announced publicly that she had borne a baby for a fee. "It's the father's child," she is reported to have said. "I'm only growing it for him." Since then there have been an estimated 500 to 700 babies born by contract, and several firms are now engaged in matching would-be adoptive parents and willing surrogates.

Are these contracts legal? Most states have laws prohibiting baby selling: the offering, giving, or receiving anything of value for placing a child for adoption. But whether surrogate mother contracts are baby selling or just another form of private adoption has yet to be settled in the courts. Even if the contracts are proven to be legal, serious questions remain about whether they are enforceable—whether, for instance, a mother who decides to keep the baby when it is born can be forced to give it up. The 1987–88 Baby M case in New Jersey, which was played out in the glare of publicity, illustrated how divisive such court battles can be. In the end, the court declared the contract illegal but awarded custody of Baby M to her father and adoptive mother, William and Elizabeth Stern. Her natural mother, Mary Beth Whitehead, has visitation rights.

When any unusual social arrangement is introduced, people tend to see it either as a continuation of already existing patterns or as something completely novel, and therefore suspect. Those who support the idea of surrogate mothers see it as similar to other practices in which a child is reared by someone other than its genetic parents. They believe that, as long as the child is wanted and cared for, the practice is acceptable—even desirable—as is expressed in the following selection by John A. Robertson.

Those who oppose the practice point not only to the legal uncertainties but also to the psychological and family stresses that will face the children, the surrogate, and the adoptive family. According to the view expressed in the selection by Herbert T. Krimmel, it is unethical to produce children in order to give them up and to encourage the view of children as commodities.

YES   John A. Robertson

SURROGATE MOTHERS:
NOT SO NOVEL AFTER ALL

All reproduction is collaborative, for no man or woman reproduces alone. Yet the provision of sperm, egg, or uterus through artificial insemination, embryo transfer, and surrogate mothers makes reproduction collaborative in another way. A third person provides a genetic or gestational factor not present in ordinary paired reproduction. As these practices grow, we must confront the ethical issues raised and their implications for public policy.

Collaborative reproduction allows some persons who otherwise might remain childless to produce healthy children. However, its deliberate separation of genetic, gestational, and social parentage is troublesome. The offspring and participants may be harmed, and there is a risk of confusing family lineage and personal identity. In addition, the techniques intentionally manipulate a natural process that many persons want free of technical intervention. Yet many well-accepted practices, including adoption, artificial insemination by donor (AID), and blended families (families where children of different marriages are raised together) intentionally separate biologic and social parenting, and have become an accepted thread in the social fabric. Should all collaborative techniques be similarly treated? When, if ever, are they ethical? Should the law prohibit, encourage, or regulate them, or should the practice be left to private actors? Surrogate motherhood—the controversial practice by which a woman agrees to bear a child conceived by artificial insemination and to relinquish it at birth to others for rearing—illustrates the legal and ethical issues arising in collaborative reproduction generally.

AN ALTERNATIVE TO AGENCY ADOPTIONS

Infertile couples who are seeking surrogates hire attorneys and sign contracts with women recruited through newspaper ads. The practice at present probably involves at most a few hundred persons. But repeated attention on *Sixty Minutes* and the *Phil Donahue Show,* and in the popular press is likely to engender more demand, for thousands of infertile couples might find surrogate mothers the answer to their reproductive needs. What began as an enterprise involving a few lawyers and doctors in Michigan, Kentucky, and California is now a national phenomenon. There are surrogate mother centers in Maryland, Arizona, and several other states, and even a surrogate mother newsletter.

Surrogate mother arrangements occur within a tradition of family law that gives the gestational mother (and her spouse, if one exists) rearing rights and obligations. (However, the presumption that the husband is the father can be challenged, and a husband's obligations to his wife's child by AID will usually require his consent.)[1] Although no state has legislation directly on the subject of surrogate motherhood, independently arranged adoptions are lawful in most states. It is no crime to agree to bear a child for another, and then relinquish it for adoption. However, paying the mother a fee for adoption beyond medical expenses is a crime in some states, and in others will prevent the adoption.[2] Whether termination and transfer of parenting rights will be legally recognized depends on the state. Some states, like Hawaii and Florida, ask few questions and approve independent adoptions very quickly. Others, like Michigan and Kentucky, won't allow surrogate mothers to terminate and assign rearing rights to another if a fee has been paid, or even allow a paternity determination in favor of the sperm donor. The enforcibility of surrogate contracts has also not been tested, and it is safe to assume that some jurisdictions will not enforce them. Legislation clarifying many of these questions has been proposed in several states, but has not yet been enacted.

Even this brief discussion highlights an important fact about surrogate motherhood and other collaborative reproductive techniques. They operate as an alternative to the non-market, agency system of allocating children for adoption, which has contributed to long queues for distributing healthy white babies. This form of independent adoption is controlled by the parties and planned before conception, and enables both the father and mother of the adopted child to be selected in advance.

Understood in these terms, the term "surrogate mother," which means substitute mother, is a misnomer. The natural mother, who contributes egg and uterus, is not so much a substitute mother as a substitute spouse who carries a child for a man whose wife is infertile. Indeed, it is the adoptive mother who is the surrogate mother for the child, since she parents a child borne by another. What, if anything, is wrong with this arrangement? Let us look more closely at its benefits and harms before discussing public policy.

ALL THE PARTIES CAN BENEFIT

Reproduction through surrogate mothering is a deviation from our cultural norms of reproduction, and to many persons it seems immoral or wrong. But surrogate mothering may be good for the parties involved.

Surrogate contracts meet the desire of a husband and wife to rear a healthy child, and more particularly, a child with one partner's genes. The need could arise because the wife has an autosomal dominant or sex-linked genetic disorder, such as hemophilia. More likely, she is infertile and the couple feels a strong need to have children. For many infertile couples the inability to conceive is a major personal problem causing marital conflict and filling both partners with anguish and self-doubt. It may also involve multiple medical work-ups and possibly even surgery. If the husband and wife have sought to adopt a child, they may have been told either that they do not qualify or to join the queue of couples waiting several years for agency adoptions (the wait has grown longer due to birth control, abortion, and the greater willingness of illegitimate mothers to keep their children[3]). For couples exhausted and frustrated by these efforts, the surrogate arrangement seems a Godsend. While the intense desire to have a child often appears selfish, we must not lose sight of the deep-seated psychosocial and biological roots of the desire to generate children.[4]

The arrangement may also benefit the surrogate. Usually women undergo pregnancy and childbirth because they want to rear children. But some women want to have the experience of bearing and birthing a child without the obligation to rear. Phillip Parker, a Michigan psychiatrist who has interviewed over 275 surrogate applicants, finds that the decision to be a surrogate springs from several motives.[5] Most women willing to be surrogates have already had children, and many are married. They choose the surrogate role primarily because the fee provides a better economic opportunity than alternative occupations, but also because they enjoy being pregnant and the respect and attention it draws. The surrogate experience may also be a way to master, through reliving, guilt they feel from past pregnancies that ended in abortion or adoption. Some surrogates may also feel pleased or satisfied, as

organ donors do, that they have given the "gift of life" to another couple.[6]

The child born of a surrogate arrangement also benefits. Indeed, but for the surrogate contract, this child would not have been born at all. Unlike the ordinary agency or independent adoption, where a child is already conceived or brought to term, the conception of this child occurs solely as a result of the surrogate agreement. Thus even if the child does suffer identity problems, as adopted children often do, because they are not able to know their mother, this child has benefited, or at least has not been wronged, for without the surrogate arrangement, she would not have been born at all.[7]

BUT PROBLEMS EXIST TOO

Surrogate mothering is also troublesome. Many people think that it is wrong for a woman to conceive and bear a child that she does not intend to raise, particularly if she receives a fee for her services. There are potential costs to the surrogate and her family, the adoptive couple, the child, and even society at large from satisfying the generative needs of infertile couples in this way.

The couple must be willing to spend about $20,000–25,000, depending on lawyers' fees and the supply of and demand for surrogate mothers. (While this price tag makes the surrogate contract a consumption item for the middle classes, it is not unjust to poor couples, for it does not leave them worse off than they were.) The couple must also be prepared to experience, along with the adjustment and demands of becoming parents, the stress and anxiety of participating in a novel social relationship that many still consider immoral or deviant. What do they tell their friends or family? What do they tell the child? Will the child have contact with the mother? What is the couple's relationship with the surrogate and her family during the pregnancy and after? Without established patterns for handling these questions, the parties may experience confusion, frustration, and embarrassment.

A major source of uncertainty and stress is likely to be the surrogate herself. In most cases she will be a stranger, and may never even meet the couple. The lack of a preexisting relation between the couple and surrogate and the possibility that they live far apart enhance the possibility of mistrust. Is the surrogate taking care of herself? Is she having sex with others during her fertile period? Will she contact the child afterwards? What if she demands more money to relinquish the child? To allay these anxieties, the couple could try to establish a relationship of trust with the surrogate, yet such a relationship creates reciprocal rights and duties and might create demands for an undesired relationship after the birth. Even good lawyering that specifies every contingency in the contract is unlikely to allay uncertainty and anxiety about the surrogate's trustworthiness.

The surrogate may also find the experience less satisfying than she envisioned. Conceiving the child may require insemination efforts over several months at inconvenient locations. The pregnancy and birth may entail more pain, unpleasant side effects, and disruption than she expected. The couple may be more intrusive or more aloof than she wishes. As the pregnancy advances and the birth nears, the surrogate may find it increasingly difficult to remain detached by thinking of the child as "theirs" rather than "hers." Relinquishing the baby after birth may be considerably more disheartening and disappointing than she anticipated. Even if informed of this possibility in advance, she may be distressed for several weeks with feelings of loss, depression, and sleep disturbance.[8] She may feel angry at the couple for cutting off all contact with her once the baby is delivered, and guilty at giving up her child. Finally, she will have to face the loss of all contact with "her" child. As the reality of her situation dawns, she may regret not having bargained harder for access to "her baby."

As with the couple, the surrogate's experience will vary with the expectations, needs, and personalities of the parties , the course of the pregnancy, and an advance understanding of the problems that can arise. The surrogate should have a lawyer to protect her interests. Often, however, the couple's lawyer will end up advising the surrogate. Although he has recruited the surrogate, he is paid by and represents the couple. By disclosing his conflicting interest, he satisfies legal ethics, but he may not serve the interests of the surrogate as well as independent counsel.

HARMS TO THE CHILD

Unlike embryo transfer, gene therapy, and other manipulative techniques (some of which are collaborative), surrogate arrangements do not pose the risk of physical harm to the offspring. But there is the risk of psychosocial harm. Surrogate mothering, like adoption and artificial insemination by donor (AID), deliberately separates genetic and gestational from social parentage. The mother who begets, bears, and births does not parent. This separation can pose a problem for the child who discovers it. Like adopted and AID children, the child may be strongly motivated to learn the absent parent's identity and to establish a relationship, in this case with the mother and her family. Inability to make that connection, especially inability to learn who the mother is, may affect the child's self-esteem, create feelings of rootlessness, and leave the child thinking she had been rejected due to some personal fault.[9] While this is a serious concern, the situation is tolerated when it arises with AID and adoptive children. Intentional conception for adoption—the essence of surrogate mothering—poses no different issue.

The child can also be harmed if the adoptive couple are not fit parents. After all, a willingness to spend substantial money to fulfill a desire to rear children is no guarantee of good parenting. But then neither is reproduction by paired mates who wish intensely to have a child. The nonbiologic parent may resent or reject the child, but the same possibility exists with adoption, AID, or ordinary reproduction.

There is also the fear, articulated by such commentators as Leon Kass and Paul Ramsey,[10] that collaborative reproduction confuses the lineage of children and destroys the meaning of family as we know it. In surrogate mothering, as with sperm or ovum or womb donors, the genetic and gestational mother does not rear the child, though the biologic father does. What implications does this hold for the family and the child's lineage?

The separation of the child from the genetic or biologic parent in surrogate mothering is hardly unique. It arises with adoption, but surrogate arrangements are more closely akin to AID or blended families, where at least one parent has a bloodtie to the child and the child will know at least one genetic parent. He may, as adopted children often do, have intense desires to learn his biologic mother's identity and seek contact with her and her family. Failure to connect with biologic roots may cause suffering. But the fact that adoption through surrogate mother contracts is planned before conception does not increase the chance of identity confusion, lowered self esteem, or the blurring of lineage that occurs with adoption or AID.

The greatest chance of confusing family lines arises if the child and couple establish relations with the surrogate and the surrogate's family. If that unlikely event occurs, questions about the child's relations with the surrogate's spouse, parents, and other children can arise. But these issues are not unique. Indeed, they are increasingly common with the growth of blended families. Surrogate mothering in a few instances may lead to a new variation on blended families, but its threat to the family is trivial compared to the rapid changes in family structure now occurring for social, economic, and demographic reasons.

In many cases surrogate motherhood and other forms of collaborative reproduction may shore up, rather than undermine, the traditional family by enabling couples who would otherwise be childless to have children. The practice of employing others to assist in child rearing—including wet-nurses, neonatal ICU nurses, day-care workers, and babysitters—is widely accepted. We also tolerate assistance in the form of sperm sales and donation of egg and gestation (adoption). Surrogate mothering is another method of assisting people to undertake childrearing, and thus serves the purposes of the marital union. It is hard to see how its planned nature obstructs that contribution.

USING BIRTH FOR SELFISH ENDS

A basic fear about the new reproductive technologies is that they manipulate a natural physiologic process involved in the creation of human life. When one considers the potential power that resides in our ability to manipulate the genes of embryos, the charges of playing God or arrogantly tampering with nature, and the dark Huxleyian vision of genetically engineered babies decanted from bottles are not surprising. While *Brave New World* is the standard text for this fear, the 1982 film *Bladerunner* also evokes it. Trycorp, a genetic engineering corporation, manufactures "replicants," who resemble human beings in most respects, including their ability to remember their childhoods, but who are programmed to die in four years. In portraying the replicants' struggle for a long life and full human status, the film raises a host of ethical issues relevant to the issue of gene manipulation, from the meaning of personhood to the duties we have in "fabricating" people to make them as whole and healthy as possible.

Such fears, however, are not a sufficient reason to stop splicing genes or relieving infertility through external fertilization.[11] In any event they have no application to surrogate mothering, which does not alter genes or even manipulate the embryo. The only technological aid is a syringe to inseminate and a thermometer to determine when ovulation occurs. Although embryo manipulation would occur if the surrogate received the fertilized egg of another woman, the qualms about surrogate mothering stem less from its potential for technical manipulation, and more from the attitude that it reflects toward the body and mother-child relations. Mothers bear and give up

children for adoption rather frequently when the conception is unplanned. But here the mother conceives the child for that purpose, deliberately using her body for a fee to serve the needs of others. It is the cold willingness to use her body as a baby-making machine and deny the mother-child gestational bonds that bothers. (Ironically, the natural bond may turn out to be deeper and stronger than the surrogate imagined.)

Since the transfer of rearing duties from the natural gestational mother to others is widely accepted, the unwillingness of the surrogate mother to rear her child cannot in itself be wrong. As long as she transfers rearing responsibility to capable parents, she is not acting irresponsibly. Still, some persons take a deontological position that it is wrong to use the reproductive process for ends other than the good of the child.[12] But the mere presence of selfish motives does not render reproduction immoral, as long as it is carried out in a way that respects the child's interests. Otherwise most pregnancies and births would be immoral, for people have children to serve individual ends as well as the good of the child. In terms of instrumentalism, surrogate mothering cannot be distinguished from most other reproductive situations, whether AID, adoption, or simply planning a child to experience the pleasures of parenthood.

In this vein the problems that can arise when a defective child is born are cited as proof of the immorality of surrogate mothering. The fear is that neither the contracting couple nor the surrogate will want the defective child. In one recent case (*New York Times*, January 28, 1983, p. 18) a dispute arose when none of the parties wanted to take a child born with microcephaly, a condition related to mental retardation. The contracting man claimed on the basis of blood typing that the baby was not his, and thus was not obligated under the contract to take it, or to pay the surrogate's fee. It turned out that the surrogate had borne her husband's child, for she had unwittingly become pregnant by him before being artificially inseminated by the contracting man. The surrogate and her husband eventually assumed responsibility for the child.

An excessively instrumental and callous approach to reproduction when a less than perfect baby is born is not unique to surrogate mothering. Similar reactions can occur whenever married couples have a defective child, as the Baby Doe controversy, which involved the passive euthansia of a child with Down's syndrome, indicates. All surrogate mothering is not wrong because in some instances a defective newborn will be rejected. Nor is it clear that this reaction is more likely in surrogate mothering than in conventional births for it reflects common attitudes toward handicapped newborns more than alienation inherent in the surrogate arrangement.

As with most situations, "how" something is done is more important than the mere fact of doing it. The morality of surrogate mothering thus depends on how the duties and responsibilities of the role are carried out, rather than on the mere fact that a couple produces a child with the aid of a collaborator.

NOTES

The author gratefully acknowledges the comments of Rebecca Dresser, Mark Frankel, Inga Markovits, Phillip Parker, Bruce Russell, John Sampson, and Ted Schneyer on earlier drafts.

1. People v. Sorenson, 68 Cal. 2d 280, 437 P.2d 495; Walter Wadlington. "Artificial Insemination: The Dangers of a Poorly Kept Secret," *Northwestern Law Review* 64 (1970), 777.

2. See, for example, Michigan Statutes Annotated, 27.3178 (555.54)(555.69).

3. William Landes and Eleanor Posner, "The Economics of the Baby Shortage," *Journal of Legal Studies* 7 (1978), 323.

4. See Erik Erikson, *The Life Cycle Completed* (New York: Norton, 1980), pp. 122-124.

5. Phillip Parker, "Surrogate Mother's Motivations: Initial Findings," *American Journal of Psychiatry* 140:1 (January 1983), 117-118; Phillip Parker, "The Psychology of Surrogate Motherhood: A Preliminary Report of a Longitudinal Pilot Study" (unpublished). See also Dava Sobel, "Surrogate Mothers: Why Women Volunteer," *New York Times*, June 25, 1981, p. 18.

6. Mark Frankel, "Surrogate Motherhood: An Ethical Perspective," pp. 1-2. (Paper presented at Wayne State Symposium on Surrogate Motherhood, Nov. 20, 1982.)

7. See John Robertson, "In Vitro Conception and Harm to the Unborn," 8 *Hastings Center Report* 8 (October 1978), 13-14; Michael Bayles, "Harm to the Unconceived," *Philosophy and Public Affairs* 5 (1976), 295.

8. A small, uncontrolled study found these effects to last some 4-6 weeks. Statement of Nancy Reame, R.N. at Wayne State University, Symposium on Surrogate Motherhood, Nov. 20, 1982.

9. Betty Jane Lifton, *Twice Born: Memoirs of an Adopted Daughter* (New York: Penguin, 1977); L. Dusky, "Brave New Babies," *Newsweek*, Dec. 6, 1982, p. 30.

10. Leon Kass, "Making Babies—the New Biology and the Old Morality," *The Public Interest* 26 (1972), 18; "Making Babies Revisited," *The Public Interest* 54 (1979), 32; Paul Ramsey, *Fabricated Man: The Ethics of Genetic Control* (New Haven: Yale University Press, 1970).

11. The President's Commission for the Study of Ethical Problems in Medicine and Biomedical and Behavioral Research, *Splicing Life: The Social and Ethical Issues of Genetic Engineering with Human Beings* (Washington, D.C., 1982), pp. 53-60.

12. Herbert Krimmel, Testimony before California Assembly Committee on Judiciary, Surrogate Parenting Contracts (November 14, 1982), pp. 89-96.

NO   Herbert T. Krimmel

THE CASE
AGAINST SURROGATE PARENTING

Is it ethical for someone to create a human life with the intention of giving it up? This seems to be the primary question for both surrogate mother arrangements and artificial insemination by donor (AID), since in both situations a person who is providing germinal material does so only upon the assurance that someone else will assume full responsibility for the child they help to create.

THE ETHICAL ISSUE

In analyzing the ethics of surrogate mother arrangements, it is helpful to begin by examining the roles the surrogate mother performs. First, she acts as a procreator in providing an ovum to be fertilized. Second, after her ovum has been fertilized by the sperm of the man who wishes to parent the child, she acts as host to the fetus, providing nurture and protection while the newly conceived individual develops.

In this second role as host I see no insurmountable moral objections to the functions she performs. Her actions are analogous to those of a foster mother or of a wet-nurse who cares for a child when the natural mother cannot or does not do so. Using a surrogate mother as a host for the fetus when the biological mother cannot bear the child is no more morally objectionable than employing others to help educate, train or otherwise care for a child. Except in extremes, where the parent abdicates or delegates responsibilities for a child for trivial reasons, the practice would not seem to raise a serious moral issue.

I would argue, however that the first role that the surrogate mother performs—providing germinal material to be fertilized—does pose a major ethical problem. The surrogate mother provides her ovum, and enters into a surrogate mother arrangement, with the clear understanding that she is to avoid responsibility for the life she creates. Surrogate mother arrangements are designed to separate in the mind of the surrogate mother the decision to

From Herbert T. Krimmel, "The Case Against Surrogate Parenting," *Hastings Center Report* (October 1983). Copyright © 1983 by The Hastings Center. Reprinted by permission.

have and raise that child. The cause of this disassociation is some other benefit she will receive, most often money.[1] In other words, her desire to create a child is born of some motive other than the desire to be a parent. This separation of the decision to create a child from the decision to parent it is ethically suspect. The child is conceived not because he is wanted by his biological mother, but because he can be useful to someone else. He is conceived in order to be given away.

At their deepest level, surrogate mother arrangements involve a change in motive for creating children: from a desire to have them for their own sake, to a desire to have them because they can provide her some other benefit. The surrogate mother creates a child with the intention to abdicate parental responsibilities. Can we view this as ethical? My answer is no. I will try to explain why by analyzing various situations in which surrogate mother arrangements might be used.

WHY MOTIVE MATTERS

Let's begin with the single parent. A single woman might use AID, or a single man might use a surrogate mother arrangement, if she or he wanted a child but did not want to be burdened with a spouse.[2] Either practice would intentionally deprive the child of a mother or a father. This, I assert, is fundamentally unfair to the child.

Those who disagree might point to divorce or to the death of a parent as situations in which a child is deprived of one parent and must rely solely or primarily upon the other. The comparison, however, is inapt. After divorce or the death of a parent, a child may find herself with a single parent due to cir-cumstances that were unfortunate, unintended, or undesired. But when surrogate mother arrangements are used by a single parent, depriving the child of a second parent is one of the intended and desired effects. It is one thing to ask how to make the best of a bad situation when it is thrust upon a person. It is different altogether to ask whether one may intentionally set out to achieve the same result. The morality of identical results (for example, killings) will often times differ depending upon whether the situation is invited by, or involuntarily thrust upon, the actor. Legal distinctions following and based upon this ethical distinction are abundant. The law of self-defense provides a notable example.[3]

Since a woman can get pregnant if she wishes whether or not she is married, and since there is little that society can do to prevent women from creating children even if their intention is to deprive them of a father, why should we be so concerned with single men using surrogate mother arrangements if they too want a child but not a spouse? To say that women can intentionally plan to be unwed mothers is not to condone the practice. Besides, society will hold the father liable in a paternity action if he can be found and identified, which indicates some social concern that people should not be able to abdicate the responsibilities that they incur in generating children. Otherwise, why do we condemn the proverbial sailor with a pregnant girl in every port?

In many surrogate mother arrangements, of course, the surrogate mother will not be transferring custody of the child to a single man, but to a couple: the child's biological father and a stepmother, his wife. What are the ethics of surrogate mother arrangements when the child is taken into a two-parent family? Again, surrogate mother arrangements and AID pose similar ethical questions: The surrogate mother transfers her parental responsibilities to the wife of the biological father, while with AID the sperm donor relinquishes his interest in the child to the husband of the biological mother. In both cases the child is created with the intention of transferring the responsibility for its care to a new set of parents. The surrogate mother situation is more dramatic than AID since the transfer occurs after the child is born, while in the case of AID the transfer takes place at the time of the insemination even before the child is yet in being. Nevertheless, the ethical point is the same: creating children for the purpose of transferring them. For a surrogate mother the question remains: is it ethical to create a child for the purpose of transferring it to the wife of the biological father?

At first blush this looks to be little different from the typical adoption, for what is an adoption other than a transfer of responsibility from one set of parents to another? The analogy is misleading, however, for two reasons. First, it is difficult to imagine anyone conceiving children for the purpose of putting them up for adoption. And, if such a bizarre event were to occur, I doubt if we would look upon it with moral approval. Most adoptions arise either because an undesired conception is brought to term, or because the parents wanted to have the child, but find that they are unable to provide for it because of some unfortunate circumstances that develop after conception.

Second, even if surrogate mother arrangements were to be classified as a type of adoption, not all offerings of children for adoption are necessarily moral. For example, would it be moral for parents to offer their three-year-old for adoption because they are bored with the child? Would it be moral for a couple to offer for adoption their newborn female baby because they wanted a boy?

Therefore, even though surrogate mother arrangements may in some superficial ways be likened to adoption, one must still ask whether it is ethical to separate the decision to create children from the desire to have them. I would answer no. The procreator should desire the child for its own sake, and not as a means of attaining some other end. Even though one of the ends may be stated altruistically as an attempt to bring happiness to an infertile couple, the child is still being used by the surrogate. She creates it not because she desires it, but because she desires to get something from it.

To sanction the use and treatment of human beings as means to the achievement of other goals instead of as ends in themselves is to accept an ethic with a tragic past, and to establish a precedent with a dangerous future. Already the press has reported the decision of one couple to conceive a child for the purpose of using it as a bone marrow donor for its sibling (*Los Angeles Times*, April 17, 1979, p. 1–2). And the bioethics literature contains articles seriously considering whether we should clone human beings to serve as an inventory of spare parts for organ transplants[4] and articles that foresee the use of comatose human beings as self-replenishing blood banks and manufacturing plants for human hormones.[5] How far our society is willing to proceed down this road is uncertain, but it's clear that the first step to all these practices is the acceptance of the same principle that the Nazis attempted to use to justify their medical experiments at the Nuremberg War Crimes Trials: that human beings may be used as means to the achievement of other worthy goals, and need not be treated solely as ends in themselves.[6]

But why, it might be asked, is it so terrible if the surrogate mother does not desire the child for its own sake, when under the proposed surrogate mother arrangements there will be a couple eagerly desiring to have the child and to be its parents? That this argument may not be entirely accurate will be illustrated in the following section, but the basic reply is that creating a child without desiring it fundamentally changes the way we look at children—instead of viewing them as unique individual personalities to be desired in their own right, we may come to view them as commodities or items of manufacture to be desired because of their utility. A recent newspaper account describes the business of an agency that matches surrogate mothers with barren couples as follows:

> Its first product is due for delivery today. Twelve others are on the way and an additional 20 have been ordered. The "company" is Surrogate Mothering Ltd. and the "product" is babies.[7]

The dangers of this view are best illustrated by examining what might go wrong in a surrogate mother arrangement, and most important, by viewing how the various parties to the contract may react to the disappointment of their expectations.

WHAT MIGHT GO WRONG

Ninety-nine percent of the surrogate mother arrangements may work out just fine; the child will be born normal, and the adopting parents (that is, the biological father and his wife) will want it. But, what happens when, unforeseeably, the child is born deformed? Since many defects cannot be discovered prenatally by amniocentesis or other means, the situation is bound to arise.[8] Similarly, consider what would happen if the biological father were to die before the birth of the child. Or if the "child" turns out to be twins or triplets. Each of these instances poses an inevitable situation where the adopting parents may be unhappy with the prospect of getting the child or children. Although legislation can mandate that the adopting parents take the child or children in whatever condition they come or whatever the situation, provided the surrogate mother has abided by all the contractual provisions of the surrogate mother arrangement, the important point for our discussion is the attitude that the surrogate mother or the adopting parent might have. Consider the example of the deformed child.

When I participated in the Surrogate Parent Foundation's inaugural symposium in November 1981, I was struck by the attitude of both the surrogate mothers and the adopting parents to these problems. The adopting parents worried, "Do we have to take such a child?" and the surrogate mothers said in response, "Well, we don't want to be stuck with it." Clearly, both groups were anxious not to be responsible for the "undesirable child" born of the surrogate mother arrangement. What does this portend?

It is human nature that when one pays money, one expects value. Things that one pays for have a way of becoming viewed as commodities. Unavoidable in surrogate mother arrangements are questions such as: "Did I get a good one?" We see similar behavior with respect to the adoption of children: comparatively speaking, there is no shortage of black, Mexican-American, mentally retarded, or older children seeking homes; the shortage is in attractive, intelligent-looking Caucasian babies.[9] Similarly, surrogate mother arrangements involve more than just the desire to have a child. The desire is for a certain type of child.

But, it may be objected, don't all parents voice these same concerns in the normal course of having children? Not exactly. No one doubts or minimizes the pain and disappointment parents feel when they learn that their child is born with some genetic or congenital birth defect. But this is different from the surrogate mother situation, where neither the surrogate mother nor the adopting parents may feel responsible, and both sides may feel that they have a legitimate excuse not to assume responsibility for the child. The surrogate mother might blame the biological father for having "defective sperm," as the adopting parents might blame the surrogate mother for a "defective ovum" or for improper care of the fetus during pregnancy. The point is that the adopting parents desire a normal child, not *this* child in any condition, and the surrogate mother doesn't want it in any event. So both sides will feel threatened by the birth of an "undesirable child." Like bruised fruit in the produce bin of a supermarket, this child is more likely to become an object of avoidance than one of desire.

Certainly, in the natural course of having children a mother may doubt whether she wants a child if the father has died before its birth; parents may shy away from a defective infant, or be distressed at the thought of multiple births. Nevertheless, I believe they are more likely to accept these contingencies as a matter of fate. I do not think this is the case with surrogate mother arrangements. After all, in the surrogate mother arrangement the adopting parents can blame someone outside the marital relationship. The surrogate mother has been hosting this child all along, and she is delivering it. It certainly *looks* far more like a commodity than the child which arrives in the natural course within the family unit.

A DANGEROUS AGENDA

Another social problem, which arises out of the first, is the fear that surrogate mother arrangements will fall prey to eugenic concerns.[10] Surrogate mother contracts typically have clauses requiring genetic tests of the fetus and stating that the surrogate mother must have an abortion (or keep the child herself) if the child does not meet these tests.[11]

In the last decade we have witnessed a renaissance of interest in eugenics. This, coupled with advances in biomedical technology, has created a host of abuses and new moral problems. For example, genetic counseling clinics now face a dilemma: amniocentesis, the same procedure that identifies whether a fetus suffers from certain genetic defects, also discloses the sex of a fetus. Genetic counseling clinics have reported that even when the fetus is normal, a disproportionate number of mothers abort female children.[12] Aborting normal fetuses simply because the prospective parents desire children of a certain sex is one result of viewing children as commodities. The recent scandal at the Repository for Germinal Choice, the so-called "Nobel Sperm Bank," provides another chilling example. Their first "customer" was, unbeknownst to them, a woman who "had lost custody of two other children because they were abused in an effort to 'make them smart.' "[13] Of course, these and similar evils may occur whether or not surrogate mother arrangements are allowed by law. But to the extent that these arrangements are part of the milieu that promotes the view of children as commodities, they contribute to these problems. There is nothing wrong with striving for betterment, as long as it does not result in intolerance to that which is not perfect. But I fear that the latter attitude will become prevalent.

Sanctioning surrogate mother arrangements can also exert pressures upon the family structure. First, as was noted earlier, there is nothing technically to prevent the use of surrogate mother arrangements by single males desiring to become parents and, indeed, single females can already do this with AID or even without it. But even if legislation were to limit the use of the surrogate mother arrangement to infertile couples, other pressures would make themselves felt: namely the intrusion of a third adult into the marital community.[14] I do not think that society is ready to accept either single parenting or quasi-adulterous arrangements as normal.

Another stress on the family structure arises within the family of the surrogate mother. When the child is surrendered to the adopting parents it is removed not only from the surrogate mother, but also from her family. They too have interests to be considered. Do not the siblings of that child have an interest in the fact that their little baby brother has been "given" away?[15] One woman, the mother of a medical student who had often donated sperm for artificial insemination, expressed her feelings to me eloquently. She asked, "I wonder how many grandchildren I have that I have never seen and never been able to hold or cuddle."

Intrafamily tensions can also be expected to result in the family of the adopting parents due to the asymmetry of relationship the adopting parents will have toward the child. The adopting mother has no biological relationship to the child, whereas the adopting father is also the child's biological father. Won't this unequal biological claim on the child be used as a wedge in child-rearing arguments? Can't we imagine the father saying, "Well, he is my son, not yours"? What if the couple eventually gets divorced? Should custody in a subsequent divorce between the adopting mother and the biological father be treated simply as a normal child custody dispute in any other divorce? Or should the biological relationship between father and child weigh more heavily? These questions do not arise in typical adoption situations since both parents are equally unrelated biologically to the child. Indeed, in adoption there is symmetry. The surrogate mother situation is more analogous to second marriages, where the children of one party by a prior marriage are adopted by the new spouse. Since asymmetry in second marriage situations causes problems, we can anticipate similar difficulties arising from surrogate mother arrangements.

There is also the worry the offspring of a surrogate mother arrangement will be deprived of important information about his or her heritage. This also happens with adopted children or children conceived by AID,[16] who lack information about their biological parents, which could be important to them medically. Another less popularly recognized problem is the danger of half-sibling marriages,[17] where the child of the surrogate mother unwittingly falls in love with a half sister or brother. The only way to avoid these problems is to dispense with the confidentiality of parental records; however, the natural parents may not always want their identity disclosed.

The legalization of surrogate mother arrangements may also put undue pressure upon poor women to use their bodies in this way to support themselves and their families. Analogous problems have arisen in the past with the use of paid blood donors.[18] And occasionally the press reports someone desperate enough to offer to sell an eye or some other organ.[19] I believe that certain things should be viewed as too important to be sold as commodities, and I hope that we have advanced from the time when parents raised children for profitable labor, or found themselves forced to sell their children.

While many of the social problems I have outlined here have their analogies in other present-day occurrences such as divorced families or in adoption, every addition is hurtful. Legalizing surrogate mother arrangements will increase the frequency of these problems, and due to its dramatic nature is more likely to put stress on our society's shared moral values.[20]

NOTES

1. Phillip J. Parker, "Motivation of Surrogate Mothers: Initial Findings," *American Journal of Psychiatry* 140:1 (January 1983), 117–18; see also Doe v. Kelley, Circuit Court of Wayne County Michigan (1980) reported in 1980 Rep. on Human Reproduction and Law II-A-1.

2. See, e.g., C.M. v. C.C., 152 N.J. Supp. 160, 377 A.2d 821 (1977); "Why She Went to 'NobelSperm Bank' for Child," *Los Angeles Herald Examiner*, Aug. 6, 1982, p. A9; "Womb for Rent," *Los Angeles Herald Examiner*, Sept. 21, 1981, p. A3.

3. See also Richard McCormick, "Reproductive Technologies: Ethical Issues" in *Encyclopedia of Bioethics*, edited by Walter Reich, Vol. 4 (New York: The Free Press, 1978) pp. 1454, 1459; Robert

Snowden and G.D. Mitchell, *The Artificial Family* (London: George Allen & Unwin, 1981), p. 71.

4. See, e.g., Alexander Peters, "The Brave New World: Can the Law Bring Order Within Traditional Concepts of Due Process?" *Suffolk Law Review* 4 (1970), 894, 901–02; Roderic Gorney, "The New Biology and the Future of Man," *UCLA Law Review* 15 (1968), 273, 302; J.G. Castel, "Legal Implications of Biomedical Science and Technology in the Twenty-First Century," *Canadian Bar Review* 51 (1973), 119, 127.

5. See Harry Nelson, "Maintaining Dead to Serve as Blood Makers Proposed: Logical, Sociologist Says," *Los Angeles Times*, February 26, 1974; Hans Jonas, "Against the Stream: Comments on the Definition and Redefinition of Death," in *Philosophical Essays: From Ancient Creed to Technological Man* (Chicago: University of Chicago Press, 1974), pp. 132–40.

6. See Leo Alexander, "Medical Science under Dictatorship," *New England Journal of Medicine* 241:2 (1949), 39; United States v. Brandt, Trial of the Major War Criminals, International Military Tribunal: Nuremberg, 14 November 1945–1 October 1946.

7. Bob Dvorchak, "Surrogate Mothers: Pregnant Idea Now a Pregnant Business," *Los Angeles Herald Examiner*, December 27, 1983, p. A1.

8. "Surrogate's Baby Born with Deformities Rejected by All," *Los Angeles Times*, January 22, 1983, p. 1–17; "Man Who Hired Surrogate Did Not Father Ailing Baby," *Los Angeles Herald Examiner*, February 3, 1983, p. A-6.

9. See, e.g., Adoption in America, Hearing before the Subcommittee on Aging, Family and Human Services of the Senate Committee on Labor and Human Resources, 97th Congress, 1st Session (1981), p. 3 (comments of Senator Jeremiah Denton and p. 3 (statement of Warren Master, Acting Commissioner of Administration for Children, Youth and Families, HHS.

10. Cf. "Discussion: Moral, Social and Ethical Issues," in *Law and Ethics of A.I.D. and Embryo Transfer* (1973) (comments of Himmelweit); reprinted in Michael Shapiro and Roy Spece, *Bioethics and Law* (St. Paul: West Publishing Company, 1981), p. 548.

11. See, e.g., Lane (Newsday), "Womb for Rent," *Tucson Citizen* (Weekender), June 7, 1980, p. 3; Susan Lewis, "Baby Bartering? Surrogate Mothers Pose Issues for Lawyers, Courts," *The Los Angeles Daily Journal*, April 20, 1981; see also Elaine Markoutsas, "Women Who Have Babies for Other Women," *Good Housekeeping* 96 (April 1981), 104.

12. See Morton A. Stenchever, "An Abuse of Prenatal Diagnosis," *Journal of the American Medical Association* 221 (1972), 408; Charles Westoff and Ronald R. Rindfus, "Sex Preselection in the United States: Some Implications," *Science* 184

(1974), 633, 636; see also Phyllis Battelle, "Is it a Boy or a Girl?" *Los Angeles Herald Examiner*, Oct. 8, 1981, p. A17.

13. "2 Children Taken from Sperm Bank Mother," *Los Angeles Times*, July 14, 1982; p. 1–3; "The Sperm-Bank Scandal," *Newsweek* 24 (July 26, 1982).

14. See Helmut Thielicke, *The Ethics of Sex*, John W. Doberstein, trans. (New York: Harper & Row, 1964).

15. According to one newspaper account, when a surrogate mother informed her nine-year-old daughter that the new baby would be given away, the daughter replied: "Oh, good. If it's a girl we can keep it and give Jeffrey (her two-year-old half brother) away." "Womb for Rent," *Los Angeles Herald Examiner*, Sept. 21, 1981, p. A3.

16. See, e.g., Lorraine Dusky, "Brave New Babies?" *Newsweek* 30 (December 6, 1982). Also testimony of Suzanne Rubin before the California Assembly Committee on Judiciary, Surrogate Parenting Contracts, Assembly Publication No. 962, pp. 72–75 (November 19, 1982).

17. Regarding how this has posed an accelerating problem for children conceived through AID, see, e.g., Martin Curie-Cohen, et al., "Current Practice of Artificial Insemination by Donor in the United States," *New England Journal of Medicine* 300 (1979), 585–89.

18. See Richard M. Titmuss, *The Gift Relationship: From Human Blood to Social Policy* (New York: Random House, 1971).

19. See, e.g., "Man Desperate for Funds: Eye for Sale at $35,000," *Los Angeles Times*, February 1, 1975; "100 Answer Man's Ad for New Kidney," *Los Angeles Times*, September 12, 1974.

20. See generally Guido Calabresi, "Reflections on Medical Experimentation in Humans," *Daedalus* 98 (1969), 387–93; also see Michael Shapiro and Roy Spece, "On Being 'Unprincipled on Principle': The Limits of Decision Making 'On the Merits,' " in *Bioethics and Law*, pp. 67–71.

POSTSCRIPT

Should Women Be Allowed to Bear Babies for a Fee?

In the aftermath of the Baby M case, the Task Force on New Reproductive Practices of the New Jersey Bioethics Commission recommended that commercial surrogacy be outlawed. It did not, however, recommend criminalizing noncommercial surrogacy, that is, when a woman volunteers to bear a child for an infertile relative without a fee. The New York State Task Force on Life and the Law has declared that paying women to bear children "has the potential to undermine the dignity of women, children, and human reproduction," and it has advised the state legislators to declare surrogacy illegal. Although two states (Michigan and Florida) now ban paid surrogacy outright, and a few others (for example, Kentucky, Louisiana, and Nebraska) consider such contracts legally unenforceable, the law in most states is murky. The proposals that flooded state legislatures after the Baby M case have not led to any clarifications of the legal or ethical issues.

Concerned by the growth of the practice, the American College of Obstetricians and Gynecologists has issued ethical guidelines for its members, and it cautions physicians to avoid any surrogate mother arrangement that is likely to lead to financial exploitation of any of the parties involved. Particularly troubling for physicians is, who shall give the consent for treatment? Should consent be given by the surrogate or by the adoptive parents?

In *Between Strangers: Surrogate Mothers, Expectant Fathers, and Brave New Babies* (Harper & Row, 1989), Lori Andrews argues strongly in favor of a woman's right to enter into a binding surrogacy contract and a couple's right to require enforcement. Another argument in favor of surrogacy is Carmel Shalev's *Birth Power: The Case for Surrogacy* (Yale University Press, 1989).

Maura A. Ryan presents a countervailing view in "The Argument for Unlimited Procreative Liberty: A Feminist Critique" (*Hastings Center Report*, July/August 1990). George J. Annas, in his article "The Baby Broker Boom," *Hastings Center Report* (April 1986), warns against commercialism. See also Sherman Elias and George J. Annas, "Social Policy Considerations in Noncoital Reproduction," *Journal of the American Medical Association* (January 3, 1986, pp. 62–68).

See also Diane M. Bartels et al., eds., *Beyond Baby M: Ethical Issues in New Reproductive Technologies* (Humana Press, 1989); Janice G. Raymond, "Reproductive Gifts and Gift Giving: The Altruistic Woman," *Hastings Center Report* (November/December 1990); and Thomas A. Shannon, *Surrogate Motherhood: The Ethics of Using Human Beings* (Crossroad, 1989). Sue A. Meinke's "Surrogate Motherhood: Ethical and Legal Issues" (Scope Note #6, Kennedy Institute of Ethics, 1987) offers a good bibliography.

ISSUE 4

The Maternal-Fetal Relationship: Can Compelled Medical Treatment of Pregnant Women Be Justified?

YES: Frank A. Chervenak and Laurence B. McCullough, from "Perinatal Ethics: A Practical Method of Analysis of Obligations to Mother and Fetus," *Obstetrics and Gynecology* (September 1985)

NO: Lawrence J. Nelson and Nancy Milliken, from "Compelled Medical Treatment of Pregnant Women: Life, Liberty, and Law in Conflict," *Journal of the American Medical Association* (February 19, 1988)

ISSUE SUMMARY

YES: Physician Frank A. Chervenak and philosopher Laurence B. McCullough argue that respect for maternal autonomy is not an absolute ethical principle and that physicians' obligations to honor the autonomy of the mother must be weighed against obligations to promote the best interests of the fetus.

NO: Philosopher Lawrence J. Nelson and physician Nancy Milliken believe that the decision of a competent woman to forgo medical treatment to benefit her fetus should not be overridden, even if others disagree with her choice.

"Mother and baby are both doing fine!" These happy words mark the end of a successful pregnancy and the beginning of a new life. Most pregnancies proceed normally, without medical or ethical complications. The exceptions, however, pose difficult problems.

Consider, for example, the cases of Jessie Mae Jefferson, Angela Carder, and Pamela Rae Stewart. In 1981 Mrs. Jefferson refused, on religious grounds, to agree to a cesarean section her doctors said was necessary to save the life of her baby. The hospital and the Georgia Department of Human Resources appealed to the Georgia courts, which awarded temporary custody to the agency. The fetus, the court said, was not receiving proper parental care, and a cesarean section was authorized. But before the operation could take place, Mrs. Jefferson gave birth naturally to a healthy baby.

Angela Carder was a 27-year-old pregnant woman dying of bone cancer. After she was admitted to a Washington (D.C.) hospital in a terminal condition, the hospital decided to try to save the life of the unborn child through a cesarean section. The operation would surely hasten Angela's death, and the likelihood that a 26-week-old fetus would survive was slim. Even though Angela's family and her physician objected, and Angela herself did not want the operation, the District of Columbia Court ordered that it be performed. The baby died two hours after birth, and Angela died two days later, with the surgery a contributing factor in her death.

Pamela Rae Stewart was brought to trial in 1986 in California after the birth and death of her son. She had been warned by her doctor to seek medical attention at the first sign of bleeding and not to have sex with her husband or to take any drugs. However, she disregarded the warnings and the baby was born with severe brain damage and died six weeks after birth. Ms. Stewart was charged with violating a criminal statute prohibiting a parent from denying "necessary clothing, food, shelter, or medical attention or other remedial care for his or her child." Her husband was not charged. The case was eventually thrown out on the grounds that the statute was not intended to apply to a mother's refusal to obey doctor's orders.

These cases illustrate some of the situations in which conflicts about decision-making in pregnancy may occur. Although these are typically called "maternal-fetal" conflicts, they are actually conflicts between pregnant women and medical and legal professionals over the preferred course of action or inaction. They are not cases in which mothers intentionally harm fetuses, but cases in which they disagree with or are unable to follow through with advice on preventing harm to fetuses.

In addition to forced cesareans and transfusions and prosecution for failure to heed medical advice resulting in birth damage, the use of illegal drugs or alcohol during pregnancy is becoming relatively common as a basis for court action. Other situations have been suggested as possibilities for legal intervention: failure to seek prenatal care, failure to consent to intra-uterine fetal therapy, and home births in high-risk pregnancies.

The following two selections explore the ethical dimensions of these troubling cases. Frank A. Chervenak and Laurence B. McCullough argue that in difficult cases, obligations based on respect for maternal autonomy must be balanced against obligations of beneficence (promoting welfare) to fetuses. In that balance, maternal autonomy may sometimes be overridden. Lawrence J. Nelson and Nancy Milliken conclude that neither society nor the medical profession should support judicially compelled treatment of pregnant women.

YES

Frank A. Chervenak and
Laurence B. McCullough

PERINATAL ETHICS: A PRACTICAL METHOD OF ANALYSIS OF OBLIGATIONS TO MOTHER AND FETUS

Protecting and promoting the best interests of the mother and the best interests of the fetus, and the child it will become, are the basic moral goals or purposes of obstetric care. These goals form the basis on which the principles of respect for autonomy and beneficence are applied in obstetric care. These principles, in turn, generate moral obligations to mother and fetus. Figure 1 illustrates how these obligations work toward the moral goals of protecting and promoting maternal and fetal best interests.

Maternal best interests are protected and promoted by both autonomy-based and beneficence-based obligations of the physician.

The fetus is incapable of having its own perspective on its best interests: Because of an insufficiently developed central nervous system, the fetus has no values or beliefs that are necessary for an individual to have his or her own perspective on his or her own best interests. Hence, there are no autonomy-based obligations to the fetus. Hence, fetal best interests in obstetric care are understood exclusively in terms of the principle of beneficence that generates the moral status of the fetus and the serious obligations owed to it.

The pregnant woman has beneficence-based obligations to the fetus because she is its moral fiduciary: She is expected to protect and promote her fetus's best interests, and those of the child it will become. The physician also has beneficence-based obligations to the fetus, to protect and promote its interest and those of the child it will become, as these are understood from medicine's perspective. From medicine's perspective, the goods to be sought for the child the fetus will become and therefore for the fetus are prevention of premature death, disease, and handicapping conditions, as well as the cure or amelioration of disease, handicapping conditions, pain, and suffering. It, therefore, may be appropriate to refer to the fetus as a patient[1,2] with the possible exception of abortion of previable fetuses.

Figure 1

Moral Obligations in Obstetric Care

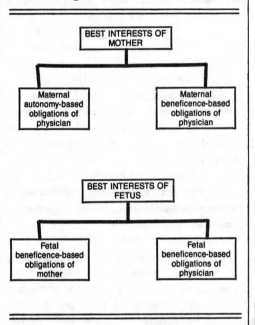

Most often, the moral obligations of a physician to a pregnant woman and her fetus work in concert as the physician and the woman agree on the plan of management that will best serve both the maternal and fetal interests. However, because autonomy-based and beneficence-based obligations to the fetus are a priori equally strong or weighty, conflicts among these moral obligations are not uncommon in obstetric care.

These conflicts can be subdivided into four groups: 1) conflicts between maternal autonomy-based obligations of physician and maternal beneficence-based obligations of physician, 2) conflicts between fetal beneficence-based obligations of mother and the fetal beneficence-based obligations of physician, 3) conflicts between maternal autonomy-based obligations of physician and fetal beneficence-based obligations of physician, and 4) conflicts between maternal beneficence-based obligations of physician and fetal beneficence-based obligations of physician.

CONFLICTS BETWEEN MATERNAL AUTONOMY-BASED OBLIGATIONS OF PHYSICIAN AND MATERNAL BENEFICENCE-BASED OBLIGATIONS OF PHYSICIAN

Meaningful communication between the obstetrician and the mother in the form of patient education and sustained attention to the patient's values and beliefs is essential for a positive synergism between autonomy-based and beneficence-based obligations and prevention of potential conflicts. A patient who is well informed about her condition and therapeutic options has a greater capacity for autonomous decision making. The obstetrician who is knowledgeable about the patient's values and preferences can better determine a management plan that would be consistent with the woman's perspective on her best interests.

On occasion, the patient and the obstetrician may conclude that different management strategies would best serve the patient's interests. A Jehovah's Witness may refuse the administration of a life-saving transfusion during cesarean section because it will jeopardize her eternal salvation; the obstetrician may assess that such refusal would jeopardize her earthly existence.[3] A young woman with her first pregnancy may insist that she have tubal ligation [sterilization]

(1) Wanted by Mom cesarean vs vaginal birth because of pain

at the time she has her cesarean section because she is certain of her choice and does not desire the risk of a second operation; the physician may feel that such a procedure would lead to possibly irreversible damage to her reproductive capabilities. In such cases the physician faces a conflict between his beneficence-based obligations, ie, to effect the management that from medicine's perspective protects and promotes the best interests of the patient, and autonomy-based obligations, ie, to implement the management plan that the patient, on the basis of a voluntary and informed choice, has determined to be in her best interests. Resolution of these conflicts depends on the moral weight these obligations assume in particular circumstances.

In some circumstances, autonomy-based obligations to the pregnant woman override beneficence-based obligations, especially when the basic beliefs and values of the woman are at stake. To override an autonomous decision that is based on such serious moral concerns in an individual's life as religious belief or self-determination of one's reproductive capabilities, would constitute an intolerable assault on personal freedom. However, fulfilling such autonomy-based obligations does not obliterate all beneficence-based obligations. The physician is still obligated under beneficence to provide all forms of medical support other than blood products to a Jehovah's Witness who refuses transfusion and to offer to help the patient with a tubal ligation obtain subsequent tubal reanastomosis if she so desires.

In some cases, beneficence-based obligations override autonomy-based obligations. This can happen when a woman's decisions are significantly reduced in their autonomy, eg, if there is a reduced ability to understand choices and make reasonable decisions, or when immediate action is necessary to preserve maternal life or health. In such circumstances, the physician is justified in acting in a way that is contrary to what the woman may indicate. A woman in her first pregnancy in labor warrants analgesia and emotional support to help deal with pain. To accede to a demand for cesarean section, when this same patient is in considerable labor pain and is very frightened as a consequence, however, would violate beneficence-based obligations to protect maternal health. Because such a request probably does not reflect her basic values and beliefs, autonomy-based obligations are diminished. Although a mother may strongly desire a low transverse cesarean section to permit vaginal delivery in subsequent pregnancies, intraoperatively, the obstetrician may realize that . . . a vertical uterine incision is necessary to avoid injury to the uterine vessels. Time constraints may not permit the physician to obtain consent for such an incision. Thus, in some cases, a woman's preferences are justifiably overridden in favor of beneficence-based obligations.

In both cases, analysis shows potential goods (avoidance of cesarean section, avoidance of possible hysterectomy) to outweigh the potential harms (maternal discomfort and psychic stress, the necessity of future cesarean sections) of nonintervention on the first case and intervention in the latter. In all cases in which beneficence-based obligations take precedence, there is an inescapable autonomy-based obligation to explain later to the woman what was done and why it was done. This is one important sense in which respect of autonomy helps to avoid dehumanized obstetric care.

Speed necessary. Verticle Uterine.
2 Methods of cesarean section. Verticle Uterine. One desired by Dr. Other by Mom. (Low transverse

CONFLICTS BETWEEN FETAL BENEFICENCE-BASED OBLIGATIONS OF MOTHER AND FETAL BENEFICENCE-BASED OBLIGATIONS OF PHYSICIAN

Usually the mother and the physician are in agreement as to what plan of management provides the greatest balance of fetal goods over harms. However, there is the potential for conflict in matters concerning the diagnosis or management of fetal disorders because the woman and the physician may have conflicting views about what is in the best interests of the fetus and the child it will become.

Such conflicts can occur in the context of fetal diagnosis and therapy. For example, some mothers may feel that because life presents many challenges, a fetus with any anomaly is best served by not being born. Their assessment may in some cases extend so far as to justify a potentially damaging invasive procedure such as fetoscopy to diagnose isolated cleft lip. The obstetrician may conclude that the risk of miscarriage and thus fetal death associated with fetoscopy is not warranted to detect a relatively minor and easily correctable cosmetic defect. If such reasoning is correct, then one could conclude that a woman who made such a choice was acting contrary to the fetus as its moral fiduciary. Hence, fetal beneficence-based obligations of the physician come to the fore. The physician should be aware of the pitfalls of condescension in such cases and opt, instead, for careful and sympathetic explanations of his or her evaluation of the fetus's best interests.

Matters become more uncertain when the condition to be diagnosed or treated is more serious for the fetus. For example, invasive fetal therapy to place a ventriculoamniotic shunt to alleviate fetal hydrocephalus involves uncertainty about risks of morbidity and mortality due to the underlying condition, the efficacy of the therapy to correct the defect, and the risks of morbidity and mortality during and after the intervention.[4] The physician and the mother in their analyses of the best interests of the fetus may reasonably weigh the various components differently. In such cases, there may be a genuine moral dilemma, ie, the necessity to choose between two courses of action with substantial moral justification. At the present time, the authors believe that there can be no decisive resolution of this moral dilemma until these levels of uncertainty are reduced. Thus, to respect a woman's decision concerning fetal therapy may be an acceptable way to resolve this dilemma.

CONFLICTS BETWEEN MATERNAL AUTONOMY-BASED OBLIGATIONS OF PHYSICIAN AND FETAL BENEFICENCE-BASED OBLIGATIONS OF PHYSICIAN

Conflicts between maternal autonomy-based obligations and fetal beneficence-based obligations are probably the most common and challenging moral conflicts faced by the obstetrician. Indeed, the morality of elective abortion presents a dilemma whereby either respect for maternal autonomy of beneficence-based obligations to the fetus must be significantly compromised. Although there is nor moral consensus for the resolution of this dilemma, Roe v. Wade has defined a legal modus vivendi whereby termination of pregnancy before fetal viability is a woman's legal right.[5]

When abortion is not an issue, ie, when the woman intends to complete her pregnancy, beneficence-based obliga-

Anencephaly – Congenital absence of the brain & spinal cord.

tions to the fetus and the child it will become assume greater importance. It is especially important that these obligations be determined on a careful, objective assessment the fetus's best interests. These obligations include such routine matters in obstetric care as providing education about the effects on the fetus of maternal cigarette, alcohol, and drug use and compassionate attempts to modify such maternal behaviors by repeated emphasis about the potential ill effects on the fetus.

In some situations, the fetus stands to benefit from maternal bed rest, hospitalization, or external fetal heart rate monitoring. In addition, certain drugs administered to the mother . . . may provide clear benefit to the fetus. Thus, it is evident that for optimal fetal outcome in many pregnancies maternal participation in the obstetric plan, with subsequent restriction on maternal autonomy, is necessary. When this cooperation is not present, conflicts between autonomy-based obligations to the mother and beneficence-based obligations to the fetus arise. The physician should discharge fetal beneficence-based obligations by vigorously attempting to persuade the woman to accept the required restrictions or treatment.

This sort of moral conflict becomes difficult to resolve when more invasive procedures are needed for fetal diagnosis or management such as . . . cesarean section in the event of well-documented fetal distress. This is because a woman may determine that the risks to her well-being are not worth taking, even though the fetus might well benefit from the proposed intervention.

The following guidelines help to negotiate such a moral conflict. The greater the likelihood that a particular intervention will clearly result in a substantial benefit for the fetus, ie, a significant decrease in morbidity and mortality, the stronger are the beneficence-based obligations to the fetus. The greater the likelihood that the fetus will be at substantial risk from the intervention, eg, increased morbidity and mortality, the weaker are fetal beneficence-based obligations. The greater the risk of harm to the mother, ie, increase in morbidity and mortality, the stronger are maternal autonomy-based obligations in those cases in which the woman refuses the intervention. These guidelines permit fetal diagnosis and treatment when the risks to the fetus are minimal, the potential benefit for the fetus is substantial, and the risks to the woman are those she should reasonably accept on behalf of her fetus.

Because the outlook for fetal anencephaly is universally dismal, beneficence-based obligations to such a fetus are minimal, and termination of pregnancy, even in the third trimester, may be acceptable.[6] By contrast, if maternal brain death were to occur, autonomy-based obligations may be overridden by fetal beneficence-based obligations, justifying sustaining maternal biologic life until fetal maturity.[7] . . .

If intrapartum fetal monitoring reveals severe bradycardia [slow heart rate] which is subsequently not responsive to conservative measures, the beneficence-based obligations to perform a cesarean section to preserve fetal life and avoid the morbidity and handicapping conditions associated with asphyxic brain damage may be so compelling as to override maternal autonomy-based obligations generated by a refusal of the procedure.[8] Respect for autonomy in such cases requires the physician in such circumstances to attempt to persuade the woman to permit the procedure by informing her that cesarean section is indeed necessary to save her child's life. A more coercive approach, eg, threatening to seek or seeking a court order, may sometimes be morally justifiable. In considering this more serious compromise to maternal autonomy, the benefit to the fetus of such action must be clear and overwhelming and the mother should be accorded respect and compassion, not degradation. Because remedies short of legal action, eg, vigorous persuasion, involve fewer negative consequences for the physician-patient relationship and maternal-infant bonding, the authors believe that such remedies are preferable on grounds of beneficence.

CONFLICTS BETWEEN MATERNAL BENEFICENCE-BASED OBLIGATIONS OF THE PHYSICIAN AND FETAL BENEFICENCE-BASED OBLIGATIONS OF THE PHYSICIAN

In modern obstetrics, conflicts exist between maternal and fetal beneficence-based obligations. The most difficult of these conflicts involve putting one party at great risk of substantial morbidity and mortality to avoid great risk of similarly grave consequences for the other. These moral conflicts can sometimes be agonizing. Maternal malignancy or abdominal ectopic gestation may necessitate termination of pregnancy as the only reliable means to save the woman's life. In other cases, potentially fetotoxic drugs . . . may be needed to prevent serious maternal disorders such as seizures. The resolution of these sorts of conflicts presents the physician with tragic choices. This is because there is no clearly convincing moral argument that the woman's life is more important than that of the fetus or that one form of serious morbidity and handicap in the mother is more grave than such morbidity and handicap in the fetus. The authors believe that to respect the pregnant woman's decisions may be an acceptable course in these tragic cases.

In summary, when obstetricians confront moral conflict in a particular case, successful clinical management requires identification of the component moral obligations of the conflict and determination of the relative weight of those obligations. This process requires thorough documentation and objective assessment of fetal and maternal best interests. A morally justified decision is consistent with what can be shown to be the weightiest obligations as the result of ethical analysis. At times, however, there is no clear resolution: The competing obligations appear to be of equal weight. It should be recognized that reasonable and conscientious people may determine the weight of moral obligations differently from others. The goal of this paper is to outline a framework that permits meaningful and serious dialogue about moral issues in clinical practice that will lead to reliable identification and, sometimes, resolution of moral conflicts in obstetric care.

REFERENCES

1. Pritchard JA, MacDonald PC: Williams Obstetrics. 16th edition. New York, Appleton-Century-Crofts, 1980, p. vii.
2. Harrison MR, Golbus MS, Filly RA: The Unborn Patient. New York, Grune & Stratton, 1984.
3. Jewett JF: Report from the Committee on Maternal Welfare: Total exsanguination. N Engl J Med 305:1218, 1981.
4. Clewell WH, Johnson ML, Meier PR, et al: A surgical approach to the treatment of fetal hydrocephalus. N Engl J Med 306:1320, 1982.

5. Roe v. Wade, 410 US 113, 1973.
6. Chervenak FA, Farley MA, Walter L, et al: When is termination of pregnancy during the third trimester morally justifiable? N Engl J Med 310:501, 1984.
7. Dillon WP, Lee RV, Tronolone MJ, et al: Life support and maternal brain death during pregnancy: JAMA 248:1089, 1982.
8. Jurow R, Paul RH: Cesarean delivery for fetal distress without maternal consent. Obstet Gynecol 63:596, 1984.

NO
Lawrence J. Nelson and
Nancy Milliken

COMPELLED MEDICAL TREATMENT OF PREGNANT WOMEN: LIFE, LIBERTY, AND LAW IN CONFLICT

As recently stated by the this committee of the American College of Obstetricians and Gynecologists, the maternal-fetal relationship is a "unique one" as it involves "two patients with access to one through the other."[1] In no other situation is the physician faced with one patient literally inside the body of another patient. Conceptually, the medical care of each can be approached independently, but practically, neither can be treated without affecting the other. Because of this unique relationship, conflicts between the interests of the woman and the fetus can arise if the former refuses treatment recommended for the benefit of the latter (eg, refusing cesarean section for documented fetal distress and anoxia [lack of oxygen]) or if she is unwilling or unable to change behaviors that potentially could harm her fetus, such as smoking, consuming alcohol, eating inadequately, or engaging in certain job-related or recreational activities. *The rest can have control over?*

Kolder et al[2] recently documented a substantial number of court-ordered obstetric procedures performed despite a woman's refusal of treatment considered necessary to preserve the life or health of the fetus. As the survey included only obstetricians directing fellowship and residency programs in maternal-fetal medicine, there certainly are instances of compelled treatment not included in their report. Other recent reports seem to confirm this.[3-5] Perhaps most important, the report by Kolder et al documented that almost half of the fellowship directors thought that judicial force should be used to impose treatment thought to be lifesaving, including surgery, on unconsenting pregnant women for the sake of the fetus. Court-ordered obstetric treatment raises a host of fundamental ethical and legal questions for physicians, pregnant women, and society—questions that have not been adequately explored in the medical literature. . . .

Lawrence J. Nelson and Nancy Milliken, "Compelled Medical Treatment of Pregnant Women: Life, Liberty, and Law in Conflict," *Journal of the American Medical Association*, vol. 259, no. 7 (February 19, 1988), pp. 1060-1066. Copyright © 1988 by the American Medical Association. Reprinted by permission.

OBSTETRICS, ETHICS, AND THE PHYSICIAN-PATIENT RELATIONSHIP

As a result of the rapid development of obstetric knowledge and technology, the physician's relationship to the fetus has changed dramatically. In part because the fetus has become the subject of many direct medical interventions, it has emerged as the obstetrician's second patient. The preface to the most recent edition of *Williams Textbook of Obstetrics* reflects this view: "Quality of life for the mother and her infant is our most important concern. Happily, we live and work in an era in which the fetus is established as our second patient with many rights and privileges comparable to those previously achieved only after birth."[6] Although this excerpt is not a description of a fetus' legal rights, it does suggest that obstetricians commonly conceptualize the fetus as a patient to whom they owe ethical duties as they would to any other patient.

The fetus has not become a patient in its own right because the goal of obstetrics has changed; that goal has always been the birth of a healthy baby to a healthy mother. Rather, medicine's means to achieve this goal have changed significantly during the past few decades. Formerly, the physician was able to treat only the mother and had to assume that in maintaining her health, the health of the fetus would be enhanced. The fetus itself was largely beyond the diagnostic and therapeutic reach of the physician. Advances in knowledge of fetal physiology and the development of new technology have enabled physicians to see the fetus in detail with ultrasound, to assess its condition with amniocentesis and fetal heart rate monitoring, and to operate on it in utero. In short, medicine's enhanced ability to treat the fetus directly has profoundly affected, perhaps even created, physicians' perception of the fetus as a separate patient. Such a perception is reinforced by clinical experience of the fetus as a technically interesting and challenging patient.

One might infer from the foregoing that it is only the new emphasis on the fetus as patient that determines the physician's ethical obligation to promote its well-being. This is not true. The physician's obligation to promote fetal health is firmly rooted in his or her ethical obligations to the pregnant woman. In seeking prenatal care, a pregnant woman is at least implicitly demonstrating that she has freely chosen to pursue a successful pregnancy. Regardless of an individual physician's conceptualization of the fetus as a separate patient, he or she is required to monitor the fetus and recommend appropriate treatment in accordance with the standard of care because of the woman's choice to bring her pregnancy to term. The failure to do so would be both ethically wrong and medical malpractice. Therefore, the fetus does not need to be seen as a second or separate obstetric patient to create a duty on the part of a physician to render it excellent care.

While the physician's relationship to the fetus has undergone significant expansion and qualitative change, the physician's relationship to a pregnant woman has a venerable history. The pregnant woman who presents for prenatal care is clearly the obstetrician's patient. Their interaction is governed by the fiduciary nature of any physician-patient relationship in which an individual patient voluntarily entrusts the physician with her medical concerns, and the physician reciprocates with the skillful application of medical knowledge to serve the patient's interests faithfully. The ethical principle of beneficence requires a physician to implement the therapy that best promotes the patient's health while minimizing potential harm. In the context of obstetrics, the physician has the responsibility to monitor the health of both the woman and the fetus and to advocate treatment intended to enhance the health of both.

In addition to the principle of beneficence, the physician is ethically obliged to recognize the principle of respect for individual autonomy. In keeping with this latter principle, all adult patients traditionally are deemed to have the right to accept or reject medical recommendations based on their personal priorities and values,[7] a right respected and protected by the law.[8-11] Like other adults, a pregnant woman must make decisions about medical care within the broader context of her life. Her responsibility to her fetus will sometimes be weighed against responsibilities to her children, husband, and others with whom she has a special relationship. Her decisions also may be influenced by a religious faith or commitments to strongly held personal values, and she may not always agree with her physician's advice.

Usually it is frustrating for physicians when patients do not follow their advice. Often it is painful when the patient's medically foolish decision results in serious damage or death. Perhaps nowhere are the physician's frustration and pain with a patient's noncompliance more excruciating than in obstetrics, where the decisions of the pregnant woman affect not only her own health but also that of her fetus. However, these feelings alone do not ethically justify ignoring or circumventing a pregnant woman's refusal to follow medical advice.

Because she is an autonomous adult, a competent pregnant woman has the same prerogative as other adults to control her own life and what will happen to her body. In addition, because conceiving and bearing a child is a highly personal and private matter, others (including physicians) should be very reluctant to substitute their value judgments in such a matter for those of the woman herself. Therefore, due to respect for an individual's autonomy and privacy, physicians should recognize and honor a competent pregnant woman's informed decision to reject medical advice about her care.

This view surely can be criticized for ignoring the value of the fetus as a being with interests separate from those of its mother. Factually, a fetus is a human life with a distinct genetic constitution that develops and possess an organ system distinct from its mother's. However, the ethical evaluation of fetal life varies dramatically within our society. Some contend that a fertilized human ovum is a human life with the same rights as any live-born man or woman.[12] Others see the fetus as at most a potential human life that receives the protection of the ethical principle forbidding harm to persons only after it lives outside of the mother's body. Still others have claimed that a fetus achieves protectable ethical status at quickening or when it reaches the point of viability.[4] A more recent view argues that the fetus gains ethical status when it has developed neurologically to the point where it has consciousness.[13] Not only is there a lack of agreement on how to value fetal life, particularly when it comes into conflict with the interests of the mother, but this disagreement is violently expressed both literally in abortion clinic bombings and figuratively in slogan slinging on both sides of the issue.

In light of this seemingly intractable controversy, it is arbitrary for a physician to resolve maternal-fetal conflict by claiming that his or her ethical evaluation of the fetus is the "right" one while the woman's is "wrong." When there is such profound disagreement, we believe that the ethically preferable course of action is to leave the determination of the weight of the fetus' interests to the mother in conflict situations. Nonetheless, it is certainly ethically permissible (perhaps even mandatory) for a physician to try to persuade a pregnant woman refusing medically indicated treatment to change her mind. Neither patient autonomy nor the doctrine of informed consent requires physicians to accept patient refusal passively and without inquiry, protest, or argument. However, the purposeful use of threats or deception to "convince" a patient to change her mind is ethically unacceptable.

LEGAL ANALYSIS
Law and Ethics

The study by Kolder et al[2] showed that a number of physicians have been willing to seek court orders compelling pregnant women to undergo treatment for the sake of their fetuses. While judicial sanction may reduce a physician's exposure to legal liability, it does not eliminate the ethical issues involved. In fact, the very decision to pursue a court order implicates important ethical values. Judicial involvement inevitably invades a woman's privacy, entails the disclosure of confidential medical and personal information, and thrusts the woman into the adversarial system, where she must defend her choices on a highly personal matter at a time when she is psychologically and physically ill-disposed to do so. Moreover, the request for a court order demonstrates the physician's willingness to use physical force against a competent adult to effect treatment, an ethically perilous course of action for a physician to adopt under any circumstances.

Furthermore, physicians cannot legitimately claim that they are compelled by the law to seek such orders. There is no affirmative legal duty on the part of the clinician to seek a court order in these circumstances.[4] Also, there is no reported case of a court imposing civil damages on any physician for failing to seek judicial review of any competent adult's refusal of treatment,[4] a finding corroborated by the study of Kolder et al.[2] Finally, the fact that a child may be able to sue his mother for prenatal injuries caused by her conduct[14,15] does not mean that the state would have the power to force her to forsake such conduct,[5] much less that a physician could be held liable for failing to force her similarly.

Persuasive arguments can be made that a pregnant woman not intending to have an abortion has an ethical obligation to accept reasonable, nonexperimental medical treatment and to behave otherwise in a manner that will benefit and not harm her fetus. Indeed, we are convinced that such an ethical obligation exists and that women should behave accordingly. Also, physicians should generally act toward their pregnant patients under the assumption that such an obligation exists and that the woman will fulfill it. Nevertheless, it is quite another matter to transform this ethical obligation into a legal duty by enforcing it with the coercive power of the law. . . .

MEDICAL AND SOCIAL POLICY

In our view, there is no compelling ethical or legal justification for requiring competent pregnant women to undergo medical treatment against their will. Others disagree and advocate the use of coercion against pregnant women in certain situations.[16,17,18] Commenting on the Kolder study, Annas[19] detected the beginning of an alliance between physicians and the courts to force pregnant women to accept medical treatment for the sake of their fetuses. Before such an alliance becomes entrenched, its assumptions, its terms, and what its operation would entail must be carefully examined.

The most plausible case for compelling a pregnant woman to undergo treatment for the sake of her fetus can be made in those situations when either the failure to provide the indicated treatment puts the fetus at great risk of serious physical harm or the treatment promises to be of significant benefit to the fetus, and the risks of the treatment itself to the mother and fetus are low or minimal. For example, Chervenak and McCullough[17] have proposed guidelines that would permit fetal diagnosis and treatment, presumably even against the mother's wishes, when "the risks [of treatment] to the fetus are minimal, the potential benefit to the fetus is substantial, and the risks to the woman are those she should reasonably accept on behalf of the fetus." In short, forced maternal treatment would be sanctioned if treatment presented substantial benefit to the fetus and low risk to the mother. This is a simple, appealing, and reasonable-sounding proposal until one tries to define its terms or apply it to clinical situations.

It is extremely difficult to identify clearly the clinical situations in which the failure to provide treatment poses a risk of harm to the fetus serious enough to warrant forcible intervention. Would only the certainty of fetal demise without intervention warrant compelled treatment, or would the risk of fetal harm be sufficient? If the risk of harm would be the relevant criterion, the degree of severity of harm sufficient to justify the undeniably serious act of forcing treatment on an unconsenting adult woman would have to be identified. The standard could be articulated as "serious harm," "grave harm," or "significant harm." However phrased, such a standard is ripe for idiosyncratic and arbitrary interpretation. Forcing women to undergo medical treatment against their will is too weighty a matter to be left to the vagaries of personal interpretation by physicians and judges. Moreover, such an inherently vague standard contains the risk of unequal treatment of women in similar medical situations.

Attempts to devise precise criteria encounter the problem of medical uncertainty. In many obstetric situations, the medical knowledge may not be available to make the correct diagnosis or to describe accurately the likelihood of occurrence of fetal harm.[5,20] For example, abnormalities on the fetal heart rate tracing may not be indicative of true fetal distress or predictive of fetal damage in the absence of medical intervention. As Kolder et al[2] rightly noted, while physicians are quick to embrace uncertainty as a justification for their errors, they are less quick to recognize its effect on patient self-determination. Furthermore, reported cases of court-ordered cesarean sections in which the woman delivered vaginally without incident despite medical predictions that she could not do so.[5,20,21] illustrate that if physicians' medical recommendations are legally enforceable, they will be allowed to be wrong, while the women involved will never be allowed to be right or wrong. As Elias and Annas[20] have observed, "It seems wrong to say that patients have the right to be wrong in all cases except pregnancy."

In addition to these difficult problems in identifying the fetal risk that would purportedly justify a decision to force medical treatment on a woman, there are similar problems in judging what constitutes an "acceptable" level of risk of harm to the mother. Using Chervenak and McCullough's term, one can justifiably be puzzled about the ability to identify those risks that a woman should "reasonably" accept for the benefit of her fetus. This formulation also fails to mention who is to decide what is "reasonable" in this context, a substantial problem given the elasticity of the term. What is one person's "serious harm" could well be "minor" to another person.

Furthermore, whoever makes this judgment will invariably have to make tricky assessments regarding maternal factors that may significantly increase the risk of the proposed intervention. For example, there is an undeniably greater risk of morbidity and mortality associated with cesarean delivery as compared with vaginal delivery.[6] These risk may significantly increase in the presence of . . . a recent myocardial infarction [heart attack] or pulmonary [lung] conditions that would complicate the administration of general anesthesia, which might be necessary in an emergency. We suggest that no one has the wisdom or ethical authority to declare what is an "acceptable" or "reasonable" risk for a woman to take if she herself is unwilling to face it.

In addition, some women refuse treatment for religious reasons.[23] For example, pregnant Jehovah's Witnesses have been known to refuse blood transfusions.[10,24,25] To force such a woman to receive blood may, in her own mind, expose her to eternal damnation as well as cause her to suffer psychological stress or rejection within her earthly community. It is important to distinguish between this situation and the routine practice of having neonates or children receive transfusions over the religious objections of their parents. A live-born child can be given a transfusion without forcibly invading the mother's body, although it does "invade" her wishes, while a transfusion done for the sake of the fetus must necessarily invade the mother's body and ignore her wishes.

Because our society values bodily integrity highly, the "geographical" difference between a live-born child and a fetus is a very significant one. Our society and its legal system go to great lengths to protect the right of persons to preserve their bodily integrity.[4] For example, the legal system does not force persons to donate organs involuntarily to others, even if they are relatives in desperate need. . . .

A policy that would permit the courts or the police to intervene in the activities of pregnant women that arguably placed their fetuses at some risk of harm must be considered in light of its potential effectiveness and what its enforcement would require. Every action a pregnant woman takes has a potential impact on her fetus, including the simplest and most common activities of daily living: eating, drinking, sexual intercourse, and physical activity (whether too much in the case of a woman at risk of preterm labor or too little in the case of women with clearly excessive weight gain). In addition, women may expose their fetuses to potential harm when they work, due to occupational hazards. Consequently, an effective public policy designed to prevent fetal harm would require extensive monitoring of and possible interference with each of these activities. This would entail an unprecedented social intrusion into the homes and private lives of pregnant women and their families.

The only plausible justification for a policy with such tremendous impact on the lives and civil liberties of pregnant women would be overwhelming need. However, it is far from clear that such need exists. Common clinical experience shows that it is an unusual woman who does not do everything within reason for the best interests of her fetus. In fact, clinicians are often impressed with the medical risks and life-style restrictions voluntarily assumed by pregnant women to ensure a good outcome for their pregnancies. In short, situations in which fetuses may die or be born damaged as a direct result of maternal behavior are likely to be rare.[20] This being so, the price of intervention to women's liberty and privacy seems too high.

We recognize that the behavior of women who are abusers of alcohol or drugs poses significant potential for fetal harm. However, there are solid reasons to doubt that a system of legal punishment or intervention would decrease the incidence of this behavior, as it is usually an addiction over which these women have little control. If anything, a system of legal coercion and punishment might drive these women away from the prenatal care that they and their fetuses especially need.

The enactment of a public policy that would compel women to avoid certain behaviors for the sake of the fetus would also drastically change the nature of the physician–pregnant woman relationship. While many physicians probably can recall a case in which they might have welcomed legal sanction to force a pregnant woman to prevent fetal harm, they may underestimate the impact of such a precedent on their relationship to all patients. The relationship between a physician and a pregnant woman would become much less one of a partnership dedicated to a common goal and more a relationship of adversaries, like police officer and criminal suspect. The ability of a pregnant woman and her physician to negotiate a better course of care when the optimal course is not chosen by the patient would become severely compromised if she could be forced to do whatever the physician recommended.[20] In addition, some pregnant women undoubtedly would refrain from seeking prenatal care or lie about their behaviors or symptoms if they knew their physicians could use the truth to force treatment on them. This, of course, would severely restrict physicians' ability to diagnose correctly and treat adequately both pregnant women and their fetuses.

The philosophical question confronting society is whether it wishes to enforce a policy that would entail on an unprecedented scale serious invasions of a woman's privacy, restriction of her civil liberties, and interference with her religious and personal beliefs. In a secular society such as ours that embraces no particular moral point of view and that attempts to encompass groups with widely divergent views on how persons should live their own lives, individuals are required to forgo "the temptation to impose by state force [their] own view of proper private morality."[26] Given the heated and intractable controversy surrounding the ethical evaluation of the fetus and the well-established interests of all adult persons in bodily integrity and self-determination, we conclude that the decision of a competent pregnant woman to forgo medical treatment likely to benefit her fetus should remain hers, even if others see her choice as unethical.

CONCLUSION

There are many troublesome questions surrounding the use of judicial force to compel pregnant women to undergo medical treatment or behavior change for the benefit of their fetuses. We believe that it is unwise, in the last analysis, to recognize fetal rights that would create an adversarial relationship between a pregnant woman and her fetus. Incompleteness of medical knowledge and the unavoidable uncertainty of medical diagnostic and therapeutic techniques make it impossible to define a clear, precise, and accurate medical model on which society could base a fair and uniformly applied legal policy that would sanction the use of force against pregnant women. There is also insufficient reason to undermine the ethical principle of patient autonomy and the legal right to self-determination and bodily integrity for a subset of our society, namely, pregnant women.

Ultimately, it is not feasible to determine in a just and fair manner which actions or inactions of a pregnant woman should warrant interventions as drastic as involuntary treatment or surgery. It is also not possible to enforce such a policy effectively without extensive and probably distasteful intrusion into the private lives of pregnant women and their families. Furthermore, it is speculative at best whether these changes would cause im-

provement in the relationship between prenatal care givers and pregnant women and in the effectiveness of prenatal care. We suspect it would in fact do quite the contrary.

We conclude that a pregnant woman who does not intend to have a legal abortion has an affirmative ethical obligation to accept reasonable, nonexperimental medical treatment for the sake of her fetus and to behave otherwise in a manner intended to benefit and not harm her fetus. This obligation is rooted in her unique and significant influence on the health and development of the human entity she voluntarily carries, an entity that will ultimately develop into a person with human rights. Nevertheless, we do not believe that this ethical obligation should be legally enforced. The attempt to do so would not itself be ethical, practically effective, or advantageous for society or the individual. In fact, such legal enforcement would create more harm than it could prevent. Thus, the interventionist "solution" to the problem of maternal-fetal conflict is worse than the original problem.

Finally, we endorse the goal of enhancing fetal health. Physicians will play an essential role in achieving this goal by fulfilling their ethical obligations to pregnant women. This will include monitoring the health of pregnant women and their fetuses and recommending treatment to maximize the prospects of both. While physicians have an ethical obligation to respect the decisions of an informed, competent pregnant woman, they may ethically be an advocate for the fetus when the pregnant woman is making her choices. This advocacy may include the use of persuasion to try to influence the woman to do the "right" thing but not the use of threats, lies, or physical force. Because most prenatal care relationships between physicians and pregnant women last several months, there is an opportunity to anticipate conflicts and spend additional time to ensure that a pregnant woman's fears or misinformation, which may prevent her from doing what is best for her pregnancy, can be addressed and corrected.

If society and the medical profession are truly interested in enhancing fetal health, their efforts should be directed toward increasing the availability and quality of voluntary prenatal care for all pregnant women and the availability of drug and alcohol rehabilitation programs and other social services for those pregnant women who need them and discouraging physicians from running to the courthouse for an order forcing a woman to accept treatment she does not want. John Stuart Mill has said, "Mankind are greater gainers by suffering each other to live as seems good to themselves, than by compelling each to live as seems good to the rest."[27] We agree: society will, in the end, gain far more by allowing each pregnant woman to live as seems good to her, rather than by compelling each to live as seems good to the rest of us.

The preparation on this article was assisted in part by a grant from the Robert Wood Johnson Foundation, Princeton, NJ. The opinions expressed herein are those of the authors and do not necessarily represent the views of the Foundation.

REFERENCES

1. Gianelli DM: ACOG issues guidelines on maternal, fetal rights. *American Medical News*, Aug 28, 1987, p. 7.
2. Kolder VE, Gallagher J, Parsons MT: Court-ordered obstetrical interventions. *N Engl J Med* 1987; 316:1192–1196.
3. Gallagher J: Prenatal invasions and interventions: What's wrong with fetal rights. *Harv Women's Law J* 1987; 10:9–58.
4. Nelson LJ, Buggy BP, Weil CJ: Forced medical treatment of pregnant women: 'Compelling each to live as seems good to the rest.' *Hastings Law J* 1986; 37:703–763.
5. Rhoden N: The judge in the delivery room: The emergence of court-ordered cesareans. *Calif Law Rev* 1986; 74:1951–2030.
6. Pritchard JA, MacDonald PC, Gant NF: *Williams Obstetrics.* East Norwalk, Conn, Appleton-Century-Crofts, 1985, pp. xi, 867–871.
7. Jonsen AR, Siegler M, Winslade WJ: *Clinical Ethics.* New York, Macmillan Publishing Co Inc, 1986, pp. 47–51.
8. *Bouvia vs Superior Court,* 179 Cal App 3d 1127 (Cal App 1986).
9. *Bartling vs Superior Court,* 163 Cal App 3d 1986 (Call App 1984).
10. *Mercy Hospital vs Jackson,* 510 A 2d 562 (Md 1986).
11. *Satz vs Perlmutter,* 379 So 2d 359 (Fla 1980).
12. Congregation for the Doctrine of the Faith: *Instruction on Respect for Human Life in Its Origin and on the Dignity of Procreation.* Vatican City, Vatican Polyglot Press, 1987.
13. Gertler GB: Brain birth: A proposal for defining when a fetus is entitled to human life status. *South Calif Law Rev* 1986; 59:1061–1078.
14. *Grodin vs Grodin,* 301 NW 2d 869 (Mich App 1980).
15. *Stallman vs Youngquist,* 504 NE 2d 920 (Ill App 1987).
16. Robertson JA: Legal issues in fetal therapy. *Semin Perinatol* 1985; 9:136–142.
17. Chervenak FA, McCullough LB: Perinatal ethics: A practical analysis of obligations to mother and fetus. *Obstet Gynecol* 1985; 66: 442–446.
18. Mathieu D: Respecting liberty and preventing harm: Limits of state intervention in prenatal choice. *Harv J Law Public Policy* 1985; 8:19–52.
19. Annas GJ: Protecting the liberty of pregnant patients. *N Engl J Med* 1987; 316:1213–1214.
20. Elias E, Annas GJ: *Reproductive Genetics and the Law.* Chicago, Year Book Medical Publishers Inc, 1987, pp. 118– 120, 253–262.
21. *In re Baby Jeffries,* No. 14004 (Jackson Cty P Ct Mich, May 24, 1982).
22. Fletcher JC: Ethical considerations in and beyond experimental fetal therapy. *Semin Perinatol* 1985; 9:130–135.
23. *Jefferson vs Griffin Spalding County Hospital Authority,* 274 SE 2d 457 (Ga 1981).
24. *Raleigh Fitkin–Paul Morgan Memorial Hospital vs Anderson,* 201 A 2d 537, (NJ 1964), cert denied, 377 US 984.

25. *In re Application of Jamaica Hospital*, 491 NYS 2d 898 (NY Sup Ct 1985).

26. Englehardt HT Jr: Introduction, in Bondeson W, Englehardt HT, Spicker S, et al (eds): *Abortion and the Status of the Fetus*. Dordrecht, the Netherlands, D Reidel Publishing Co, 1983, pp. xi–xxxii.

27. Mill JS: On liberty, in Warnock M (ed): *Utilitarianism and Other Writings*. New York, World Publishers, 1962, pp. 126–250.

POSTSCRIPT

The Maternal-Fetal Relationship: Can Compelled Medical Treatment of Pregnant Women Be Justified?

In April 1990 the District of Columbia Court of Appeals overturned the lower court's decision in the case of Angela Carder. In the appeal decision, the majority ruled that the lower court had not followed proper procedures in determining Ms. Carder's competency. It did not decide whether or in what circumstances "the state's interest [in preserving life] can ever prevail over the interests of a pregnant patient." It did, however, emphasize that the patient's confirmed wishes must be followed in "virtually all cases." In November 1990 George Washington University Medical Center announced a new policy intended to ensure that ethically difficult decisions on how to treat severely ill pregnant women and their fetuses will be made by the women, their families, and doctors, and not by the courts.

Cases involving pregnant drug-using women have been handled in different ways. A jury in Illinois refused to charge a mother with involuntary manslaughter for causing the death of her newborn baby by using cocaine before she gave birth. On the other hand, two Michigan women have been ordered to stand trial on a charge usually restricted to drug dealers: delivering cocaine to a minor. The minors in this instance were newborn infants, and the drug was allegedly delivered through the umbilical cord in the minute or two before delivery. Nationwide, there have been about 35 cases, but only one conviction, and even that case is on appeal because the woman had tried to obtain drug treatment and was turned away.

In November 1990 the Board of Trustees of the American Medical Association recommended adoption of a statement that opposes judicial intervention or compelled medical treatment, unless there are exceptional circumstances. One of the principles states: "The physician's duty is to provide appropriate information, such that the pregnant woman may make an informed and thoughtful decision, not to dictate the woman's decision" (*Journal of the American Medical Association*, November 28, 1990).

For legal and ethical analyses opposing forced treatment, see Martha A. Field, "Controlling the Woman to Protect the Fetus," *Law, Medicine, & Health Care* (Summer 1989), and George J. Annas, "Foreclosing the Use of Force: A. C. Reversed," *Hastings Center Report* (July/August 1990).

Frank A. Chervenak and Laurence B. McCullough provide some practical assistance to physicians in implementing their ethical framework in "Clinical Guides to Preventing Ethical Conflict between Pregnant Women and Their Physicians," *American Journal of Obstetrics and Gynecology* (February 1990). Jeffrey Parness argues for strengthening the criminal law to prevent "crimes against the fetus" in "Crime Against the Unborn: Protecting and Respecting the Potentiality of Human Life," *Harvard Journal on Legislation* (Winter 1985).

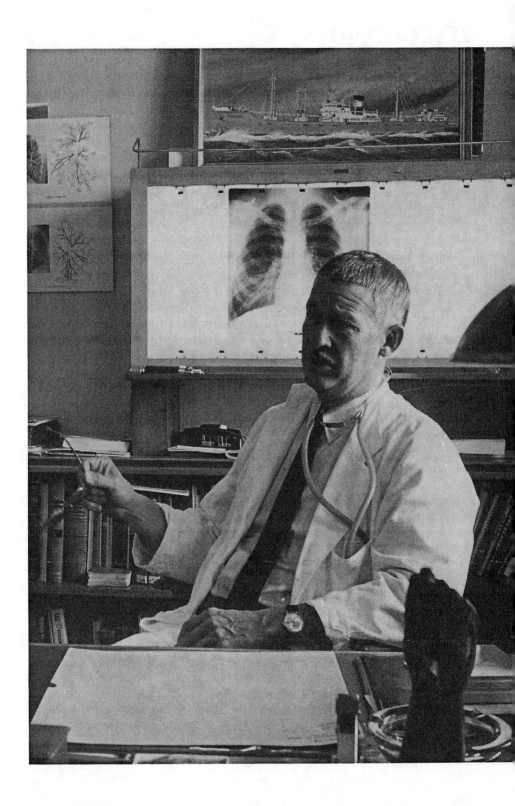

PART 2

Decisions About Death

What are the ethical responsibilities associated with death? Doctors are sworn "to do no harm," but this proscription is open to many different interpretations. Death is a natural event that can, in some instances, put an end to suffering. Is it ethically necessary to prolong life at all times under all circumstances? If not, is the quality of life a valid criterion for determining if a life should be prolonged? Medical personnel often face these agonizing questions and must decide matters of literal life and death. Even the question of whether or not to tell terminally ill patients the truth about their conditions has great ethical implications. The right of an individual to decide his or her own fate conflicts with society's interest in maintaining the value of human life. This conflict is apparent in the matter of physician-assisted suicide. This section examines some of these anguishing questions.

Is It Ethical to Withhold the Truth from
   Dying Patients?

Is Physician-Assisted Suicide Ethical?

Is It Ever Morally Right to Withhold
   Food and Water from Dying
   Patients?

ISSUE 5

Is It Ethical to Withhold the Truth From Dying Patients?

YES: Bernard C. Meyer, from "Truth and the Physician," in E. Fuller Torrey, ed., *Ethical Issues in Medicine* (Little, Brown, 1968)

NO: Sissela Bok, from *Lying: Moral Choice in Public and Private Life* (Pantheon Books, 1978)

ISSUE SUMMARY

YES: Physician Bernard C. Meyer argues that physicians must use discretion in communicating bad news to patients. Adherence to a rigid formula of truth telling fails to appreciate the differences in patients' readiness to hear and understand the information.

NO: Philosopher Sissela Bok challenges the traditional physician's view by arguing that the harm resulting from disclosure is less than they think and is outweighed by the benefits, including the important one of giving the patient the right to choose among treatments.

In his powerful short story "The Death of Ivan Ilych," Leo Tolstoy graphically portrays the physical agony and the social isolation of a dying man. However, "[w]hat tormented Ivan Ilych most was the deception, the lie, which for some reason they all accepted, that he was not dying but was simply ill, and that he only need keep quiet and undergo a treatment and then something very good would result." Instrumental in setting up the deception is Ilych's doctor, who reassures him to the very end that all will be well. Hearing the banal news from his doctor once again, "Ivan Ilych looks at him as much as to say: 'Are you really never ashamed of lying?' But the doctor does not wish to understand this question. . . ."

Unlike many of the ethical issues discussed in this volume, which have arisen as a result of modern scientific knowledge and technology, the question of whether to tell dying patients the truth is an old and persistent one. But this debate has been given a new urgency because medical practices today are so complex that it is often difficult to know just what the "truth" really is. A dying patient's life can often be prolonged, although at great financial and personal cost, and many people differ over the definition of a terminal illness.

What must be balanced in this decision are two significant principles of ethical conduct: the obligation to tell the truth and the obligation not to harm others. Moral philosophers, beginning with Aristotle, have regarded truth as either an absolute value or one that, at the very least, is preferable to deception. The great nineteenth-century German philosopher Immanuel Kant argued that there is no justification for lying (although some later commentators feel that his absolutist position has been overstated). Other philosophers have argued that deception is sometimes justified. For example, Henry Sidgwick, an early twentieth-century British philosopher, believed that it was entirely acceptable to lie to invalids and children to protect them from the shock of the truth. Although the question has been debated for centuries, no clear-cut answer has been reached. In fact, the case of a benevolent lie to a dying patient is often given as the prime example of an excusable deception.

If moral philosophers cannot agree, what guidance is there for the physician torn between the desire for truth and the desire to protect the patient from harm (and the admittedly paternalistic conviction that the doctor knows best what will harm the patient)? None of the early medical codes and oaths offered any advice to physicians on what to tell patients, although they were quite explicit about the physician's obligation to keep confidential whatever a patient revealed. The American Medical Association's (AMA) 1847 "Code of Ethics" did endorse some forms of deception by noting that the physician has a sacred duty "to avoid all things which have a tendency to discourage the patient and to depress his spirits." The most recent (1980) AMA "Principles of Medical Ethics" say only that "A physician shall deal honestly with patients and colleagues. . . ." However, the American Hospital Association's "Patient's Bill of Rights," adopted in 1972, is more specific: "The patient has the right to obtain from his physician complete current information concerning his diagnosis, treatment, and prognosis in terms the patient can reasonably be expected to understand. When it is not medically advisable to give such information to the patient, the information should be made available to an appropriate person in his behalf."

In the following selections, Bernard C. Meyer argues for an ethic that transcends the virtue of uttering truth for truth's sake. He believes that the physician's prime responsibility is contained in the Hippocratic Oath—"So far as possible, do no harm." Sissela Bok counters with evidence that physicians often misread patients' wishes and that withholding the truth can often harm them more than disclosure.

YES

Bernard C. Meyer

TRUTH AND THE PHYSICIAN

Truth does not do so much good in this world as the semblance of it does harm.
La Rochefoucauld

Among the reminiscences of his Alsatian boyhood, my father related the story of the local functionary who was berated for the crude and blunt manner in which he went from house to house announcing to wives and mothers news of battle casualties befalling men from the village. On the next occasion, mindful of the injunctions to be more tactful and to soften the impact of his doleful message, he rapped gently on the door and, when it opened, inquired, "Is the widow Schmidt at home?"

Insofar as this essay is concerned with the subject of truth it is only proper to add that when I told this story to a colleague, he already knew it and claimed that it concerned a woman named Braun who lived in a small town in Austria. By this time it would not surprise me to learn that the episode is a well-known vignette in the folklore of Tennessee where it is attributed to a woman named Smith or Brown whose husband was killed at the battle of Shiloh. Ultimately, we may find that all three versions are plagiarized accounts of an occurrence during the Trojan War.

COMMUNICATION BETWEEN PHYSICIAN AND PATIENT

Apocryphal or not, the story illustrates a few of the vexing aspects of the problem of conveying unpalatable news, notably the difficulty of doing so in a manner that causes a minimum amount of pain, and also the realization that not everyone is capable of learning how to do it. Both aspects find their application in the field of medicine where the imparting of the grim facts of diagnosis and prognosis is a constant and recurring issue. Nor does it seem likely that for all our learning we doctors are particularly endowed with superior talents and techniques for coping with these problems. On the contrary, for reasons to be given later, there is cause to believe that in not a few instances, elements in his own psychological makeup may cause the physician to be singularly ill-equipped to be the bearer of bad tidings. It should be observed, moreover, that until comparatively recent times, the subject of communication between physician and patient received little attention in medical curriculum and medical literature.

Within the past decade or so, coincident with an expanded recognition of the significance of emotional factors in all medical practice, an impressive number of books and articles by physicians, paramedical personnel, and others have been published, attesting to both the growing awareness of the importance of the subject and an apparent willingness to face it. An especially noteworthy example of this trend was provided by a three-day meeting in February, 1967, sponsored by the New York Academy of Sciences, on the subject of *The Care of Patients with Fatal Illness.* The problem of communicating with such patients and their families was a recurring theme in most of the papers presented.

Both at this conference and in the literature, particular emphasis has been focused on the patient with cancer, which is hardly surprising in light of its frequency and of the extraordinary emotional reactions that it unleashes not only in the patient and in his kinsmen but in the physician himself. At the same time, it should be noted that the accent on the cancer patient or the dying patient may foster the impression that in less grave conditions this dialogue between patient and physician hardly warrants much concern or discussion. Such a view is unfounded, however, and could only be espoused by someone who has had the good fortune to escape the experience of being ill and hospitalized. Those less fortunate will recall the emotional stresses induced by hospitalization, even when

the condition requiring it is relatively banal.

A striking example of such stress may sometimes be seen when the patient who is hospitalized, say, for repair of an inguinal hernia, happens to be a physician. All the usual anxieties confronting a prospective surgical subject tend to become greatly amplified and garnished with a generous sprinkling of hypochondriasis in the physician-turned-patient. Wavering unsteadily between these two roles, he conjures up visions of all the complications of anesthesia, of wound dehiscence or infection, of embolization, cardiac arrest, and whatnot that he has ever heard or read about. To him, lying between hospital sheets, clad in impersonal hospital clothes, divested of his watch and the keys to his car, the hospital suddenly takes on a different appearance from the place he may have known in a professional capacity. Even his colleagues—the anesthetist who will put him to sleep or cause a temporary motor and sensory paralysis of the lower half of his body, and the surgeon who will incise it—appear different. He would like to have a little talk with them, a very professional talk to be sure, although in his heart he may know that the talk will also be different. And if they are in tune with the situation, they too know that it will be different, that beneath the restrained tones of sober and factual conversation is the thumping anxiety of a man who seeks words of reassurance. With some embarrassment he may introduce his anxieties with the phrase, "I suppose this is going to seem a little silly, but . . ."; and from this point on he may sound like any other individual confronted by the ordeal of surgical experience.[1] Indeed, it would appear that under these circumstances, to say nothing of more ominous ones, most people, regardless of their experience, knowledge, maturity or sophistication, are assailed by more or less similar psychological pressures, from which they seek relief not through pharmacological sedation, but through the more calming influence of the spoken word.

Seen in this light the question of what to tell the patient about his illness is but one facet of the practice of medicine as an art, a particular example of that spoken and mute dialogue between patient and physician which has always been and will always be an indispensable ingredient in the therapeutic process. How to carry on this dialogue, what to say and when to say it, and what not to say, are questions not unlike those posed by an awkward suitor; like him, those not naturally versed in this art may find themselves discomfited and needful of the promptings of some Cyrano who will whisper those words and phrases that ultimately will wing their way to soothe an anguished heart.

EMOTIONAL REACTIONS OF PHYSICIAN

The difficulties besetting the physician under these circumstances, however, cannot be ascribed simply to his mere lack of experience or innate eloquence. For like the stammering suitor, the doctor seeking to communicate with his patient may have an emotional stake in his message. When that message contains an ominous significance, he may find himself too troubled to use words wisely, too ridden with anxiety to be kind, and too depressed to convey hope. An understanding of such reactions touches upon a recognition of some of the several psychological motivations that have led some individuals to choose a medical career. There is evidence that at times that choice has been dictated by what might be viewed as counterphobic forces. Having in childhood experienced recurring brushes with illness and having encountered a deep and abiding fear of death and dying, such persons may embrace a medical career as if it will confer upon them a magical immunity from a repetition of those dreaded eventualities; for them the letters M.D. constitute a talisman bestowing upon the wearer a sense of invulnerability and a pass of safe conduct through the perilous frontiers of life. There are others for whom the choice of a career dedicated to helping and healing appears to have arisen as a reaction formation against earlier impulses to wound and to destroy.[2] For still others among us, the practice of medicine serves as the professional enactment of a long-standing rescue fantasy.

It is readily apparent in these examples (which by no means exhaust the catalogue of motives leading to the choice of a medical career) that confrontation by the failure of one's efforts and by the need to announce it may unloose a variety of inner psychological disturbances: faced by the gravely ill or dying patient the "counterphobic" doctor may feel personally vulnerable again; the "reaction-formation" doctor, evil and guilty; and the "rescuer," worthless and impotent. For such as these, words cannot come readily in their discourse with the seriously or perilously ill. Indeed, they may curtail their communications; and, what is no less meaningful to their patients, withdraw their physical presence. Thus the patient with inoperable cancer and his family may discover that the physician, who at a more hopeful moment in the course of the illness had been both articulate and supportive, has become remote both in his speech and in his behavior. Nor is the patient uncomprehending of the significance of the change in his doctor's attitude. Observers have recorded the verbal expressions of patients who sensed the feelings of futility and depression in their physicians. Seeking to account for their own reluctance to ask questions (a reluctance based partly upon their own disinclination to face a grim reality), one such patient said, "He looked so tired." Another stated, "I don't want to upset him because he has tried so hard to help me"; and another, "I know he feels so badly already and is doing his best" (Abrams, 1966). To paraphrase a celebrated utterance, one might suppose that these remarks were dictated by the maxim: "Ask not what your doctor can do for you; ask what you can do for your doctor."[3]

ADHERENCE TO A FORMULA

In the dilemma created both by a natural disinclination to be a bearer of bad news and by those other considerations already cited, many a physician is tempted to abandon personal judgment and authorship in his discourse with his patients, and to rely instead upon a set formula which he employs with dogged and indiscriminate consistency. Thus, in determining what to say to patients with cancer, there are exponents of standard policies that are applied routinely in seeming disregard of the overall clinical picture and of the personality or psychological makeup of the patient. In general, two such schools of thought prevail; i.e., those that always tell and those that never do. Each of these is amply supplied with statistical anecdotal evidence proving the correctness of the policy. Yet

even if the figures were accurate—and not infrequently they are obtained via a questionnaire, itself a rather opaque window to the human mind—all they demonstrate is that more rather than less of a given proportion of the cancer population profited by the policy employed. This would provide small comfort, one might suppose, to the patients and their families that constitute the minority of the sample.

TRUTH AS ABSTRACT PRINCIPLE

At times adherence to such a rigid formula is dressed up in the vestments of slick and facile morality. Thus a theologian has insisted that the physician has a moral obligation to tell the truth and that his withholding it constitutes a deprivation of the patient's right; therefore it is "theft, therefore unjust, therefore immoral" (Fletcher, 1954). "Can it be," he asks, "that doctors who practice professional deception would, if the roles were reversed, want to be coddled or deceived?" To which, as many physicians can assert, the answer is distinctly *yes*. Indeed so adamant is this writer upon the right of the patient to know the facts of his illness that in the event he refuses to hear what the doctor is trying to say, the latter should "ask leave to withdraw from the case, urging that another physician be called in his place."[4] (Once there were three boy scouts who were sent away from a campfire and told not to return until each had done his good turn for the day. In 20 minutes all three had returned, and curiously each one reported that he had helped a little old lady to cross a street. The scoutmaster's surprise was even greater when he learned that in each case it was the same little old lady, prompting him to inquire why it took the three of them to perform this one simple good deed. "Well, sir," replied one of the boys, "you see she really didn't want to cross the street at all.")

In this casuistry wherein so much attention is focused upon abstract principle and so little upon humanity, one is reminded of the no less specious arguments of those who assert that the thwarting of suicide and the involuntary hospitalization of the mentally deranged constitute violations of personal freedom and human right.[5] It is surely irregular for a fire engine to travel in the wrong direction on a one-way street, but if one is not averse to putting out fires and saving lives, the traffic violation looms as a conspicuous irrelevancy. No less irrelevant is the obsessional concern with meticulous definitions of truth in an enterprise where kindness, charity, and the relief of human suffering are the ethical verities. "The letter killeth," say the Scriptures, "but the spirit giveth life."

Problem of Definition

Nor should it be forgotten that in the healing arts, the matter of truth is not always susceptible to easy definition. Consider for a moment the question of the hopeless diagnosis. It was not so long ago that such a designation was appropriate for subacute bacterial endocarditis, pneumococcal meningitis, pernicious anemia, and a number of other conditions which today are no longer incurable, while those diseases which today are deemed hopeless may cease to be so by tomorrow. Experience has proved, too, the unreliability of obdurate opinions concerning prognosis even in those conditions where all the clinical evidence and the known behavior of a given disease should leave no room for doubt. To paraphrase Clemenceau, to insist that a patient is hopelessly ill may at times be worse than a crime; it may be a mistake.

Problem of Determining Patient's Desires

There are other pitfalls, moreover, that complicate the problem of telling patients the truth about their illness. There is the naive notion, for example, that when the patient asserts that what he is seeking is the plain truth he means just that. But as more than one observer has noted, this is sometimes the last thing the patient really wants. Such assertions may be voiced with particular emphasis by patients who happen to be physicians and who strive to display a professional and scientifically objective attitude toward their own condition. Yet to accept such assertions at their face value may sometimes lead to tragic consequences, as in the following incident.

A distinguished urological surgeon was hospitalized for a hypernephroma, which diagnosis had been withheld from him. One day he summoned the intern into his room, and after appealing to the latter on the basis of we're-both-doctors-and-grown-up-men, succeeded in getting the unwary younger man to divulge the facts. Not long afterward, while the nurse was momentarily absent from the room, the patient opened a window and leaped to his death.

Role of Secrecy in Creating Anxiety

Another common error is the assumption that until someone has been formally told the truth he doesn't know it. Such self-deception is often present when parents feel moved to supply their pubertal children with the sexual facts of life. With much embarrassment and a good deal of backing and filling on the subjects of eggs, bees, and babies, sexual information is imparted to a child who often not only already knows it but is uncomfortable in hearing it from that particular source. There is indeed a general tendency to underestimate the perceptiveness of children not only about such matters but where graver issues, notably illness and death, are concerned. As a consequence, attitudes of secrecy and overprotection designed to shield children from painful realities may result paradoxically in creating an atmosphere that is saturated with suspicion, distrust, perplexity, and intolerable anxiety. Caught between trust in their own intuitive perceptions and the deceptions practiced by the adults about them, such children may suffer greatly from a lack of opportunity of coming to terms emotionally with some of the vicissitudes of existence that in the end are inescapable. A refreshing contrast to this approach has been presented in a paper entitled "Who's Afraid of Death on a Leukemia Ward?" (Vernick and Karon, 1965). Recognizing that most of the children afflicted with this disease had some knowledge of its seriousness, and that all were worried about it, the hospital staff abandoned the traditional custom of protection and secrecy, providing instead an atmosphere in which the children could feel free to express their fears and their concerns and could openly acknowledge the fact of death when one of the group passed away. The result of this measure was immensely salutary.

Similar miscalculations of the accuracy of inner perceptions may be noted in dealing with adults. Thus, in a study entitled "Mongolism: When Should Parents Be Told?" (Drillien and Wilkinson, 1964), it was found that in nearly half the cases the mothers declared they had real-ized before being told that something was seriously wrong with the child's development, a figure which obviously excludes the mothers who refused consciously to acknowledge their suspicions. On the basis of their findings the authors concluded that a full explanation given in the early months, coupled with regular support thereafter, appeared to facilitate the mother's acceptance of and adjustment to her child's handicap.

A pointless and sometimes deleterious withholding of truth is a common practice in dealing with elderly people. "Don't tell Mother" often seems to be an almost reflex maxim among some adults in the face of any misfortune, large or small. Here, too, elaborate efforts at camouflage may backfire, for, sensing that he is being shielded from some ostensibly intolerable secret, not only is the elderly one deprived of the opportunity of reacting appropriately to it, but he is being tacitly encouraged to conjure up something in his imagination that may be infinitely worse.

Discussion of Known Truth

Still another misconception is the belief that if it is certain that the truth is known it is all right to discuss it. How mistaken such an assumption may be was illustrated by the violent rage which a recent widow continued to harbor toward a friend for having alluded to cancer in the presence of her late husband. Hearing her outburst one would have concluded that until the ominous word had been uttered, her husband had been ignorant of the nature of his condition. The facts, however, were different, as the unhappy woman knew, for it had been her husband who originally had told the friend what the diagnosis was.

DENIAL AND REPRESSION

The psychological devices that make such seeming inconsistencies of thought and knowledge possible are the mechanisms of repression and denial. It is indeed the remarkable capacity to bury or conceal more or less transparent truth that makes the problem of telling it so sticky and difficult a matter, and one that is so unsusceptible to simple rule-of-thumb formulas. For while in some instances the maintenance of denial may lead to severe emotional distress, in others it may serve as a merciful shield. For example,

A physician with a reputation for considerable diagnostic acumen developed a painless jaundice. When, not surprisingly, a laparotomy revealed a carcinoma of the head of the pancreas, the surgeon relocated the biliary outflow so that postoperatively the jaundice subsided. This seeming improvement was consistent with the surgeon's explanation to the patient that the operation had revealed a hepatitis. Immensely relieved, the patient chided himself for not having anticipated the "correct" diagnosis. "What a fool I was!" he declared, obviously alluding to an earlier, albeit unspoken, fear of cancer.

Among less sophisticated persons the play of denial may assume a more primitive expression. Thus a woman who had ignored the growth of a breast cancer to a point where it had produced spinal metastases and paraplegia, attributed the latter to "arthritis" and asked whether the breast would grow back again. The same mental mechanism allowed another woman to ignore dangerous rectal bleeding by ascribing it to menstruation, although she was well beyond the menopause.

In contrast to these examples is a case reported by Winkelstein and Blacher of a man who, awaiting the report of a cervical node biopsy, asserted that if it showed cancer he wouldn't want to live, and that if it didn't he wouldn't believe it (Winkelstein and Blacher, 1967). Yet despite this seemingly unambiguous willingness to deal with raw reality, when the chips were down, as will be described later, this man too was able to protect himself through the use of denial.

From the foregoing it should be self-evident that what is imparted to a patient about his illness should be planned with the same care and executed with the same skill that are demanded by any potentially therapeutic measure. Like the transfusion of blood, the dispensing of certain information must be distinctly indicated, the amount given consonant with the needs of the recipient, and the type chosen with the view of avoiding untoward reactions. This means that only in selected instances is there any justification for telling a patient the precise figures of his blood pressure, and that the question of revealing interesting but asymptomatic congenital anomalies should be considered in light of the possibility of evoking either hypochondriacal ruminations or narcissistic gratification.

Under graver circumstances the choices of confronting the physician rest upon more crucial psychological issues. In principle, we should strive to make the patient sufficiently aware of the facts of his condition to facilitate his participation in the treatment without at the same time giving him cause to believe that such participation is futile. "The indispensable ingredient of this therapeutic approach," write Stehlin and Beach, "is free communication between [physician] and patient, in which the latter is sustained by hope within a framework of reality" (Stehlin and Beach, 1966). What this may mean in many instances is neither outright truth nor outright falsehood but a carefully modulated formulation that neither overtaxes human credulity nor invites despair. Thus a sophisticated woman might be expected to reject with complete disbelief the notion that she has had to undergo mastectomy for a benign cyst, but she may at the same time accept postoperative radiation as a prophylactic measure rather than as evidence of metastasis.

A doctor's wife was found to have ovarian carcinoma with widespread metastases. Although the surgeon was convinced she would not survive for more than three or four months, he wished to try the effects of radiotherapy and chemotherapy. After some discussion of the problem with a psychiatrist, he addressed himself to the patient as follows: to his surprise, when examined under the microscope the tumor in her abdomen proved to be cancerous; he fully believed he had removed it entirely; to feel perfectly safe, however, he intended to give her radiation and chemical therapies over an indeterminate period of time. The patient was highly gratified by his frankness and proceeded to live for nearly three more *years*, during which time she enjoyed an active and a productive life.

A rather similar approach was utilized in the case of Winkelstein and Blacher previously mentioned (Winkelstein and Blacher, 1967). In the presence of his wife the patient was told by the resident surgeon, upon the advice of the psychiatrist, that the biopsy of the cervical node showed cancer; that he had a cancerous growth in the abdomen; that it was the type of cancer that responds well to chemotherapy; that if the latter produced any discomfort he would receive medication for its relief; and finally that the doctors were very

hopeful for a successful outcome. The patient, who, it will be recalled, had declared he wouldn't want to live if the doctors found cancer, was obviously gratified. Immediately he telephoned members of his family to tell them the news, gratuitously adding that the tumor was of low-grade malignancy. That night he slept well for the first time since entering the hospital and he continued to do so during the balance of his stay. Just before leaving he confessed that he had known all along about the existence of the abdominal mass but that he had concealed his knowledge to see what the doctors would tell him. Upon arriving home he wrote a warm letter of thanks and admiration to the resident surgeon.

It should be emphasized that although in both of these instances the advice of a psychiatrist was instrumental in formulating the discussion of the facts of the illness, it was the surgeon, not the psychiatrist, who did the talking. The importance of this point cannot be exaggerated, for since it is the surgeon who plays the central and crucial role in such cases, it is to him, and not to some substitute mouthpiece, that the patient looks for enlightenment and for hope. As noted earlier, it is not every surgeon who can bring himself to speak in this fashion to his patient; and for some there may be a strong temptation to take refuge in a sterotyped formula, or to pass the buck altogether. The surgical resident, in the last case cited, for example, was both appalled and distressed when he was advised what to do. Yet he steeled himself, looked the patient straight in the eye and spoke with conviction. When he saw the result, he was both relieved and gratified. Indeed, he emerged from the experience a far wiser man and a better physician.

THE DYING PATIENT

The general point of view expressed in the foregoing pages has been espoused by others in considering the problem of communicating with the dying patient. Aldrich stresses the importance of providing such persons with an appropriately timed opportunity of selecting acceptance or denial of the truth in their efforts to cope with their plight (Aldrich, 1963). Weisman and Hackett believe that for the majority of patients it is likely that there is neither complete acceptance nor total repudiation of the imminence of death (Weismann and Hackett, 1961). "To deny this 'middle knowledge' of approaching death," they assert,

> . . . is to deny the responsiveness of the mind to both internal perceptions and external information. There is always a psychological sampling of the physiological stream; fever, weakness, anorexia, weight loss and pain are subjective counterparts of homeostatic alteration. . . . If to this are added changes in those close to the patient, the knowledge of approaching death is confirmed.

Other observers agree that a patient who is sick enough to die often knows it without being told, and that what he seeks from his physician are no longer statements concerning diagnosis and prognosis, but earnest manifestations of his unwavering concern and devotion. As noted earlier, it is at such times that for reason of their own psychological makeup some physicians become deeply troubled and are most prone to drift away, thereby adding, to the dying patient's physical suffering, the suffering that is caused by a sense of abandonment, isolation, and emotional deprivation.

In contrast, it should be stressed that no less potent than morphine nor less effective than an array of tranquilizers is the steadfast and serious concern of the physician for those often numerous and relatively minor complaints of the dying patient. To this beneficent manifestation of psychological denial, which may at times attain hypochondriacal proportions, the physician ideally should respond in kind, shifting his gaze from the lethal process he is now helpless to arrest to the living being whose discomfort and distress he is still able to assuage. In these, the final measures of the dance of life, it may then appear as if both partners had reached a tacit and a mutual understanding, an unspoken pledge to ignore the dark shadow of impending death and to resume those turns and rhythms that were familiar figures in a more felicitious past. If in this he is possessed of enough grace and elegance to play his part the doctor may well succeed in fulfilling the assertion of Oliver Wendell Holmes that if one of the functions of the physician is to assist at the coming in, another is to assist at the going out.

If what has been set down here should prove uncongenial to some strict moralists, one can only observe that there is a hierarchy of morality, and that ours is a profession which traditionally has been guided by a precept that transends the virtue of uttering truth for truth's sake; that is, "So far as possible, do no harm." Where it concerns the communication between the physician and his patient, the attainment of this goal demands an ear that is sensitive to both what is said and what is not said, a mind that is capable of understanding what has been heard, and a heart that can respond to what has been understood. Here, as in many difficult human enterprises, it may prove easier to learn the words than to sing the tune.

We did not dare to breathe a prayer
Or give our anguish scope!
Something was dead in each of us,
And what was dead was Hope!

Oscar Wilde,
The Ballad of Reading Gaol

NOTES

1. It should be observed, however, that while the emotional conflicts of the sick doctor may contribute to the ambiguity of his position, that ambiguity may be abetted by the treating physician, who in turn may experience difficulty in assigning to his ailing colleague the unequivocal status of patient. Indeed the latter may be more or less tacitly invited to share the responsibility in the diagnosis and care of his own illness to a degree that in some instances he is virtually a consultant on his own case.

A similar lack of a clear-cut definition of role is not uncommon when members of a doctor's family are ill. Here a further muddying of the waters may be caused by the time-honored practice of extending so-called courtesy—i.e., free care—to physicians and their families, a custom which, however well intentioned, may place its presumed beneficiaries in a moral straitjacket that discourages them from making rather ordinary demands on the treating physician, to say nothing of discharging him. It is not surprising that the care of physicians and their families occasionally evokes an atmosphere of bitterness and rancor.

2. The notion that at heart some doctors are killers is a common theme in literature. It is claimed that when in a fit of despondency Napoleon Bonaparte declared he should have been a physician, Talleyrand commented: *"Toujours assassin."*

3. This aspect of the patient-doctor relationship has not received the attention it deserves. Moreover, aside from being a therapeutic success, there are other ways in which his patients may support the doctor's psychological needs. His self-esteem, no less than his economic well-being, may be nourished by an ever-growing roster of devoted patients, particularly when the latter include celebrities and other persons of prominence. How important this can be may be judged by the not too uncommon indiscretions perpetrated by some physicians (and sometimes by their wives) in leaking confidential matters pertaining to their practice, notably the identity of their patients.

4. The same writer relaxes his position when it concerns psychiatric patients. Here he would sanction the withholding of knowledge "precisely because he may prevent the patient's recovery by revealing it." But in this, too, the writer is in error, in double error, it would seem, for, first, it is artificial and inexact to make a sharp distinction between psychiatric and nonpsychiatric patterns—the seriously sick and the dying are not infrequently conspicuously emotionally disturbed: and second, because it may at times be therapeutically advisable to acquaint the psychiatric patient with the facts of his illness.

5. Proponents of these views have seemingly overlooked the unconscious elements in human behavior and thought. Paradoxical though it may seem, the would-be suicide may wish to live: what he seeks to destroy may be restricted to that part of the self that has become burdensome or hateful. By the same token, despite his manifest combativeness, a psychotic individual is often inwardly grateful for the restraints imposed upon his dangerous aggression. There can be no logical objection to designating such persons as "prisoners," as Szasz would have it, provided we apply the same term to breathless individuals who are "incarcerated" in oxygen tents.

REFERENCES

Abrams, R.D. The patient with cancer—His changing pattern of communication. *New Eng. J. Med.* 274:317, 1966.

Aldrich, C.K. The dying patient's grief. *J.A.M.A.* 184:329, 1963.

Drillien, C.M., and Wilkinson, E.M. Mongolism: When should parents be told? *Brit. Med. J.* 2:1306, 1964.

Fletcher, J. *Morals and Medicine.* Princeton: Princeton University Press, 1954.

Stehlin, J.S., and Beach, K.A. Psychological aspects of cancer therapy. *J.A.M.A.* 197:100, 1966.

Vernick, J., and Karon, M. Who's afraid of death on a leukemia ward? *Amer. J. Dis. Child,* 109:393, 1965.

Weisman, A.D., and Hackett, T. Predilection to death: Death and dying as a psychiatric problem. *Psychosom. Med.* 23:232, 1961.

Winkelstein, C., and Blacher, R. Personal communication, 1967.

NO

Sissela Bok

LIES TO THE SICK AND DYING

DECEPTION AS THERAPY

A forty-six-year-old man, coming to a clinic for a routine physical check-up needed for insurance purposes, is diagnosed as having a form of cancer likely to cause him to die within six months. No known cure exists for it. Chemotherapy may prolong life by a few extra months, but will have side effects the physician does not think warranted in this case. In addition, he believes that such therapy should be reserved for patients with a chance for recovery or remission. The patient has no symptoms giving him any reason to believe that he is not perfectly healthy. He expects to take a short vacation in a week.

For the physician, there are now several choices involving truthfulness. Ought he to tell the patient what he has learned, or conceal it? If asked, should he deny it? If he decides to reveal the diagnosis, should he delay doing so until after the patient returns from his vacation? Finally, even if he does reveal the serious nature of the diagnosis, should he mention the possibility of chemotherapy and his reasons for not recommending it in this case? Or should he encourage every last effort to postpone death?

In this particular case, the physician chose to inform the patient of his diagnosis right away. He did not, however, mention the possibility of chemotherapy. A medical student working under him disagreed; several nurses also thought that the patient should have been informed of this possibility. They tried, unsuccessfully, to persuade the physician that this was the patient's right. When persuasion had failed, the student elected to disobey the doctor by informing the patient of the alternative of chemotherapy. After consultation with family members, the patient chose to ask for the treatment.

Doctors confront such choices often and urgently. What they reveal, hold back, or distort will matter profoundly to their patients. Doctors stress with corresponding vehemence their reasons for the distortion or concealment:

not to confuse the sick person needlessly, or cause what may well be unnecessary pain or discomfort, as in the case of the cancer patient; not to leave a patient without hope, as in those many cases where the dying are not told the truth about their condition; or to improve the chances of cure, as where unwarranted optimism is expressed about some form of therapy. Doctors use information as part of the therapeutic regimen; it is given out in amounts, in admixtures, and according to timing believed best for patients. Accuracy, by comparison, matters far less.

Lying to patients has, therefore, seemed an especially excusable act. Some would argue that doctors, and *only* doctors, should be granted the right to manipulate the truth in ways so undesirable for politicians, lawyers, and others. Doctors are trained to help patients; their relationship to patients carries special obligations, and they know much more than laymen about what helps and hinders recovery and survival.

Even the most conscientious doctors, then, who hold themselves at a distance from the quacks and the purveyors of false remedies, hesitate to forswear all lying. Lying is usually wrong, they argue, but less so than allowing the truth to harm patients. B. C. Meyer echoes this very common view:

> [O]urs is a profession which traditionally has been guided by a precept that transcends the virtue of uttering truth for truth's sake, and that is, "so far as possible, do no harm."

Truth, for Meyer, may be important, but not when it endangers the health and well-being of patients. This has seemed self-evident to many physicians in the past—so much so that we find very few mentions of veracity in the codes and oaths and writings by physicians through the centuries. This absence is all the more striking as other principles of ethics have been consistently and movingly expressed in the same documents. . . .

Given such freedom, a physician can decide to tell as much or as little as he wants the patient to know, so long as he breaks no law. In the case of the man mentioned at the beginning of this chapter, some physicians might feel justified in lying for the good of the patient, others might be truthful. Some may conceal alternatives to the treatment they recommend; others not. In each case, they could appeal to the A.M.A. Principles of Ethics. A great many would choose to be able to lie. They would claim that not only can a lie avoid harm for the patient, but that it is also hard to know whether they have been right in the first place in making their pessimistic diagnosis; a "truthful" statement could therefore turn out to hurt patients unnecessarily. The concern for curing and for supporting those who cannot be cured then runs counter to the desire to be completely open. This concern is especially strong where the prognosis is bleak; even more so when patients are so affected by their illness or their medication that they are more dependent than usual, perhaps more easily depressed or irrational.

Physicians know only too well how uncertain a diagnosis or prognosis can be. They know how hard it is to give meaningful and correct answers regarding health and illness. They also know that disclosing their own uncertainty or fears can reduce those benefits that depend upon faith in recovery. They fear, too, that revealing grave risks, no matter how unlikely it is that these will come about, may exercise the pull of the "self-fulfilling prophecy." They dislike being the bearers of uncertain or bad news as much as anyone else. And last, but not least, sitting down to discuss an illness truthfully and sensitively may take much-needed time away from other patients.

These reasons help explain why nurses and physicians and relatives of the sick and dying prefer not to be bound by rules that might limit their ability to suppress, delay, or distort information. This is not to say that they necessarily plan to lie much of the time. They merely want to have the freedom to do so when they believe it wise. And the reluctance to see lying prohibited explains, in turn, the failure of the codes and oaths to come to grips with the problems of truth-telling and lying.

But sharp conflicts are now arising. Doctors no longer work alone with patients. They have to consult with others much more than before; if they choose to lie, the choice may not be met with approval by all who take part in the care of the patient. A nurse expresses the difficulty which results as follows:

> From personal experience I would say that the patients who aren't told about their terminal illness have so many verbal and mental questions unanswered that many will begin to realize that their illness is more serious than they're being told. . . .

The doctor's choice to lie increasingly involves coworkers in acting a part they find neither humane nor wise. The fact that these problems have not been carefully thought through within the medical profession, nor seriously addressed in medical education, merely serves to intensify the conflicts. Different doctors then respond very differently to patients in exactly similar predicaments. The friction is increased by the fact that relatives often disagree even where those giving medical care to a patient are in accord on how to approach the patient. Here again, because physicians have not worked out to common satisfaction the question of whether relatives have the right to make such requests, the problems are allowed to be haphazardly resolved by each physician as he sees fit.

THE PATIENT'S PERSPECTIVE

The turmoil in the medical profession regarding truth-telling is further augmented by the pressures that patients themselves now bring to bear and by empirical data coming to light. Challenges are growing to the three major arguments for lying to patients: that truthfulness is impossible; that patients do not want bad news; and that truthful information harms them.

The first of these arguments . . . confuses "truth" and "truthfulness" so as to clear the way for occasional lying on grounds supported by the second and third arguments. At this point, we can see more clearly that it is a strategic move intended to discourage the question of truthfulness from carrying much weight in the first place, and thus to leave the choice of what to say and how to say it up to the physician. To claim that "since telling the truth is impossible, there can be no sharp distinction between what is true and what is false" is to try to defeat objections to lying before even discussing them. One need only imagine how such an argument would be received, were it made by a car salesman or a real estate dealer, to see how fallacious it is.

In medicine, however, the argument is supported by a subsidiary point: even if people might ordinarily understand what is spoken to them, patients are often not in a position to do so. This is where paternalism enters in. When we buy cars or houses, the paternalist will argue, we need to have all our wits about us; but when we are ill, we cannot always do so. We need help in making choices, even if help can be given only by keeping us in the dark. And the physician is trained and willing to provide such help.

It is certainly true that some patients cannot make the best choices for themselves when weakened by illness or drugs. But most still can. And even those who are incompetent have a right to have someone—their guardian or spouse perhaps—receive the correct information. The paternalistic assumption of superiority to patients also carries great dangers for physicians themselves—it risks turning to contempt. The following view was recently expressed in a letter to a medical journal:

> As a radiologist who has been sued, I have reflected earnestly on advice to obtain Informed Consent but have decided to "take the risks without informing the patient" and trust to "God, judge, and jury" rather than evade responsibility through a legal gimmick. . . .
>
> [I]n a general radiologic practice many of our patients are uninformable and we would never get through the day if we had to obtain their consent to every potentially harmful study. . . .

The argument which rejects informing patients because adequate truthful information is impossible in itself or because patients are lacking in understanding, must itself be rejected when looked at from the point of view of patients. They know that liberties granted to the most conscientious and altruistic doctors will be exercised also in the "Medicaid Mills"; that the choices thus kept from patients will be exercised by not only

competent but incompetent physicians; and that even the best doctors can make choices patients would want to make differently for themselves.

The second argument for deceiving patients refers specifically to giving them news of a frightening or depressing kind. It holds that patients do not, in fact, generally want such information, that they prefer not to have to face up to serious illness and death. On the basis of such a belief, most doctors in a number of surveys stated that they do not, as a rule, inform patients that they have an illness such as cancer.

When studies are made of what patients desire to know, on the other hand, a large majority say that they *would* like to be told of such a diagnosis. All these studies need updating and should be done with larger numbers of patients and non-patients. But they do show that there is generally a dramatic divergence between physicians and patients on the factual question of whether patients want to know what ails them in cases of serious illness such as cancer. In most of the studies, over 80 percent of the persons asked indicated that they would want to be told.

Sometimes this discrepancy is set aside by doctors who want to retain the view that patients do not want unhappy news. In reality, they claim, the fact that patients say they want it has to be discounted. The more someone asks to know, the more he suffers from fear which will lead to the denial of the information even if it is given. Informing patients is, therefore, useless; they resist and deny having been told what they cannot assimilate. According to this view, empirical studies of what patients say they want are worthless since they do not probe deeply enough to uncover this universal resistance to the contemplation of one's own death.

This view is only partially correct. For some patients, denial is indeed well established in medical experience. A number of patients (estimated at between 15 percent and 25 percent) will give evidence of denial of having been told about their illness, even when they repeatedly ask and are repeatedly informed. And nearly everyone experiences a period of denial at some point in the course of approaching death. Elisabeth Kübler-Ross sees denial as resulting often from premature and abrupt information by a stranger who goes through the process quickly to "get it over with." She holds that denial functions as a buffer after unexpected shocking news, permitting individuals to collect themselves and to mobilize other defenses. She describes prolonged denial in one patient as follows:

> She was convinced that the X-rays were "mixed up"; she asked for reassurance that her pathology report could not possibly be back so soon and that another patient's report must have been marked with her name. When none of this could be confirmed, she quickly asked to leave the hospital, looking for another physician in the vain hope "to get a better explanation for my troubles." This patient went "shopping around" for many doctors, some of whom gave her reassuring answers, other of whom confirmed the previous suspicion. Whether confirmed or not, she reacted in the same manner; she asked for examination and reexamination. . . .

But to say that denial is universal flies in the face of all evidence. And to take any claim to the contrary as "symptomatic" of deeper denial leaves no room for reasoned discourse. There is no way that such universal denial can be proved true or false. To believe in it is a metaphysical belief about man's condition, not a statement about what patients do and do not want. It is true that we can never completely understand the possibility of our own death, any more than being alive in the first place. But people certainly differ in the degree to which they can approach such knowledge, take it into account in their plans, and make their peace with it.

Montaigne claimed that in order to learn both to live and to die, men have to think about death and be prepared to accept it. To stick one's head in the sand, or to be prevented by lies from trying to discern what is to come, hampers freedom—freedom to consider one's life as a whole, with a beginning, a duration, an end. Some may request to be deceived rather than to see their lives as thus finite; others reject the information which would require them to do so; but most say that they want to know. Their concern for knowing about their condition goes far beyond mere curiosity or the wish to make isolated personal choices in the short time left to them; their stance toward the entire life they have lived, and their ability to give it meaning and completion, are at stake. In lying or withholding the facts which permit such discernment, doctors may reflect their own fears (which, according to one study, are much stronger than those of laymen) of facing questions about the meaning of one's life and the inevitability of death.

Beyond the fundamental deprivation that can result from deception, we are also becoming increasingly aware of all that can befall patients in the course of their illness when information is denied or distorted. Lies place them in a position where they no longer participate in choices concerning their own health, including the choice of whether to be a "patient" in the first place. A terminally ill person who is not informed that his illness is incurable and that he is near death cannot make decisions about the end of his life: about whether or not to enter a hospital, or to have surgery; where and with whom to spend his last days; how to put his affairs in order—these most personal choices cannot be made if he is kept in the dark, or given contradictory hints and clues.

It has always been especially easy to keep knowledge from terminally ill patients. They are most vulnerable, least able to take action to learn what they need to know, or to protect their autonomy. The very fact of being so ill greatly increases the likelihood of control by others. And the fear of being helpless in the face of such control is growing. At the same time, the period of dependency and slow deterioration of health and strength that people undergo has lengthened. There has been a dramatic shift toward institutionalization of the aged and those near death. (Over 80 percent of Americans now die in a hospital or other institution.)

Patients who are severely ill often suffer a further distancing and loss of control over their most basic functions. Electrical wiring, machines, intravenous administration of liquids, all create new dependency and at the same time new distance between the patient and all who come near. Curable patients are often willing to undergo such procedures; but when no cure is possible, these procedures merely intensify the sense of distance and uncertainty and can even become a substitute for comforting human acts. Yet those who suffer in this way often fear to seem troublesome by complaining. Lying to them, perhaps for the most charitable of purposes, can then

cause them to slip unwittingly into subjection to new procedures, perhaps new surgery, where death is held at bay through transfusions, respirators, even resuscitation far beyond what most would wish.

Seeing relatives in such predicaments has caused a great upsurge of worrying about death and dying. At the root of this fear is not a growing terror of the *moment* of death, or even the instants before it. Nor is there greater fear of *being* dead. In contrast to the centuries of lives lived in dread of the punishments to be inflicted after death, many would now accept the view expressed by Epicurus, who died in 270 B.C.:

> Death, therefore, the most awful of evils, is nothing to us, seeing that, when we are, death is not come, and, when death is come, we are not.

The growing fear, if it is not of the moment of dying nor of being dead, is of all that which now precedes dying for so many: the possibility of prolonged pain, the increasing weakness, the uncertainty, the loss of powers and chance of senility, the sense of being a burden. This fear is further nourished by the loss of trust in health professionals. In part, the loss of trust results from the abuses which have been exposed—the Medicaid scandals, the old-age home profiteering, the commercial exploitation of those who seek remedies for their ailments; in part also because of the deceptive practices patients suspect, having seen how friends and relatives were kept in the dark; in part, finally, because of the sheer numbers of persons, often strangers, participating in the care of any one patient. Trust which might have gone to a doctor long known to the patient goes less easily to a team of strangers, no matter how expert or well-meaning.

It is with the working out of all that *informed consent** implies and the information it presupposes that truth-telling is coming to be discussed in a serious way for the first time in the health professions. Informed consent is a farce if the information provided is distorted or withheld. And even complete information regarding surgical procedures or medication is obviously useless unless the patient also knows what the condition is that these are supposed to correct.

Bills of rights for patients, similarly stressing the right to be informed, are now gaining acceptance. This right is not new, but the effort to implement it is. Nevertheless, even where patients are handed the most elegantly phrased Bill of Rights, their right to a truthful diagnosis and prognosis is by no means always respected.

The reason why even doctors who recognize a patient's right to have information might still not provide it brings us to the third argument against telling all patients the truth. It holds that the information given might hurt the patient and that the concern for the right to such information is therefore a threat to proper health care. A patient, these doctors argue, may wish to commit suicide after being given discouraging news, or

*The law requires that inroads made upon a person's body take place only with the informed voluntary consent of that person. The term "informed consent" came into common use only after 1960, when it was used by the Kansas Supreme Court in Nathanson vs. Kline, 186 Kan. 393, 350, p. 2d, 1093 (1960). The patient is now entitled to full disclosure of risks, benefits, and alternative treatments to any proposed procedure, both in therapy and in medical experimentation, except in emergencies or when the patient is incompetent, in which case proxy consent is required.

suffer a cardiac arrest, or simply cease to struggle, and thus not grasp the small remaining chance for recovery. And even where the outlook for a patient is very good, the disclosure of a minute risk can shock some patients or cause them to reject needed protection such as a vaccination or antibiotics.

The factual basis for this argument has been challenged from two points of view. The damages associated with the disclosure of sad news or risks are rarer than physicians believe; and the *benefits* which result from being informed are more substantial, even measurably so. Pain is tolerated more easily, recovery from surgery is quicker, and cooperation with therapy is greatly improved. The attitude that "what you don't know won't hurt you" is proving unrealistic; it is what patients do not know but vaguely suspect that causes them corrosive worry.

It is certain that no answers to this question of harm from information are the same for all patients. If we look, first, at the fear expressed by physicians that informing patients of even remote or unlikely risks connected with a drug prescription or operation might shock some and make others refuse the treatment that would have been best for them, it appears to be unfounded for the great majority of patients. Studies show that very few patients respond to being told of such risks by withdrawing their consent to the procedure and that those who do withdraw are the very ones who might well have been upset enough to sue the physician had they not been asked to consent before hand. It is possible that on even rarer occasions especially susceptible persons might manifest physical deterioration from shock; some physicians have even asked whether patients who die after giving informed consent to an operation, but before it actually takes place, somehow expire because of the information given to them. While such questions are unanswerable in any one case, they certainly argue in favor of caution, a real concern for the person to whom one is recounting the risks he or she will face, and sensitivity to all signs of distress.

The situation is quite different when persons who are already ill, perhaps already quite weak and discouraged, are told of a very serious prognosis. Physicians fear that such knowledge may cause the patients to commit suicide, or to be frightened or depressed to the point that their illness takes a downward turn. The fear that great numbers of patients will commit suicide appears to be unfounded. And if some do, is that a response so unreasonable, so much against the patient's best interest that physicians ought to make it a reason for concealment or lies? Many societies have allowed suicide in the past; our own has decriminalized it; and some are coming to make distinctions among the many suicides which ought to be prevented if at all possible, and those which ought to be respected.

Another possible response to very bleak news is the triggering of physiological mechanisms which allow death to come more quickly—a form of giving up or of preparing for the inevitable, depending on one's outlook. Lewis Thomas, studying responses in humans and animals, holds it not unlikely that:

... there is a pivotal movement at some stage in the body's reaction to injury or disease, maybe in aging as well, when the organism concedes that it is finished and the time for dying is at hand, and at this moment the events that lead to death are launched, as a coordinated mechanism. Functions are then shut off, in sequence, irreversibly, and, while this is going on, a neural mechanism, held ready for this occasion, is switched on. . . .

Such a response may be appropriate, in which case it makes the moments of dying as peaceful as those who have died and been resuscitated so often testify. But it may also be brought on inappropriately, when the organism could have lived on, perhaps even induced malevolently, by external acts intended to kill. Thomas speculates that some of the deaths resulting from "hexing" are due to such responses. Levi-Strauss describes deaths from exorcism and the casting of spells in ways which suggest that the same process may then be brought on by the community.

It is not inconceivable that unhappy news abruptly conveyed, or a great shock given to someone unable to tolerate it, could also bring on such a "dying response," quite unintended by the speaker. There is every reason to be cautious and to try to know ahead of time how susceptible a patient might be to the accidental triggering—however rare—of such a response. One has to assume, however, that most of those who have survived long enough to be in a situationwhere their informed consent is asked have a very robust resistance to such accidental triggering of processes leading to death.

When, on the other hand, one considers those who are already near death, the "dying response" may be much less inappropriate, much less accidental, much less unreasonable. In most societies, long before the advent of modern medicine, human beings have made themselves ready for death once they felt its approach. Philippe Aries describes how many in the Middle Ages prepared themselves for death when they "felt the end approach." They awaited death lying down, surrounded by friends and relatives. They recollected all they had lived through and done, pardoning all who stood near their deathbed, calling on God to bless them, and finally praying. "After the final prayer all that remained was to wait for death, and there was no reason for death to tarry."

Modern medicine, in its valiant efforts to defeat disease and to save lives, may be dislocating the conscious as well as the purely organic responses allowing death to come when it is inevitable, thus denying those who are dying the benefits of the traditional approach to death. In lying to them, and in pressing medical efforts to cure them long past the point of possible recovery, physicians may thus rob individuals of an autonomy few would choose to give up.

Sometimes, then, the "dying response" is a natural organic reaction at the time when the body has no further defense. Sometimes it is inappropriately brought on by news too shocking or given in too abrupt a manner. We need to learn a great deal more about this last category, no matter how small. But there is no evidence that patients in general will be debilitated by truthful information about their condition.

Apart from the possible harm from information, we are coming to learn much more about the benefits it can bring patients. People follow instructions more carefully if they know what their disease is and why they are asked to take medication; any benefits from those procedures are therefore much more likely to come about.* Similarly, people recover faster from surgery and tolerate pain with less medication if they understand what ails them and what can be done for them.**

RESPECT AND TRUTHFULNESS

Taken all together, the three arguments defending lies to patients stand on much shakier ground as a counterweight to the right to be informed than is often thought. The common view that many patients cannot understand, do not want, and may be harmed by, knowledge of their condition, and that lying to them is either morally neutral or even to be recommended, must be set aside. Instead, we have to make a more complex-comparison. Over against the right of patients to knowledge concerning themselves, the medical and psychological benefits to them from this knowledge, the unnecessary and sometimes harmful treatment to which they can be subjected if ignorant, and the harm to physicians, their profession, and other patients from deceptive practices, we have to set a severely restricted and narrowed paternalistic view—that *some* patients cannot understand, *some* do not want, and *some* may be harmed by, knowledge of their

*Barbara S. Hulka, J. C. Cassel, et al. "Communication, Compliance, and Concordance between Physicians and Patients with Prescribed Medications," *American Journal of Public Health*, Sept. 1976, pp. 847–53. The study shows that of the nearly half of all patients who do not follow the prescriptions of the doctors (thus foregoing the intended effect of these prescriptions), many will follow them if adequately informed about the nature of their illness and what the proposed medication will do.

**See Lawrence D. Egbert, George E. Batitt, et al., "Reduction of Postoperative Pain by Encouragement and Instruction of Patients," *New England Journal of Medicine*, 270, pp. 825–27, 1964.

See also: Howard Waitzskin and John D. Stoeckle, "The Communication of Information about Illness," *Advances in Psychosomatic Medicine*, Vol. 8, 1972, pp. 185–215.

condition, and that they ought not to have to be treated like everyone else if this is not in their best interest.

Such a view is persuasive. A few patients openly request not to be given bad news. Others give clear signals to that effect, or are demonstrably vulnerable to the shock or anguish such news might call forth. Can one not in such cases infer implied consent to being deceived?

Concealment, evasion, withholding of information may at times be necessary. But if someone contemplates lying to a patient or concealing the truth, the burden of proof must shift. It must rest, here, as with all deception, on those who advocate it in any one instance. They must show why they fear a patient may be harmed or how they know that another cannot cope with the truthful knowledge. A decision to deceive must be seen as a very unusual step, to be talked over with colleagues and others who participate in the care of the patient. Reasons must be set forth and debated, alternatives weighed carefully. At all times, the correct information must go to *someone* closely related to the patient.

POSTSCRIPT

Is It Ethical to Withhold the Truth From Dying Patients?

In its 1983 report, *Making Health Care Decisions*, the President's Commission for the Study of Ethical Problems in Medicine and Biomedical and Behavioral Research cited evidence from a survey it conducted indicating that 94 percent of the public would "want to know everything" about a diagnosis and prognosis, and 96 percent would want to know specifically about a diagnosis of cancer. To the question, "If you had a type of cancer that usually leads to death in less than a year, would you want your doctor to give you a realistic estimate of how long you had to live, or would you prefer that he not tell you?" Eighty-five percent said that they would want the realistic estimate. However, when physicians were asked a similar question about what they would disclose to a patient, only 13 percent would give a "straight, statistical prognosis," and a third said that they would not give a definite time period but would stress that it wouldn't be a long one. Physicians, it appears, are more reluctant to tell the truth than the public (at least when faced with a hypothetical choice) is to hear it. Dennis H. Novack et al., "Physicians' Attitudes Toward Using Deception to Resolve Difficult Ethical Problems," *Journal of the American Medical Association* (May 26, 1989), reports on a survey recently conducted by a group from the Brown University Program in Medicine. Researchers found that 87 percent of 109 physicians "indicated that deception is acceptable on rare occasions."

For a strong defense of the patient's right to know the truth, see Robert M. Veatch, *Death, Dying, and the Biological Revolution* (Yale, 1976), chapter 6. A philosophical argument with a different view is Donald Van DeVeer's article, "The Contractual Argument for Withholding Information," *Philosophy and*

Public Affairs (Winter 1980). See also Mark Sheldon, "Truth Telling in Medicine," *Journal of the American Medical Association* (February 5, 1982), and Thurstan B. Brewin, "Truth, Trust, and Paternalism," *The Lancet* (August 31, 1985).

Two books that stress the importance of communication in the doctor-patient relationship are Jay Katz, *The Silent World of Doctor and Patient* (The Free Press, 1984) and Eric J. Cassell, *Talking with Patients*, 2 vols. (MIT Press, 1985). Susan J. Barnes edited a symposium called "Perspectives on J. Katz, *The Silent World of Doctor and Patient*," which appeared in the *Western New England Law Review* (vol. 9, no. 1, 1987). See also Sissela Bok, *Lying: Moral Choice in Public and Private Life* (Vintage Books, 1978).

ISSUE 6

Is Physician-Assisted Suicide Ethical?

YES: Sidney H. Wanzer et al., from "The Physician's Responsibility Toward Hopelessly Ill Patients: A Second Look," *The New England Journal of Medicine* (March 30, 1989)

NO: David Orentlicher, from "Physician Participation in Assisted Suicide," *Journal of the American Medical Association* (October 6, 1989)

ISSUE SUMMARY

YES: Physician Sidney H. Wanzer and a group of nine other physicians believe that it is not immmoral for a physician to assist in the rational suicide of a terminally ill person.

NO: Physician and lawyer David Orentlicher argues that treatment designed to bring on death, by definition, does not heal and is therefore fundamentally inconsistent with the physician's role.

Since the early 1980s physicians, lawyers, philosophers, and judges have examined questions about withholding life-sustaining treatment. Their deliberations have resulted in a broad consensus that competent adults have the right to make decisions about their medical care, even if those decisions seem unjustifiable to others and even if they result in death. Furthermore, the right of individuals to name others to carry out their prior wishes or to make decisions if they should become incompetent is now well established. Thirty-eight states now have legislation allowing advance directives (commonly known as "living wills").

The debate in specific cases continues (see, for example, the issue on withholding food and nutrition), but on the whole, patients' rights to self-determination have been bolstered by 80 or more legal cases, dozens of reports, and statements made by medical society and other organizations.

As often occurs in bioethical debate, the resolution of one issue only highlights the lack of resolution about another. There is clearly no consensus about either euthanasia or physician-assisted suicide.

Like truth telling, euthanasia is an old problem given new dimensions by the ability of modern medical technology to prolong life. The word itself is Greek (literally, *happy death*) and the Greeks wrestled with the question of whether, in some cases, people would be better off dead. But the Hippocratic Oath in this instance was clear: "I will neither give a deadly drug to anybody if asked for it, nor will I make a suggestion to that effect." On the other hand, if the goal of medicine is not simply to prolong life but to reduce suffering, at some point the question of what measures should be taken or withdrawn will inevitably arise. The problem is: When death is inevitable, how far should one go in hastening it?

The majority of cases in which euthanasia is raised as a possibility are among the most difficult ethical issues to resolve, for they involve the conflict between a physician's duty to preserve life and the burden on the patient and the family that is created by fulfilling that duty. One common distinction is between *active* euthanasia (that is, some positive act such as administering a lethal injection) and *passive* euthanasia (that is, an inaction such as deciding not to administer antibiotics when the patient has a severe infection). Another common distinction is between *voluntary* euthanasia (that is, the patient wishes to die and consents to the action that will make it happen) and *involuntary*—or better, *nonvoluntary*—euthanasia (that is, the patient is unable to consent, perhaps because he or she is in a coma).

The two selections that follow take up one aspect of this large issue: the question of whether physicians may ethically assist in a hopelessly ill patient's suicide. A group of physicians headed by Sidney H. Wanzer concludes that it is not immoral for a physician to assist in the rational suicide of a terminally ill person, even though that act deviates from the physician's traditional role of care-giver. David Orentlicher asserts that deeply rooted medical traditions and the guiding principles of medical practice prohibit physicians from assisting in suicide.

YES

Sidney H. Wanzer et al.

THE PHYSICIAN'S RESPONSIBILITY TOWARD HOPELESSLY ILL PATIENTS

TREATING THE DYING PATIENT—THE IMPORTANCE OF FLEXIBLE CARE

The care of the dying is an art that should have its fullest expression in helping patients cope with the technologically complicated medical environment that often surrounds them at the end of life. The concept of a good death does not mean simply the withholding of technological treatments that serve only to prolong the act of dying. It also requires the art of deliberately creating a medical environment that allows a peaceful death. Somewhere between the unacceptable extremes of failure to treat the dying patient and intolerable use of aggressive life-sustaining measures, the physician must seek a level of care that optimizes comfort and dignity.

In evaluating the burdens and benefits of treatment for the dying patient—whether in the hospital, in a nursing home, or at home—the physician needs to formulate a flexible and adjustable care plan, tailoring treatment to the patient's changing needs as the disease progresses. Such plans contrast sharply with the practice, frequent in medicine, in which the physician makes rounds and prescribes, leaving orders for nurses and technicians, but not giving continual feedback and adjustment. The physician's actions on behalf of the patient should be appropriate, with respect to both the types of treatments and the location in which they are given. Such actions need to be adjusted continually to the individual patient's needs, with the physician keeping primarily in mind that the benefits of treatment must outweigh the burdens imposed.

When the patient lacks decision-making capacity, discussing the limitation of treatment with the family becomes a major part of the treatment plan. The principle of continually adjusted care should guide all these decisions.

Pain and Suffering

The principle of continually adjusted care is nowhere more important than in the control of pain, fear, and suffering. The hopelessly ill patient must have whatever is necessary to control pain. One of the most persuasive causes of anxiety among patients, their families, and the public is the perception that physicians' efforts toward the relief of pain are sadly deficient. Because of this perceived professional deficiency, people fear that needless suffering will be allowed to occur as patients are dying.[1] To a large extent, we believe such fears are justified.

In the patient whose dying process is irreversible, the balance between minimizing pain and suffering and potentially hastening death should be struck clearly in favor of pain relief. Narcotics or other pain medications should be given in whatever dose and by whatever route is necessary for relief. It is morally correct to increase the dose of narcotics to whatever dose is needed, even though the medication may contribute to the depression of respiration or blood pressure, the dulling of consciousness, or even death, provided the primary goal of the physician is to relieve suffering. The proper dose of pain medication is the dose that is sufficient to relieve pain and suffering, even to the point of unconsciousness. . . . To allow a patient to experience unbearable pain or suffering is unethical medical practice.

Legal Concerns

The principles of medical ethics are formulated independently of legal decisions, but physicians may fear that decisions about the care of the hopelessly ill will bring special risks of criminal charges and prosecution. Although no medical decision can be immune from legal scrutiny, courts in the United States have generally supported the approaches advocated here.[2-5] The physician should follow these principles without exaggerated concern for legal consequences, doing whatever is necessary to relieve pain and bring comfort, and adhering to the patient's wishes as much as possible. To withhold any necessary measure of pain relief in a hopelessly ill person out of fear of depressing respiration or of possible legal repercussions is unjustifiable. Good medical practice is the best protection against legal liability.

Preparing for Death

As sickness progresses toward death, measures to minimize suffering should be intensified. Dying patients may require palliative care of an intensity that rivals even that of curative efforts. Keeping the patient clean, caring for the skin, preventing the formation of bed sores, treating neuropsychiatric symptoms, controlling peripheral and pulmonary edema, aggressively reducing nausea and vomiting, using intravenous medications, fighting the psychosocial forces that can lead to family fragmentation—all can tax the ingenuity and equanimity of the most skilled health professionals. Even though aggressive curative techniques are no longer indicated, professionals and families are still called on to use intensive measures—extreme responsibility, extraordinary sensitivity, and heroic compassion.

In training programs for physicians, more attention needs to be paid to these aspects of care. Progress has been made in persuading house staff and attending physicians to discuss do-not-resuscitate (DNR) orders and to include clear orders and notes in the chart about limits on life-sustaining therapies, but patients are too rarely cared for directly by the physician at or near the time of death. Usually it is nurses who care for patients at this time. In a few innovative training programs, most notably at the University of Oregon, the hands-on aspects of care of the dying are addressed,[6] and such techniques should be presented at all training institutions.

ASSISTED SUICIDE

If care is administered properly at the end of life, only the rare patient should be so distressed that he or she desires to commit suicide. Occasionally, however, all fails. The doctor, the nurse, the family, and the patient may have done everything possible to relieve the distress occasioned by a terminal illness, and yet the patient perceives his or her situation as intolerable and seeks assistance in bringing about death. Is it ever justifiable for the physician to assist suicide in such a case?

Some physicians, believing it to be the last act in a continuum of care provided for the hopelessly ill patient, do assist patients who request it, either by prescribing sleeping pills with knowledge of their intended use or by discussing the required doses and methods of administration with the patient. The frequency with which such actions are undertaken is unknown, but they are certainly not rare. Suicide differs from euthanasia in that the act of bringing on death is performed by the patient, not the physician.

The physician who considers helping a patient who requests assistance with suicide must determine first that the patient is indeed beyond all help and not merely suffering from a treatable depression of the sort common in people with terminal illnesses. Such a depression requires therapeutic intervention. If there is no treatable component to the depression and the patient's pain or suffering is refractory to treatment, then the wish for suicide may be rational. If such a patient acts on the wish for death and actually commits suicide, it is ethical for a physician who knows the patient well to refrain from an attempt at resuscitation.

Even though suicide itself is not illegal, helping a person commit suicide is a crime in many states, either by statute or under common law. Even so, we know of no physician who has ever been prosecuted in the United States for prescribing pills in order to help a patient commit suicide.[7] However, the potential illegality of this act is a deterrent, and apart from that, some physicians simply cannot bring themselves to assist in suicide or to condone such action.

Whether it is bad medical practice or immoral to help a hopelessly ill patient commit a rational suicide is a complex issue, provoking a number of considerations. First, as their disease advances, patients may lose their decision-making capacity because of the effects of the disease or the drug treatment. Assisting such patients with suicide comes close to performing an act of euthanasia. Second, patients who want a doctor's assistance with suicide may be unwilling to endure their terminal illness because they lack information about what is ahead. Even when the physician explains in careful detail the availability of the kind of flexible, continually adjusted care described here, the patient may still opt out of that treatment plan and reject the physician's efforts to ease the dying process. Also, what are the physician's obligations if a patient who retains decision-making capacity insists that family members not be told of a suicide plan? Should the physician insist on obtaining the family's consent? Finally, should physicians acknowledge their role in a suicide in some way—by obtaining consultation, or in writing? Physicians who act in secret become isolated and cannot consult colleagues or ethics committees for confirmation that the patient has made a rational decision. If contacted, such colleagues may well object and even consider themselves obligated to report the physician to the Board of Medical Licensure or to the prosecutor. The impulse to maintain secrecy gives the lie to the moral intuition that assistance with suicide is ethical.

It is difficult to answer such questions, but all but two of us (J.v.E. and E.H.C.) believe that it is not immoral for a physician to assist in the rational suicide of a terminally ill person. However, we recognize that such an act represents a departure from the principle of continually adjusted care that we have presented. As such, it should be considered a separate alternative and not an extension of the flexible approach to care that we have recommended. Clearly, the subject of assisted suicide deserves wide and open discussion.

REFERENCES

1. Angell M. The quality of mercy. N Engl J Med 1982; 306:98–9.
2. Bartling v. Superior Court (Glendale Adventist Medical Center), 163 Cal. App. 3d 186, 209 Cal. Rptr. 220 (Ct. App. 1984).
3. Bouvia v. Superior Court (Glenchur), 179 Cal. App. 3d 1127, 225 Cal. Rptr. 297 (Ct. App. 1986), review denied (Cal. June 5, 1986).
4. Brophy v. New England Sinai Hosp., Inc., 398 Mass. 417, 497, N.E. 2d 626 (1986).
5. In re Culham, No. 87-340537-AC (Mich. Cir. Ct., Oakland County, Dec. 15, 1987) (Breck J.)
6. Tolle SW, Hickham DH, Larson EB, Benson JA. Patient death and housestaff stress. Clin Res 1987; 35:762A. abstract.
7. Glantz LH. Withholding and withdrawing treatment: the role of the criminal law. Law Med Health Care 1987–88; 15:231–41.

NO

David Orentlicher

PHYSICIAN PARTICIPATION IN ASSISTED SUICIDE

Should a physician be able to assist the suicide of a hopelessly ill patient? A panel of distinguished physicians, brought together by the Society for the Right to Die and writing in the *New England Journal of Medicine*, says yes.[1] Deeply rooted medical traditions and the guiding principles of medical practice, however, say no.

According to 10 of the panel's 12 members, if a hopelessly ill patient believes his or her condition is intolerable, then it should be permissible for a physician to provide the patient with the medical means and the medical knowledge to commit suicide.[1] For example, the physician could prescribe sleeping pills for the patient and indicate how many pills there are in a lethal dose.[1]

Assisted suicide, then, differs from euthanasia in the extent to which the physician participates in the process. In assisted suicide, the patient performs the life-ending act under the physician's guidance, while in euthanasia, the physician administers the death-causing drug or other agent.

The panel's endorsement of assisted suicide appears to reflect an increasing willingness by society to condone assisted suicide or even euthanasia. In the Netherlands, for example, euthanasia under limited circumstances is practiced openly and commonly, with the support of the Dutch Medical Association, a government commission, and court decisions.[2] Euthanasia is permitted in the Netherlands when four conditions are satisfied: there is intolerable suffering with no prospect of improvement; the patient is mentally competent to choose euthanasia; the patient requests euthanasia voluntarily, repeatedly, and consistently over a reasonable period of time; and two physicians, one of whom has not participated in the patient's care, agree that euthanasia is appropriate.[1,2] According to estimates, 5000 to 10000 of the Dutch die by euthanasia each year.[1]

In the United States, anecdotal evidence suggests that assisted suicide is infrequently but increasingly being performed, particularly by patients with acquired immunodeficiency syndrome (*New York Times.* May 24, 1989:A1). In

From David Orentlicher, "Physician Participation in Assisted Suicide," *Journal of the American Medical Association*, vol. 262, no. 13 (October 6, 1989), pp. 1844-1845. Copyright © 1989 by the American Medical Association. Reprinted by permission.

addition, public opinion polls indicate that the majority of Americans believe that assisted suicide should be permitted (*New York Times*. May 24, 1989:A1).[2]

Society's increasing support for assisted suicide is demonstrated by trends in law enforcement. Even though assisted suicide is prohibited by law (*New York Times*. May 24, 1989:A1), there apparently have been no cases in which a physician was prosecuted for providing a patient with the medical means to take his or her own life.[1,3]

Advocates of assisted suicide suggest that it is a natural extension of the principle that hopelessly ill patients may refuse life-prolonging medical care. However, assisted suicide is not easily justified by the concerns underlying that principle.

Society has increasingly recognized the right of hopelessly ill patients to decline life-sustaining treatments because these treatments often serve only to prolong suffering and because the right of personal autonomy entitles each person to decide for him or herself whether to accept medical care.[4] Theoretically, these justifications could also support a hopelessly ill patient's right to commit suicide. Suicide would put an end to suffering that could be considered needless, and it would be a fulfillment of the patient's desires.[2] However, it is quite another question whether the physician should provide the medical means to carry out the suicide.

Ordinarily, a physician provides medical care for two reasons: to sustain life and to relieve suffering.[5] Occasionally, in the process of trying to sustain life or relieve suffering, a treatment may cause the patient to die. For example, a small percentage of patients will not survive coronary bypass surgery. Or, the dose of morphine necessary to ease pain in a terminally ill patient may impair the patient's ability to breathe. Performance of the surgery or administration of the morphine is nevertheless permissible because the primary purpose of the treatment is a valid one.[6] In assisted suicide, on the other hand, the primary purpose of the treatment is to cause death. And, as recognized by the American Medical Association's Council on Ethical and Judicial Affairs, in its opinion on euthanasia, that purpose has no role in the professional responsibilities of the physician.[6] Indeed, from the time of Hippocrates, the principles of medical ethics have instructed physicians to refuse their patients' requests for death-causing treatments.

This long-standing rejection of assisted suicide reflects a number of concerns with assisted suicide. A patient contemplating assisted suicide will naturally want to discuss that possibility with his or her physician. If the physician appears sympathetic to the patient's interest in suicide, it may convey the impression that the physician feels assisted suicide is a desirable alternative. Such an impression may not be very comforting to the patient.[7] Moreover, if the patient decides to reject suicide, will the patient have the same degree of confidence in the physician's commitment to his or her care as previously? In short, assisted suicide might seriously undermine an essential element of the patient-physician relationship, the patient's trust that the physician is wholeheartedly devoted to caring for the patient's health.

More troubling, as Prof Yale Kamisar has observed, is the possibility that the hopelessly ill patient will not feel entirely free to resist a suggestion from the physician that suicide would be appropriate, particularly since it comes from the person whose medical judgment the patient relies on. Patients who are enfeebled by disease and devoid of hope may choose assisted suicide not because they are really tired of life but because they think others are tired of them.[7] Some patients, moreover, may feel an obligation to choose death to spare their families the emotional and financial burden of their care. Other patients may succumb to the repeated signals from society that it would prefer to spend its limited resources on other compelling needs.

Finally, assisted suicide is problematic in terms of its implementation. For many patients, the progression of disease will result in the impairment of decision-making capacity, either from the effects of the disease itself or those of drug treatment.[1] Consequently, it may be difficult to ensure that a competent decision is being made. Even with competent patients, physicians may have trouble deciding whether a reliable decision has been made. At what point in the contemplation of suicide by the patient, for example, can the physician be confident that the patient has made a firm decision to end his or her life? What if the patient has changed his or her mind previously? Finally, the patient's apparently rational decision to commit suicide may reflect a mental depression that should be treated.

Not surprisingly, many of the arguments against assisted suicide could also be used to oppose the withdrawal of artificial life supports; the two have much in common. Nevertheless, for most people there is a clearly and viscerally felt distinction between acting to hasten death and refraining from delaying death.

An important explanation for the distinction lies in the fact that withdrawal of treatment permits death to take its natural course while assisted suicide short-circuits the dying process.

The distinction may also be articulated in terms of the relationship between the sick and those who try to help them. As Dr Leon Kass has written, physicians serve the needs of patients not because patients exercise self-determination but because patients are sick.[8] Thus, for example, a patient may not insist on a treatment that the physician feels is inconsistent with sound medical practices. What the sick need and are entitled to seek from the efforts of physicians is health. Accordingly, physicians provide medical treatments to the sick to make them well, or as well as they can become. Treatment designed to bring on death, by definition, does not heal and is therefore fundamentally inconsistent with the physician's role in the patient-physician relationship.

The withdrawal of life support, on the other hand, does not violate the nature of the patient-physician relationship. While the physician has a duty to care for those who want to be healed, there should not be an obligation, or even an option, to impose treatment on those for whom it is unwelcome.

The distinction between acting to hasten death and refraining from delaying death also reflects an element of pragmatism. If patients were not entitled to refuse life-prolonging treatment, it would be difficult to define their corollary obligation to obtain medical care. Would a patient dying of cancer have to accept a regimen of chemotherapy that might prolong life for several months but would be painful, nauseating, and debilitating? Would patients have to remain hospitalized during the final stages of their illnesses if to return home to die would shorten their lives by days or weeks? If these obligations would not be appropriate, then there must be a right to decline at least some life-sustaining treatments. And, if that right exists, who, other than the patient, is in a position to assess whether the ability of a particular treatment to prolong life is outweighed by the burdens of the treatment?

Suicide by the hopelessly ill may someday be sanctioned. However, much more thought needs to be given before involving physicians in the process and compromising their essential role as healers.

REFERENCES

1. Wanzer SH, Federman DD, Edelstein SJ, et al. The physician's responsibility toward hopelessly ill patients: a second look. *N Engl J Med.* 1989; 320:844–849.

2. Angell M. Euthanasia. *N Engl J Med.* 1988; 319:1348–1350.

3. Meyers DW. *Medico-legal Implications of Death and Dying,* §7.12. Rochester, NY: Lawyers Co-Operative Publishing Co; 1981.

4. President's Commission for the Study of Ethical Problems in Medicine and Biomedical and Behavioral Research. *Deciding to Forego Life-Sustaining Treatment.* Washington, DC: Government Printing Office; 1983.

5. *Current Opinions of the Council on Ethical and Judicial Affairs of the American Medical Association—1989: Withholding or Withdrawing Life-Prolonging Treatment.* Chicago, Ill: American Medical Association; 1989.

6. *Report of the Council on Ethical and Judicial Affairs of the American Medical Association: Euthanasia.* Chicago, Ill: American Medical Association; 1989.

7. Kamisar Y. Some non-religious views against proposed 'mercy-killing' legislation. *Minn Law Rev.* 1958; 42:969–1042.

8. Kass LR. Neither for love nor money: why doctors must not kill. *Public Interest.* 1989; 94:25–46.

POSTSCRIPT

Is Physician-Assisted Suicide Ethical?

In June 1990 Janet Adkins, a 54-year-old Oregon woman who had been diagnosed with Alzheimer's disease, killed herself in a van in a Michigan suburb. The manner in which she died created a national furor, because it depended on a suicide device built by Dr. Jack Kevorkian, a physician. Dr. Kevorkian inserted an intravenous device in her arm and dripped salt water through it. Then Mrs. Adkins herself pressed a button that stopped the salt water and replaced it with the drug used to induce unconsciousness in executions. The machine then injected potassium chloride, which killed her. Many states (but not Michigan) have laws specifically prohibiting assisting in suicide.

A similar furor was touched off by publication in the *Journal of the American Medical Association* (January 8, 1988) of an anonymous short account of a gynecology resident's decision to inject morphine into Debbie, a 20-year-old patient dying of ovarian cancer whose only words were: "Let's get this over with."

Both these cases illustrate the continuing highly charged debate over the proper role of physicians in dealing with patients who explicitly or implicitly want to end their lives. For the reaction to "It's Over, Debbie," including critiques of the journal's decision to publish an anonymous and unverified story, see the series of articles in the *Journal of the American Medical Association* (April 8, 1988). The American Medical Association's official position, reaffirmed in 1982, is that a physician "should not intentionally cause death."

In Great Britain the Working Party on the Ethics of Prolonging Life and Assisting Death of the Institute of Medical Ethics supports a doctor's decision to assist "if the need to relieve intense and unceasing pain or distress caused by an incurable illness greatly outweighs the benefit to the patient of further prolonging his life" (*The Lancet*, September 8, 1990).

Suicide and Euthanasia: Historical and Contemporary Themes, edited by Baruch A. Brody (Kluwer, 1989) includes essays on a range of views. Another collection is Robert N. Wennberg, *Terminal Choices: Euthanasia, Suicide, and the Right to Die* (Eermans, 1989).

In "Neither for Love nor Money: Why Doctors Must Not Kill," *Public Interest* (Winter 1989), Leon R. Kass argues forcefully that physician ethics do not permit assisting patients to die. The opposite view is expressed by Philip J. Miller in "Death with Dignity and the Right to Die: Sometimes Doctors Have a Duty to Hasten Death," *Journal of Medical Ethics* (June 1987). A *Hastings Center Report* Special Supplement (January/February 1989) entitled "Mercy, Murder, and Morality: Perspectives on Euthanasia" contains, among other articles, a harsh critique of practice in the Netherlands. In response (*Hastings Center Report*, November/December 1989), the General Assembly of the Dutch Society of Health Law, the Board of the Dutch Society for Voluntary Euthanasia, and others defend the procedures.

ISSUE 7

Is It Ever Morally Right to Withhold Food and Water from Dying Patients?

YES: Joanne Lynn and James F. Childress, from "Must Patients Always Be Given Food and Water?" *Hastings Center Report* (October 1983)

NO: Gilbert Meilaender, from "On Removing Food and Water: Against the Stream," *Hastings Center Report* (December 1984)

ISSUE SUMMARY

YES: Physician Joanne Lynn and professor of religious studies James F. Childress claim that nutrition and hydration are not morally different from other life-sustaining medical treatments that may be withheld or withdrawn, according to the patient's best interest.

NO: Professor of religion Gilbert Meilaender asserts that removing the ordinary human care of feeding aims to kill and is morally wrong.

The landmark *Quinlan* decision in 1976 affirmed the right of a patient to refuse life-sustaining treatment and the right of a parent or guardian to make that same decision for an incompetent patient. But Karen Ann Quinlan's parents wanted only to remove her from a respirator; they did not even consider the removal of a nasogastric tube through which she was artificially fed for the next ten years until her death.

The question of whether food and water must always be provided reached the public arena in a series of legal cases that began in 1981. In that year Robert Nejdl and Neil Barber, two Los Angeles physicians, were charged with murder for taking Clarence Herbert, their patient who had suffered severe brain damage after an operation, off a respirator and then, when he continued to breathe, removing all artificial nutrition. The charges were dropped, and the court ruled in 1983 that artificial feeding was like any other medical treatment and could be withheld with consent of the patient or family.

Also in 1981 in Danville, Illinois, the parents and physician of newborn conjoined twins (often called Siamese twins) decided not to feed the infants. The courts disagreed and feeding and other treatments were given. But in 1982, in Bloomington, Indiana, another newborn—with Down's syndrome, a genetic disease that results in mild to severe mental retardation—was not given surgery to correct a defect of his esophagus and was not fed. The baby's death led to a series of governmental regulations.

In a series of other cases, the courts have grappled with the same problem but have come up with different answers. In New Jersey, in the 1983 case of Claire Conroy, the court ruled, after her death, that food and nutrition could be withheld from a nursing home patient as long as a series of complicated procedures were followed to prevent abuse. In Massachusetts, in the 1986 case of Paul Brophy, a firefighter in a persistent vegetative state, the court ruled that feeding could not be withdrawn, despite the unanimous wishes of the family and the judgment of several physicians that he would never recover. A New Jersey court also held, in the case of Nancy Jobes, a 31-year-old woman in a persistent vegetative state, that feeding tubes could not be removed in the nursing home if the staff disagreed, but could be removed at home.

The most groundbreaking decision since *Quinlan* is the case of Nancy Cruzan, a 33-year-old Missouri woman who has been in a persistent vegetative state since an automobile accident in 1983. State courts refused to honor her parents' request to remove artificial nutrition and hydration, so they appealed to the Supreme Court. In June 1990 the Court ruled that it was not unconstitutional for Missouri to require very high standards of evidence that Nancy herself would have refused this treatment. Since those standards had not been met, the parents' request could be denied. In this case the Supreme Court sent a clear message that individuals' prior decisions to refuse treatment could be honored, but these decisions had to be "clear and convincing."

The ethical question centers on whether artificial nutrition and hydration is ordinary care, which must be provided for every patient, or a medical treatment like antibiotics or a respirator, which can be withheld if it is not in the patient's best interests. The symbolic value of feeding a dying patient must be weighed against the likely benefit to the patient.

In the following selections, Joanne Lynn and James F. Childress provide three circumstances when, in their view, it would be ethical to withhold fluids and nutrition: when the procedures would be futile in achieving improved nutritional and fluid levels; when the improvement, though achievable, would not benefit the patient; and when the burden of receiving the treatment outweights the benefits. Gilbert Meilaender sees a willingness to provide food and drink "even when the struggle against death has been lost" as "the last evidence we can offer that . . . we are willing to love to the very point of death."

YES

Joanne Lynn and
James F. Childress

MUST PATIENTS ALWAYS BE GIVEN FOOD AND WATER?

Many people die from the lack of food or water. For some, this lack is the result of poverty or famine, but for others it is the result of disease or deliberate decision. In the past, malnutrition and dehydration must have accompanied nearly every death that followed an illness of more than a few days. Most dying patients do not eat much on their own, and nothing could be done for them until the first flexible tubing for instilling food or other liquid into the stomach was developed about a hundred years ago. Even then, the procedure was so scarce, so costly in physician and nursing time, and so poorly tolerated that it was used only for patients who clearly could benefit. With the advent of more reliable and efficient procedures in the past few decades, these conditions can be corrected or ameliorated in nearly every patient who would otherwise be malnourished or dehydrated. In fact, intravenous lines and nasogastric tubes have become common images of hospital care.

Providing adequate nutrition and fluids is a high priority for most patients, both because they suffer directly from inadequacies and because these deficiencies hinder their ability to overcome other diseases. But are there some patients who need not receive these treatments? . . .

The answer in any real case should acknowledge the psychological contiguity between feeding and loving and between nutritional satisfaction and emotional satisfaction. Yet this acknowledgement does not resolve the core question. . . .

[W]e will concentrate upon the care of patients who are incompetent to make choices for themselves. Patients who are competent to determine the course of their therapy may refuse any and all interventions proposed by others, as long as their refusals do not seriously harm or impose unfair burdens upon others.[1] A competent patient's decision regarding whether or not to accept the provision of food and water by medical means such as tube feeding or intravenous alimentation is unlikely to raise questions of harm or burden to others.

What then should guide those who must decide about nutrition for a patient who cannot decide? As a start, consider the standard by which other medical decisions are made: one should decide as the incompetent person would have if he or she were competent, when that is possible to determine, and advance that person's interests in a more generalized sense when individual preferences cannot be known.

THE MEDICAL PROCEDURES

There is no reason to apply a different standard to feeding and hydration. Surely, when one inserts a feeding tube, or creates a gastrostomy opening, or inserts a needle into a vein, one intends to benefit the patient. Ideally, one should provide what the patient believes to be of benefit, but at least the effect should be beneficial in the opinions of surrogates and caregivers.

Thus, the question becomes: is it ever in the patient's interest to become malnourished and dehydrated, rather than to receive treatment? Posing the question so starkly points to our need to know what is entailed in treating these conditions and what benefits the treatments offer.

The medical interventions that provide food and fluids are of two basic types. First, liquids can be delivered by a tube that is inserted into a functioning gastrointestinal tract, most commonly through the nose and esophagus into the stomach or through a surgical incision in the abdominal wall and directly into the stomach. The liquids used can be specially prepared solutions of nutrients or a blenderized version of an ordinary diet. The nasogastric tube is cheap; it may

lead to pneumonia and often annoys the patient and family, sometimes even requiring that the patient be restrained to prevent its removal.

Creating a gastrostomy is usually a simple surgical procedure, and, once the wound is healed, care is very simple. Since it is out of sight, it is aesthetically more acceptable and restraints are needed less often. Also, the gastrostomy creates no additional risk of pneumonia. However, while elimination of a nasogastric tube requires only removing the tube, a gastrostomy is fairly permanent, and can be closed only by surgery.

The second type of medical intervention is intravenous feeding and hydration, which also has two major forms. The ordinary hospital or peripheral IV, in which fluid is delivered directly to the bloodstream through a small needle, is useful only for temporary efforts to improve hydration and electrolyte concentrations. One cannot provide a balanced diet through the veins in the limbs: to do that requires a central line, or a special catheter placed into one of the major veins in the chest. The latter procedure is much more risky and vulnerable to infections and technical errors, and it is much more costly than any of the other procedures. Both forms of intravenous nutrition and hydration commonly require restraining the patient, cause minor infections and other ill effects, and are costly, especially since they ordinarily require the patient to be in a hospital.

None of these procedures, then, is ideal; each entails some distress, some medical limitations, and some costs. When may a procedure be foregone that might improve nutrition and hydration for a given patient? Only when the procedure and the resulting improvement in nutrition and hydration do not offer the patient a net benefit over what he or she would otherwise have faced.

Are there such circumstances? We believe that there are; but they are few and limited to the following three kinds of situations: 1. The procedures that would be required are so unlikely to achieve improved nutritional and fluid levels that they could be correctly considered futile; 2. The improvement in nutritional and fluid balance, though achievable, could be of no benefit to the patient; 3. The burdens of receiving the treatment may outweigh the benefit.

WHEN FOOD AND WATER MAY BE WITHHELD

Futile Treatment. Sometimes even providing "food and water" to a patient becomes a monumental task. Consider a patient with a severe clotting deficiency and a nearly total body burn. Gaining access to the central veins is likely to cause hemorrhage or infection, nasogastric tube placement may be quite painful, and there may be no skin to which to suture the stomach for a gastrostomy tube. Or consider a patient with severe congestive heart failure who develops cancer of the stomach with a fistula that delivers foods from the stomach to the colon without passing through the intestine and being absorbed. Feeding the patient may be possible, but little is absorbed. Intravenous feeding cannot be tolerated because the fluid would be too much for the weakened heart. Or consider the infant with infarction of all but a short segment of bowel. Again, the infant can be fed, but little if anything is absorbed. Intravenous methods can be used, but only for a short time (weeks ormonths) until their complications, in-

cluding thrombosis, hemorrhage, infections, and malnutrition, cause death.

In these circumstances, the patient is going to die soon, no matter what is done. The ineffective efforts to provide nutrition and hydration may well directly cause suffering that offers no counterbalancing benefit for the patient. Although the procedures might be tried, especially if the competent patient wanted them or the incompetent patient's surrogate had reason to believe that this incompetent patient would have wanted them, they cannot be considered obligatory. To hold that a patient must be subjected to this predictably futile sort of intervention just because protein balance is negative or the blood serum is concentrated is to lose sight of the moral warrant for medical care and to reduce the patient to an array of measurable variables.

No Possibility of Benefit. Some patients can be reliably diagnosed to have permanently lost consciousness. This unusual group of patients includes those with anencephaly, persistent vegetative state, and some preterminal comas. In these cases, it is very difficult to discern how any medical intervention can benefit or harm the patient. These patients cannot and never will be able to experience any of the events occurring in the world or in their bodies. When the diagnosis is exceedingly clear, we sustain their lives vigorously mainly for their loved ones and the community at large.

While these considerations probably indicate that continued artificial feeding is best in most cases, there may be some cases in which the family and the caregivers are convinced that artificial feeding is offensive and unreasonable. In such cases, there seems to be no adequate reason to claim that withholding food and water violates any obligations that these parties or the general society have with regard to permanently unconscious patients. Thus, if the parents of an anencephalic infant or of a patient like Karen Quinlan in a persistent vegetative state feel strongly that no medical procedures should be applied to provide nutrition and hydration, and the caregivers are willing to comply, there should be no barrier in law or public policy to thwart the plan.[2]

Disproportionate Burden. The most difficult cases are those in which normal nutritional status or fluid balance could be restored, but only with a severe burden for the patient. In these cases, the treatment is futile in a broader sense—the patient will not actually benefit from the improved nutrition and hydration. A patient who is competent can decide the relative merits of the treatment being provided, knowing the probable consequences, and weighing the merits of life under various sets of constrained circumstances. But a surrogate decision maker for a patient who is incompetent to decide will have a difficult task. When the situation is irremediably ambiguous, erring on the side of continued life and improved nutrition and hydration seems the less grievous error. But are there situations that would warrant a determination that this patient, whose nutrition and hydration could surely be improved, is not thereby well served?

Though they are rare, we believe there are such cases. The treatments entailed are not benign. Their effects are far short of ideal. Furthermore, many of the patients most likely to have inadequate food and fluid intake are also likely to suffer the most serious side effects of these therapies.

Patients who are allowed to die without artificial hydration and nutrition may well die more comfortably than patients who receive conventional amounts of intravenous hydration.[3] Terminal pulmonary edema, nausea, and mental confusion are more likely when patients have been treated to maintain fluid and nutrition until close to the time of death.

Thus, those patients whose "need" for artificial nutrition and hydration arises only near the time of death may be harmed by its provision. It is not at all clear that they receive any benefit in having a slightly prolonged life, and it does seem reasonable to allow a surrogate to decide that, for this patient at this time, slight prolongation of life is not warranted if it involves measures that will probably increase the patient's suffering as he or she dies.

Even patients who might live much longer might not be well served by artificial means to provide fluid and food. Such patients might include those with fairly severe dementia for whom the restraints required could be a constant source of fear, discomfort, and struggle. For such a patient, sedation to tolerate the feeding mechanisms might preclude any of the pleasant experiences that might otherwise have been available. Thus, a decision not to intervene, except perhaps briefly to ascertain that there are no treatable causes, might allow such a patient to live out a shorter life with fair freedom of movement and freedom from fear, while a decision to maintain artificial nutrition and hydration might consign the patient to end his or her life in unremitting anguish. If this were the case a surrogate decision maker would seem to be well justified in refusing the treatment.

INAPPROPRIATE MORAL CONSTRAINTS

Four considerations are frequently proposed as moral constraints on foregoing medical feeding and hydration. We find none of these to dictate that artificial nutrition and hydration must always be provided.

The Obligation to Provide "Ordinary" Care. Debates about appropriate medical treatment are often couched in terms of "ordinary" and "extraordinary" means of treatment. Historically, this distinction emerged in the Roman Catholic tradition to differentiate optional treatment from treatment that was obligatory for medical professionals to offer and for patients to accept.[4] These terms also appear in many secular contexts, such as court decisions and medical codes. The recent debates about ordinary and extraordinary means of treatment have been interminable and often unfruitful, in part because of a lack of clarity about what the terms mean. Do they represent the premises of an argument or the conclusion, and what features of a situation are relevant to the categorization as "ordinary" or "extraordinary"?[5]

Several criteria have been implicit in debates about ordinary and extraordinary means of treatment; some of them may be relevant to determining whether and which treatments are obligatory and which are optional. Treatments have been distinguished according to their simplicity (simple/complex), their naturalness (natural/artificial), their customariness (usual/unusual), their invasiveness (noninvasive/invasive), their chance of success (reasonable chance/futile), their balance of benefits and burdens (proportionate/disproportionate), and their ex-

pense (inexpensive/costly). Each set of paired terms or phrases in the parentheses suggests a continuum: as the treatment moves from the first of the paired terms to the second, it is said to become less obligatory and more optional.

However, when these various criteria, widely used in discussions about medical treatment, are carefully examined, most of them are not morally relevant in distinguishing optional from obligatory medical treatments. For example, if a rare, complex, artificial, and invasive treatment offers a patient a reasonable chance of nearly painless cure, then one would have to offer a substantial justification not to provide that treatment to an incompetent patient.

What matters, then, in determining whether to provide a treatment to a competent patient is not a prior determination that this treatment is "ordinary" per se, but rather a determination that the treatment is likely to provide this patient benefits that are sufficient to make it worthwhile to endure the burdens that accompany the treatment. To this end, some of the considerations listed above are irrelevant: whether a treatment is likely to succeed is an obvious example. But such considerations taken in isolation are inconclusive. Rather, the surrogate decision maker is obliged to assess the desirability to this patient of each of the options presented, including nontreatment. For most people at most times, this assessment would lead to a clear obligation to provide food and fluids.

But sometimes, as we have indicated, providing food and fluids through medical interventions may fail to benefit and may even harm some patients. Then the treatment cannot be said to be obligatory, no matter how usual and simple its provisions may be. If "ordinary" and "extraordinary" are used to convey the conclusion about the obligation to treat, providing nutrition and fluids would have become, in these cases, "extraordinary." Since this phrasing is misleading, it is probably better to use "proportionate" and "disproportionate," as the Vatican now suggests,[6] or "obligatory" and "optional."

Obviously, providing nutrition and hydration may sometimes be necessary to keep patients comfortable while they are dying even though it may temporarily prolong their dying. In such cases, food and fluids constitute warranted palliative care. But in other cases, such as a patient in a deep and irreversible coma, nutrition and hydration do not appear to be needed or helpful, except perhaps to comfort the state and family.[7] And sometimes the interventions needed for nutrition and hydration are so burdensome that they are harmful and best not utilized.

The Obligation to Continue Treatments Once Started. Once having started a mode of treatment, many caregivers find it very difficult to discontinue it. While this strongly felt difference between the ease of withholding a treatment and the difficulty of withdrawing it provides a psychological explanation of certain actions, it does not justify them. It sometimes even leads to a thoroughly irrational decision process. For example, in caring for a dying, comatose patient, many physicians apparently find it harder to stop a functioning peripheral IV than not to restart one that has infiltrated (that is, has broken through the blood vessel and is leaking fluid into surrounding tissue), especially if the only way to reestablish an IV would be to insert a central line into the heart or to do a cutdown (make an incision to gain access to the deep large blood vessels).[8]

What factors might make withdrawing medical treatment morally worse than withholding it? Withdrawing a treatment seems to be an action, which, when it is likely to end in death, initially seems more serious than an omission that ends in death. However, this view is fraught with errors. Withdrawing is not always an act: failing to put the next infusion into a tube could be correctly described as an omission, for example. Even when withdrawing is an act, it may well be morally correct and even morally obligatory. Discontinuing intravenous lines in a patient now permanently unconscious in accord with that patient's well-informed advance directive would certainly be such a case. Furthermore, the caregiver's obligation to serve the patient's interests through both acts and omissions rules out the exculpation that accompanies omissions in the usual course of social life. An omission that is not warranted by the patient's interests is culpable.

Sometimes initiating a treatment creates expectations in the minds of caregivers, patients, and family that the treatment will be continued indefinitely or until the patient is cured. Such expectations may provide a reason to continue the treatment as a way to keep a promise. However, as with all promises, caregivers could be very careful when initiating a treatment to explain the indications for its discontinuation, and they could modify preconceptions with continuing reevaluation and education during treatment. Though all patients are entitled to expect the continuation of care in the patient's best interests, they are not and should not be entitled to the continuation of a particular mode of care.

Accepting the distinction between withholding and withdrawing medical treatment as morally significant also has a very unfortunate implication: caregivers may become unduly reluctant to begin some treatments precisely because they fear that they will be locked into continuing treatments that are no longer of value to the patient. For example, the physician who had been unwilling to stop the respirator while the infant, Andrew Stinson, died over several months is reportedly "less eager to attach babies to respirators now." But if it were easier to ignore malnutrition and dehydration and to withhold treatments for these problems than to discontinue the same treatments when they have become especially burdensome and insufficiently beneficial for this patient, then the incentives would be perverse. Once a treatment has been tried, it is often much clearer whether it is of value to this patient, and the decision to stop it can be made more reliably.

The same considerations should apply to starting as to stopping a treatment, and whatever assessment warrants withholding should also warrant withdrawing.

The Obligation to Avoid Being the Unambiguous Cause of Death. Many physicians will agree with all that we have said and still refuse to allow a choice to forego food and fluid because such a course seems to be a "death sentence." In this view death seems to be more certain from malnutrition and dehydration than from foregoing other forms of medical therapy. This implies that it is acceptable to act in ways that are likely to cause death, as in not operating on a gangrenous leg, only if there remains a chance that the patient will survive. This is a comforting formulation for caregivers, to be sure, since they can thereby avoid feeling the full weight of the responsibility for the time and manner of a patient's death. However, it is not a persuasive moral argument.

First, in appropriate cases discontinuing certain medical treatments is generally accepted despite the fact that death is as certain as with nonfeeding. Dialysis in a patient without kidney function or transfusions in a patient with severe aplastic anemia are obvious examples. The dying that awaits such patients often is not greatly different from dying of dehydration and malnutrition.

Second, the certainty of a generally undesirable outcome such as death is always relevant to a decision, but it does not foreclose the possibility that this course is better than others available to this patient.[10] Ambiguity and uncertainty are so common in medical decision making that caregivers are tempted to use them in distancing themselves from direct responsibility. However, caregivers are in fact responsible for the time and manner of death for many patients. Their distaste for this fact should not constrain otherwise morally justified decisions.

The Obligation to Provide Symbolically Significant Treatment. One of the most common arguments for always providing nutrition and hydration is that it symbolizes, expresses, or conveys the essence of care and compassion. Some actions not only aim at goals, they also express values. Such expressive actions should not simply be viewed as means to ends; they should also be viewed in light of what they communicate. From this perspective food and water are not only goods that preserve life and provide comfort; they are also symbols of care and compassion. To withhold or withdraw them—to "starve" a patient—can never express or convey care.

Why is providing food and water a central symbol of care and compassion? Feeding is the first response of the community to the needs of newborns and remains a central mode of nurture and comfort. Eating is associated with social interchange and community, and providing food for someone else is a way to create and maintain bonds of sharing and expressing concern. Furthermore, even the relatively low levels of hunger and thirst that most people have experienced are decidedly uncomfortable, and the common image of severe malnutrition or dehydration is one of unremitting agony. Thus, people are rightly eager to provide food and water. Such provision is essential to minimally tolerable existence and a powerful symbol of our concern for each other.

However, *medical* nutrition and hydration, we have argued, may not always provide net benefits to patients. Medical procedures to provide nutrition and hydration are more similar to other medical procedures than to typical human ways of providing nutrition and hydration, for example, a sip of water. It should be possible to evaluate their benefits and burdens, as we evaluate any other medical procedure. Of course, if family, friends, and caregivers feel that such procedures affirm important values even when they do not benefit the patient, their feelings should not be ignored. We do not contend that there is an obligation to withhold or to withdraw such procedures (unless consideration of the patient's advance directives or current best interest unambiguously dictates that conclusion); we only contend that nutri-

tion and hydration may be foregone in some cases.

The symbolic connection between care and nutrition or hydration adds useful caution to decision making. If decision makers worry over withholding or withdrawing medical nutrition and hydration, they may inquire more seriously into the circumstances that putatively justify their decisions. This is generally salutary for health care decision making. The critical inquiry may well yield the sad but justified conclusion that the patient will be served best by not using medical procedures to provide food and fluids. . . .

REFERENCES

We are grateful to Haavi Morreim and Steven DalleMura for their helpful comments on an earlier version of this paper. We are also grateful for the instruction provided by Dr. Lynn by the staff and patients of The Washington Home and its Hospice.

1. See e.g., the President's Commission for the Study of Ethical Problems in Medicine and Biomedical and Behavioral Research, *Making Health Care Decisions* (Washington, D.C.: Government Printing Office, 1982).

2. President's Commission, *Deciding to Forego Life-Sustaining Treatment*, pp. 171–96.

3. Joyce V. Zerwekh, "The Dehydration Question," *Nursing83* (January 1983), 47–51, with comments by Judith R. Brown and Marion B. Dolan.

4. James J. McCartney, "The Development of the Doctrine of Ordinary and Extraordinary Means of Preserving Life in Catholic Moral Theology before the Karen Quinlan Case," *Linacre Quarterly* 47 (1980), 215ff.

5. President's Commission, *Deciding to Forego Life-Sustaining Treatment*, pp. 82–90. For an argument that fluids and electrolytes can be "extraordinary," see Carson Strong, "Can Fluids and Electrolytes be 'Extraordinary' Treatment?" *Journal of Medical Ethics* 7 (1981), 83–85.

6. The Sacred Congregation for the Doctrine of the Faith, *Declaration on Euthanasia*, Vatican City, May 5, 1980.

7. Paul Ramsey contends that "when a man is irreversibly in the process of dying, to feed him and to give him drink, to ease him and keep him comfortable—these are no longer given as means of preserving life. The use of a glucose drip

should often be understood in this way. This keeps a patient who cannot swallow from feeling dehydrated and is often the only remaining 'means' by which we can express our present faithfulness to him during his dying." Ramsey, *The Patient as Person* (New Haven: Yale University Press, 1970), pp. 128–29. But Ramsey's suggestion would not apply to a patient in a deep irreversible coma, and he would be willing to disconnect the IV in the Quinlan case; see Ramsey, *Ethics at the Edges of Life: Medical and Legal Intersections* (New Haven: Yale University Press, 1978), p. 275. Bernard Towers describes an appropriate approach to comfort and dignity: "When a patient is conscious to even the smallest degree, and if he appears to be thirsty and to have a swallowing reflex, and if there is no contraindication to oral fluids, his comfort and dignity would surely demand that he be given nourishing liquids, or at least water. If he lapses into coma, good nursing practice has traditionally required sponging out the mouth and moistening the lips. Now, if he lapses into deep coma and is on a dying trajectory, would we then try to 'push' fluids by mouth or nasogastric tube? If we did, dignitywould surely suffer. The 'comfort' of the patient would, of course, be unaffected if the coma were deep enough and irreversible." Towers, "Irreversible Coma and Withdrawal of Life Support: Is It Murder If the IV Line Is Disconnected?" *Journal of Medical Ethics* 8 (1982), 205.

8. See Kenneth C. Micetich, Patricia H. Steinecker, and David C. Thomasma, "Are Intravenous Fluids Morally Required for a Dying Patient?" *Archives of Internal Medicine* 143 (May 1983), 975–78.

9. Robert and Peggy Stinson, *The Long Dying of Baby Andrew* (Boston: Little, Brown and Company, 1983), p. 355.

10. A recent article discussed a hypothetical case of maintaining a dying, comatose patient on a respirator while withdrawing IV fluids. The authors contend that this approach is not ironic because withdrawal of the respirator "creates the immediate consequence of death for which we must take responsibility. It represents an extreme form of abandonment." Nevertheless, they were willing to stop IV fluids, knowing that death would occur before long. As the article's survey reported, other physicians would have provided nutrition and fluids. See Micetich, Steinecker, and Thomasma, "Are Intravenous Fluids Morally Required for a Dying Patient?"

NO

Gilbert Meilaender

ALLOWING TO DIE, OR AIMING TO KILL? ON REMOVING FOOD AND WATER: AGAINST THE STREAM

As infants we were given food and drink when we were too helpless to nourish ourselves. And for many of us a day will come before we die when we are once again too helpless to feed ourselves. If there is any way in which the living can stand by those who are not yet dead, it would seem to be through the continued provision of food and drink even when the struggle against disease has been lost. To continue to nourish the life of one who has been defeated in that battle is the last evidence we can offer that we are more than frontrunners, that we are willing to love to the very point of death.

Today this intuitive reaction is being challenged. The President's Commission for the Study of Ethical Problems in Medicine and Biomedical and Behavioral Research has suggested that for patients with permanent loss of consciousness artificial feeding interventions need not be continued.[1] A group of physicians writing in the *New England Journal of Medicine* has counseled doctors that for irreversibly ill patients whose condition warrants nothing more aggressive than general nursing care, "naturally or artificially administered hydration and nutrition may be given or withheld, depending on the patient's comfort."[2]

Court decisions . . . are contradictory,[3] but a consensus is gradually building toward the day when what we have already done in the case of some nondying infants with birth defects who were "allowed to die" by not being fed will become standard "treatment" for all patients who are permanently unconscious or suffering from severe and irreversible dementia. Those who defend this view stand ready with ethical arguents that nutrition and hydration are not "in the best interests" of such patients, but Daniel Callahan may have isolated the energizing force that is driving this consensus: "A denial of nutrition," he says, "may in the long run become the only effective way to make certain that a large number of biologically tenacious patients actually die."[4]

From Gilbert Meilaender, "On Removing Food and Water: Against the Stream," *Hastings Center Report*, vol. 14, no. 6 (December 1984). Copyright © 1984 by The Hastings Center. Reprinted by permission.

To the degree that this is true, however, the policy toward which we are moving is not merely one of "allowing to die": it is one of aiming to kill. *If* we are in fact heading in this direction, we should turn back before this policy corrupts our intellect and emotions and our capacity for moral reasoning. That stance I take to be a given, for which I shall not attempt to argue. Here I will consider only whether removal of artificial nutrition and hydration really does amount to no more than "allowing to die."

WHY FEEDING IS NOT MEDICAL CARE

The argument for ceasing to feed seems strongest in cases of people suffering from a "persistent vegetative state," those (like Karen Quinlan) who have suffered an irreversible loss of consciousness. Sidney Wanzer and his physician colleagues suggest that in such circumstances "it is morally justifiable to withhold antibiotics and artificial nutrition and hydration, as well as other forms of life-sustaining treatment, allowing the patient to die." The President's Commission advises: "Since permanently unconscious patients will never be aware of nutrition, the only benefit to the patient of providing such increasingly burdensome interventions is sustaining the body to allow for a remote possibility of recovery. The sensitivities of the family and of care giving professionals ought to determine whether such interventions are made." Joanne Lynn, a physician at George Washington University, and James Childress, a professor of religious studies at the University of Virginia, believe that "in these cases, it is very difficult to discern how any medical intervention can benefit or harm the patient."[5] But we need to ask whether the physicians are right to suggest that they seek only to allow the patient to die; whether the President's Commission has used language carefully enough in saying that nutrition and hydration of such persons is merely sustaining a *body*; whether Lynn and Childress may too readily have assumed that providing food and drink is *medical* treatment.

Should the provision of food and drink be regarded as *medical* care? It seems, rather, to be the sort of care that all human beings owe each other. All living beings need food and water in order to live, but such nourishment does not itself heal or cure disease. When we stop feeding the permanently unconscious patient, we are not withdrawing from the battle against any illness or disease; we are withholding the nourishment that sustains all life.

The President's Commission does suggest that certain kinds of care remain mandatory for the permanently unconscious patient: "The awkward posture and lack of motion of unconscious patients often lead to pressure sores, and skin lesions are a major complication. Treatment and prevention of these problems is standard nursing care and should be provided." Yet it is hard to see why such services (turning the person regularly, giving alcohol rubs, and the like) are standard nursing care when feeding is not. Moreover, if feeding cannot benefit these patients, it is far from clear how they could experience bed sores as harm.

If this is true, we may have good reason to question whether the withdrawal of nutrition and hydration in such cases is properly characterized as stopping medical treatment in order to allow a patient to die. There are circumstances in which a plausible and helpful distinction can be made between killing and allowing to die, between an aim and a foreseen but unintended consequence. And sometimes it may make excellent moral sense to hold that we should cease to provide a now useless treatment, foreseeing but not intending that death will result. Such reasoning is also useful in the ethics of warfare, but there its use must be strictly controlled lest we simply unleash the bombs while "directing our intention" to a military target that could be attacked with far less firepower. Careful use of language is also necessary lest we talk about unconscious patients in ways that obscure our true aim.

Challenging those who have argued that it is no longer possible to distinguish between combatants and noncombatants in war, Michael Walzer has pointed out that "the relevant distinction is not between those who work for the war effort and those who do not, but between those who make what soldiers need to fight and those who make what they need to live, like the rest of us."[6]

Hence, farmers are not legitimate targets in war simply because they grow the food that soldiers need to live (and then to fight). The soldiers would need the food to live, even if there were no war. Thus, as Paul Ramsey has observed, though an army may march upon its belly, bellies are not the target. It is an abuse of double-effect reasoning to justify cutting off the food supply of a nation as a way of stopping its soldiers. We could not properly say that we were aiming at the soldiers while merely foreseeing the deaths of the civilian population.

Nor can we, when withdrawing food from the permanently unconscious person, properly claim that our intention is to cease useless treatment for a dying patient. These patients are not dying, and we cease no treatment aimed at disease; rather, we withdraw the nourishment that sustains all human beings whether healthy or ill, and we do so when the only result of our action can be death. At what, other than that death, could we be aiming?

One might argue that the same could be said of turning off a respirator, but the situations are somewhat different. Remove a person from a respirator and he may die—but, then, he may also surprise us and continue to breathe spontaneously. We test to see if the patient can breathe. If he does, it is not our task—unless we are aiming at his death—now to smother him (or to stop feeding him). But deprive a person of food and water and she will die as surely as if we had administered a lethal drug, and it is hard to claim that we did not aim at her death.

I am unable—and this is a lack of insight, not of space—to say more about the analogy between eating and breathing. Clearly, air is as essential to life as food. We might wonder, therefore, whether provision of air is not also more than medical treatment. What justification could there be, then for turning off a respirator? If the person's death, due to the progress of a disease, is irreversibly and imminently at hand, then continued assistance with respiration may now be useless. But if the person is not going to die from any disease but, instead, simply needs assistance with breathing because of some injury, it is less clear to me why such assistance should not be given. More than this I am unable to say. I repeat, however, that to remove a respirator is not necessarily to aim at death; one will not go on to kill the patient who manages to breathe spontaneously. But it is difficult for me to construe removal of nutrition for permanently unconscious patients in any other way. Perhaps we only wish them dead or think they would be better off dead. There are circumstances in which such a thought is understandable. But it would still be wrong to enact that wish by aiming at their death.

SEPARATING PERSONHOOD AND BODY

Suppose that we accept the view that provision of food and water is properly termed medical treatment. Is there good reason to withhold this treatment from permanently unconscious patients? A treatment refusal needs to be justified either on the ground that the treatment is (or has now become) useless, or that the treatment (though perhaps still useful) is excessively burdensome for the patient. Still taking as our focus the permanently unconscious patient, we can consider, first, whether feeding is useless. There could be occasions on which artificial feeding would be futile. Lynn and Childress offer instances of patients who simply cannot be fed effectively, but they are not cases of permanently unconscious patients.

Yet for many people the uselessness of feeding the permanently unconscious seems self-evident. Why? Probably because they suppose that the nourishment we provide is, in the words of the President's Commission, doing no more than "sustaining the body." But we should pause before separating personhood and body so decisively. When considering other topics (care of the environment, for example) we are eager to criticize a dualism that divorces human reason and consciousness from the larger world of nature. Why not here? We can know

people—of all ranges of cognitive capacity—only as they are embodied; there is no other "person" for whom we might care. Such care is not useless if it "only" preserves bodily life but does not restore cognitive capacities. Even if it is less than we wish could be accomplished, it remains care for the embodied person.

Some will object to characterizing as persons those who lack the capacity or, even, the potential for self-awareness, for envisioning a future for themselves, for relating to other selves. I am not fully persuaded that speaking of "persons" in such contexts is mistaken, but the point can be made without using that language. Human nature has a capacity to know, to be self-aware, and to relate to others. We can share in that human nature even though we may not yet or no longer exercise all the functions of which it is capable. We share in it simply by virtue of being born into the human species. We could describe as persons all individuals sharing our common nature, all members of the species. Or we could ascribe personhood only to those human beings presently capable of exercising the characteristic human functions.

I think it better—primarily because it is far less dualistic—to understand personhood as an endowment that comes with our nature, even if at some stages of life we are unable to exercise characteristic human capacities. But the point can be made, if anyone wishes, by talking of embodied human beings rather than embodied persons. To be a human being one need not presently be exercising or be capable of exercising the functions characteristic of consciousness. Those are capacities of human nature; they are not functions that all human beings exercise. It is human beings, not just persons in that more restricted sense, whose death should not be our aim. And if this view is characterized as an objectionable "speciesism," I can only reply that at least it is not one more way by which the strong and gifted in our world rid themselves of the weak, and it does not fall prey to that abstraction by which we reify consciousness and separate it from the body.

The permanently unconscious are not dying subjects who should simply be allowed to die. But they will, of course, die if we aim at their death by ceasing to feed them. If we are not going to feed them because that would be nothing more than sustaining a body, why not bury them at once? No one, I think, recommends that. But if, then, they are still living beings who ought not be buried, the nourishment that all human beings need to live ought not be denied them. When we permit ourselves to think that care is useless if it preserves the life of the embodied human being without restoring cognitive capacity, we fall victim to the old delusion that we have failed if we cannot *cure* and that there is, then, little point to continued *care*. David Smith, a professor of religious studies at the University of Indiana, has suggested that I might be mistaken in describing the comatose person as a "nondying" patient. At least in some cases, he believes lapsing into permanent coma might be a sign that a person is trying to die. Thus, though a comatose state would not itself be sufficient reason to characterize someone as dying, it might be one of several conditions which, taken together, would be sufficient. This is a reasonable suggestion, and it might enable us to distinguish different sorts of comatose patients—the dying, for whom feeding might be useless; the nondying, for whom it would not. Even then, how-

ever, I would still be troubled by the worry I raised earlier: whether food and drink are really medical treatment that should be withdrawn when it becomes useless.

Even when care is not useless it may be so burdensome that it should be dispensed with. When that is the case, we can honestly say—and it makes good moral sense to say—that our aim is to relieve the person of a burden, with the foreseen but unintended effect of a hastened death. We should note, however, that this line of argument *cannot* be applied to the cases of the permanently unconscious. Other patients—those, for example, with fairly severe dementia— may be made afraid and uncomfortable by artificial nutrition and hydration. But this can hardly be true of the permanently unconscious. It seems unlikely that they experience the care involved in feeding them as burdensome.

Even for severely demented patients who retain some consciousness, we should be certain that we are considering the burden of the treatment, not the burden of continued existence itself. . . . That is a judgment, I think, that no one should make for another; indeed, it is hard to know exactly how one would do so. Besides, it seems evident that if the burden involved is her continued life, the point of ceasing to feed is that we aim at relieving her of that burden—that is, we aim to kill.

Having said that, I am quite ready to grant that the burden of the feeding itself may sometimes be so excessive that it is not warranted. Lynn and Childress offer examples, some of which seem persuasive. If, however, we want to assess the burden of the treatment, we should certainly not dispense with nutrition and hydration until a reasonable trial period has demonstrated that the person truly finds such care excessively burdensome.

In short, if we focus our attention on irreversibly ill adults for whom general nursing care but no more seems appropriate, we can say the following: First, when the person is permanently unconscious, the care involved in feeding can hardly be experienced as burdensome. Neither can such care be described as useless, since it preserves the life of the embodied human being (who is not a dying patient). Second, when the person is conscious but severely and irreversibly demented, the care involved in feeding, though not useless, *may* be so burdensome that it should cease. This requires demonstration during a trial period, however, and the judgment is quite different from concluding that the person's life has become too burdensome to preserve. Third, for both sorts of patients the care involved in feeding is not, in any strict sense, medical treatment, even if provided in a hospital. It gives what all need to live; it is treatment of no particular disease; and its cessation means certain death, a death at which we can only be said to aim, whatever our motive.

That we should continue to feed the permanently unconscious still seems obvious to some people, even as it was to Karen Quinlan's father at the time he sought removal of her respirator. It has not always seemed so to me, but it does now. For the permanently unconscious person, feeding is neither useless nor excessively burdensome. It is ordinary human care and is not given as treatment for any life-threatening disease. Since this is true, a decision not to offer such care can enact only one intention: to take the life of the unconscious person.

I have offered no arguments here to prove that such a life-taking intention and aim would be morally wrong, though I believe it is and that to embrace such an aim would be corrupting. If we can face the fact that withdrawing the nourishment of such persons is, indeed, aiming to kill, I am hopeful (though not altogether confident) that the more fundamental principle will not need to be argued. Let us hope that this is the case, since that more basic principle is not one that can be argued *to*; rather, all useful moral arguments must proceed *from* the conviction that it is wrong to aim to kill the innocent.

REFERENCES

1. The President's Commission for the Study of Ethical Problems in Medicine and Biomedical and Behavioral Research, *Deciding to Forego Life-Sustaining Treatment* (Washington, DC: Government Printing Office, 1982), p. 190.
2. Sidney H. Wanzer, M.D., et al., "The Physician's Responsibility Toward Hopelessly Ill Patients," *New England Journal of Medicine*, 310 (April 12, 1984) 958.
3. See a discussion of the first two cases in Bonnie Steinbock, "The Removal of Mr. Herbert's Feeding Tube," *Hastings Center Report*, 13 (October 1983) 13–16; also see George J. Annas, "The Case of Mary Hier: When Substituted Judgment Becomes Sleight of Hand," *Hastings Center Report* 14 (August 1984), 23–25.
4. Daniel Callahan, "On Feeding the Dying," *Hastings Center Report*, 13 (October 1983) 22.
5. Joanne Lynn and James Childress, "Must Patients Always Be Given Food and Water?" *Hastings Center Report*, 13 (October 1983) 18.
6. Michael Walzer, *Just and Unjust Wars* (New York: Basic Books, Inc., 1977), p. 146.

POSTSCRIPT

Is It Ever Morally Right to Withhold Food and Water from Dying Patients?

In November 1990, four months after the Supreme Court *Cruzan* decision, Nancy Cruzan's parents went back to court with new witnesses who testified that Nancy had clearly indicated that she would not want to live in a vegetative state. The state of Missouri, which had opposed the parents' decision to withdraw her feeding tube, asked to be dismissed from the case, satisified that guidelines were established to protect the patient's interests. Standards vary by state laws, with Maine, Missouri, and New York having the most stringent requirements.

Following the *Cruzan* decision, a Florida Supreme Court ruled that dying people had a right to refuse food and that guardians could make the decision for incompetent people. The case they considered involved Estelle Browning, an elderly woman who spent the last two and a half years of her life in a nursing home fed by tube even though she had signed a "living will" affirming that she did not want to be kept alive under these circumstances.

The American Medical Association's Council on Ethical and Judicial Affairs has reaffirmed that it is not unethical, under certain circumstances and with adequate safeguards, to discontinue artificial nutrition for hopelessly comatose patients (*Journal of the American Medical Association*, January 19, 1990). Some disability and right-to-life groups oppose this position. The United Handicapped Federation, a Minnesota disability rights coalition, for example, declares that "full access to nutrition and hydration . . . is the basic right of all persons . . . whether or not they are terminally ill."

The *Cruzan* case is discussed in "Prisoners of Technology: The Case of Nancy Cruzan," by Marcia Angell, *The New England Journal of Medicine* (April 26, 1990), and a series of articles, "The Court and Nancy Cruzan," *Hastings Center Report* (January/February 1990). A series of articles commenting on the decision is "*Cruzan:* Clear and Convincing?" *Hastings Center Report* (September/October 1990).

For an account of the *Brophy* case, see George J. Annas, "Do Feeding Tubes Have More Rights Than Patients?" *Hastings Center Report* (February 1986).

Daniel Callahan writes about the dangers of a routine policy of stopping food and nutrition in "Feeding the Dying Elderly," *Generations* (Winter 1985). Also see William E. May et al., "Feeding and Hydrating the Permanently Unconscious and Other Vulnerable Persons," *Issues in Law and Medicine* (Winter 1987).

On the more general issue of advance directives or "living wills," see Chris Hackler, Ray Mosely, and Dorothy E. Vanter, eds., *Advance Directives in Medicine* (Praeger, 1989), and Larry R. Churchill, "Trust, Autonomy, and Advance Directives," *Journal of Religion and Health* (Fall 1989).

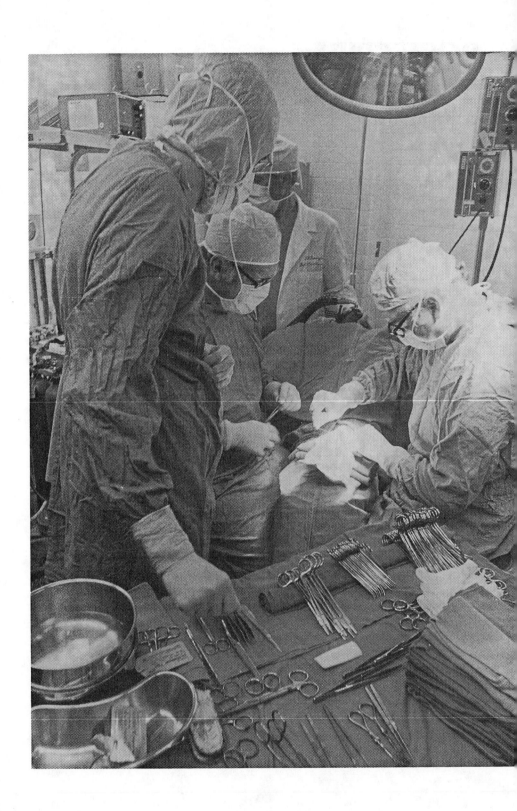

PART 3

The Doctor-Patient Relationship

While the most publicized issues in bioethics concern dramatic, life-and-death decisions, or the uses of high-technology medicine, the ordinary encounters between doctors and patients also create ethical dilemmas. The relationship between patients and practitioners is often unequal, with physicians controlling the terms. Nevertheless, physicians are obligated to serve their patients' interests. In most cases both partners share an understanding of the patient's needs and the most appropriate ways to meet them. Sometimes, however, conflicts arise, and physicians are forced to choose between their patients' interests and their own or others' interests. The issues in this section confront some of these situations, made particularly acute in the age of AIDS.

Are There Limits to Confidentiality?

Is Involuntary Commitment Wrong?

Should Surgical Patients Be Screened for HIV?

Do Physicians Have an Ethical Duty to Treat AIDS Patients?

135

ISSUE 8

Are There Limits to Confidentiality?

YES: Mark Siegler, from "Confidentiality in Medicine: A Decrepit Concept,"
The New England Journal of Medicine (December 9, 1982)

NO: Michael H. Kottow, from "Medical Confidentiality: An Intransigent
and Absolute Obligation," *Journal of Medical Ethics* (vol. 12, 1986)

ISSUE SUMMARY

YES: Physician Mark Siegler argues that confidentiality is necessarily compromised in order to ensure complete and proper medical treatment.
NO: Physician Michael H. Kottow argues that any kind of breach of patient
confidentiality causes harms that are more serious than hypothetical
benefits.

"If I tell you a secret, will you promise not to tell anyone?" This simple
question, familiar from childhood, captures two important features of human relationships: the need to confide one's fears and hopes to another
person and the need to trust that person not to reveal the secret. If the
person who receives the confidence agrees not to reveal it, he or she has
made a promise. All ethical systems place a high value on promise keeping.
    When this exchange occurs in a professional relationship—between pa-
tient and physician or therapist, client and attorney, or priest and confessor—
there is even more at stake. The professional, as part of achieving that status,
has accepted an ethical code that states that confidentiality will be maintained. One of the earliest formulations of this concept is found in the
Hippocratic Oath, which is still sworn to by all physicians: "What I may see
or hear in the course of the treatment or even outside of the treatment in
regard to the life of men, which on no account one must spread abroad, I will
keep to myself. . . ." More recently numerous codes of professional ethics,
such as those of the American Medical Association, have reaffirmed the
principle of medical confidentiality. The traditions of religious ethics and the
patients' rights movement have also strongly supported medical confidentiality.
    But no value is absolute, and some exceptions to the rule of confidentiality
are well established. For example, considerations of public health underlie
laws that require physicians to report certain contagious diseases such as
syphilis, measles, meningitis, and (most recently) acquired immunodefi-

ciency syndrome (AIDS). Similarly, a physician must report cases of gunshot wounds to the authorities, since a crime may have been committed. Physicians and social workers are required by law to report suspected cases of child abuse, so that a child who is being harmed physically or mentally can be protected.

In recent years two situations have raised questions about the limits of confidentiality. As Sissela Bok, a philosopher who has written extensively on secrets, puts it: "Does a professional owe confidentiality to clients who reveal plans or acts that endanger others directly?" The question, she says, arises equally for the lawyer whose client lets it be known that he plans a bank robbery, for the pediatrician who suspects that a mother drugs her children to keep them quiet, and for the psychiatrist whose patient reveals his violent jealousy of his wife. This last situation arose in the celebrated case of Tatiana Tarasoff, a student who was killed by a suitor she had spurned after he told a psychiatrist of his plans. The legal resolution of the case in 1976 resulted in the establishment of a "duty to protect" on the part of therapists in the state of California.

Another challenge to confidentiality arises when a person with AIDS or infection with the human immunodeficiency virus (HIV) refuses to inform his or her sexual partner of the potential risk of transmission. Is the physician or other professional who knows of this situation obligated to protect the third party and, by so doing, breach his or her primary obligation to maintain the confidentiality of the patient?

The following two selections provide the context for discussing these specific instances. Although Mark Siegler believes that confidentiality can be defended as a principle, in modern medical practice it is a matter of expediency and has inherent limits. Michael H. Kottow takes a strong stand in favor of absolute adherence to confidentiality. Confidentiality, he says, is a "brittle arrangement" that disintegrates if misdirected to pursue other goals.

YES

Mark Siegler

CONFIDENTIALITY IN MEDICINE: A DECREPIT CONCEPT

Medical confidentiality, as it has traditionally been understood by patients and doctors, no longer exists. This ancient medical principle, which has been included in every physician's oath and code of ethics since Hippocratic times, has become old, worn-out, and useless; it is a decrepit concept. Efforts to preserve it appear doomed to failure and often give rise to more problems than solutions. Psychiatrists have tacitly acknowledged the impossibility of ensuring the confidentiality of medical records by choosing to establish a separate, more secret record. The following case illustrates how the confidentiality principle is compromised systematically in the course of routine medical care.

A patient of mine . . . was transferred from the surgical intensive-care unit to a surgical nursing floor two days after . . . elective [surgery]. On the day of transfer, the patient saw a respiratory therapist writing in his medical chart . . . and became concerned about the confidentiality of his hospital records. The patient threatened to leave the hospital prematurely unless I could guarantee that the confidentiality of his hospital record would be respected.

This patient's complaint prompted me to enumerate the number of persons who had both access to his hospital record and a reason to examine it. I was amazed to learn that at least 25 and possibly as many as 100 health professionals and administrative personnel at our university hospital had access to the patient's record and that all of them had a legitimate need, indeed a professional responsibility, to open and use that chart. These persons included 6 attending physicians (the primary physician, the surgeon, the pulmonary consultant, and others); 12 house officers (medical, surgical, intensive-care unit, and "covering" house staff); 20 nursing personnel (on three shifts); 6 respiratory therapists; 3 nutritionists; 2 clinical pharmacists; 15 students (from medicine, nursing, respiratory therapy, and clinical pharmacy); 4 unit secretaries; 4 hospital financial officers; and 4 chart reviewers (utilization review, quality assurance review, tissue review, and

From Mark Siegler, "Confidentiality in Medicine: A Decrepit Concept," *The New England Journal of Medicine*, vol. 307, no. 24 (December 9, 1982), pp. 1518-1521. Copyright © 1982 by the Massachusetts Medical Society. Reprinted by permission.

insurance auditor). It is of interest that this patient's problem was straightforward, and he therefore did not require many other technical and support services that the modern hospital provides. For example, he did not need multiple consultants and fellows, such specialized procedures as dialysis, or social workers, chaplains, physical therapists, occupational therapists, and the like.

Upon completing my survey I reported to the patient that I estimated that at least 75 health professionals and hospital personnel had access to his medical record. I suggested to the patient that these people were all involved in providing or supporting his health-care services. They were, I assured him, working for him. Despite my reassurances the patient was obviously distressed and retorted, "I always believed that medical confidentiality was part of a doctor's code of ethics. Perhaps you should tell me just what you people mean by 'confidentiality'!"

TWO ASPECTS OF MEDICAL CONFIDENTIALITY

Confidentiality and Third-Party Interests

Previous discussions of medical confidentiality usually have focused on the tension between a physician's responsibility to keep information divulged by patients secret and a physician's legal and moral duty, on occasion, to reveal such confidences to third parties, such as families, employers, public-health authorities, or police authorities. In all these instances, the central question relates to the stringency of the physician's obligation to maintain patient confidentiality when the health, well-being, and safety of identifiable others or of society in general would be threatened by a failure to reveal information about the patient. The tension in such cases is between the good of the patient and the good of others.

Confidentiality and the Patient's Interest

As the example above illustrates, further challenges to confidentiality arise because the patient's personal interest in maintaining confidentiality comes into conflict with his personal interest in receiving the best possible health care. Modern high-technology health care is available principally in hospitals (often, teaching hospitals), requires many trained and specialized workers (a "health-care team"), and is very costly. The existence of such teams means that information that previously had been held in confidence by an individual physician will now necessarily be disseminated to many members of the team. Furthermore, since health-care teams are expensive and few patients can afford to pay such costs directly, it becomes essential to grant access to the patient's medical record to persons who are responsible for obtaining third-party payment. These persons include chart reviewers, financial officers, insurance auditors, and quality-of-care assessors. Finally, as medicine expands from a narrow, disease-based model to a model that encompasses psychological, social, and economic problems, not only will the size of the health-care team and medical costs increase, but more sensitive information (such as one's personal habits and financial condition) will now be included in the medical record and will no longer be confidential.

The point I wish to establish is that hospital medicine, the rise of health-care teams, the existence of third-party insurance programs, and the expanding limits of medicine all appear to be responses to the wishes of people for better and more comprehensive medical care. But each of these developments necessarily modifies our traditional understanding of medical confidentiality.

THE ROLE OF CONFIDENTIALITY IN MEDICINE

Confidentiality serves a dual purpose in medicine. In the first place, it acknowledges respect for the patient's sense of individuality and privacy. The patient's most personal physical and psychological secrets are kept confidential in order to decrease a sense of shame and vulnerability. Secondly, confidentiality is important in improving the patient's health care—a basic goal of medicine. The promise of confidentiality permits people to trust (i.e., have confidence) that information revealed to a physician in the course of a medical encounter will not be disseminated further. In this way patients are encouraged to communicate honestly and forthrightly with their doctors. This bond of trust between patient and doctor is vitally important both in the diagnostic process (which relies on an accurate history) and subsequently in the treatment phase, which often depends as much on the patient's trust in the physician as it does on medications and surgery. These two important functions of confidentiality are as important now as they were in the past. They will not be supplanted entirely either by improvements in medical technology or by recent changes in relations between some patients and doctors toward a rights-based, consumerist model.

POSSIBLE SOLUTIONS TO THE CONFIDENTIALITY PROBLEM

First of all, in all nonbureaucratic, noninstitutional medical encounters—that is, in the millions of doctor-patient encounters that take place in physicians' offices, where more privacy can be preserved—meticulous care should be taken to guarantee that patients' medical and personal information will be kept confidential.

Secondly, in such settings as hospitals or large-scale group practices, where many persons have opportunities to examine the medical record, we should aim to provide access only to those who have "a need to know." This could be accomplished through such administrative changes as dividing the entire record into several sections—for example, a medical and financial section—and permitting only health professionals access to the medical information.

The approach favored by many psychiatrists—that of keeping a psychiatric record separate from the general medical record—is an understandable strategy but one that is not entirely satisfactory and that should not be generalized. The keeping of separate psychiatric records implies that psychiatry and medicine are different undertakings and thus drives deeper the wedge between them and between physical and psychological illness. Furthermore, it is often vitally important for internists or surgeons to know that a patient is being seen by a psychiatrist or is taking a particular medication. When separate records are kept, this information may not be available. Finally, if generalized, the practice of keeping a separate psychiatric record could lead to the unacceptable consequence of having a separate record for each type of medical problem.

Patients should be informed about what is meant by "medical confidentiality." We should establish the distinction between information about the patient that generally will be kept confidential regardless of the interest of third parties and information that will be exchanged among members of the health-care team in order to provide care for the patient. Patients should be made aware of the large number of persons in the modern hospital who require access to the medical record in order to serve the patient's medical and financial interests.

Finally, at some point most patients should have an opportunity to review their medical record and to make informed choices about whether their entire record is to be available to everyone or whether certain portions of the record are privileged and should be accessible only to their principal physician or to others designated explicitly by the patient. This approach would rely on traditional informed-consent procedural standards and might permit the patient to balance the personal value of medical confidentiality against the personal value of high-technology, team health care. There is no reason that the same procedure should not be used with psychiatric records instead of the arbitrary system now employed, in which everything related to psychiatry is kept secret.

AFTERTHOUGHT: CONFIDENTIALITY AND INDISCRETION

There is one additional aspect of confidentiality that is rarely included in discussions of the subject. I am referring here to the wanton, often inadvertent, but avoidable exchanges of confidential information that occur frequently in hospital rooms, elevators, cafeterias, doctors' offices, and at cocktail parties. Of course, as more people have access to medical information about the patient the potential for this irresponsible abuse of confidentiality increases geometrically.

Such mundane breaches of confidentiality are probably of greater concern to most patients than the broader issue of whether their medical records may be entered into a computerized data bank or whether a respiratory therapist is reviewing the results of an arterial blood gas determination. Somehow, privacy is violated and a sense of shame is heightened when intimate secrets are revealed to people one knows or is close to—friends, neighbors, acquaintances, or hospital roommates—rather than when they are disclosed to an anonymous bureaucrat sitting at a computer terminal in a distant city or to a health professional who is acting in an official capacity.

I suspect that the principles of medical confidentiality, particularly those reflected in most medical codes of ethics, were designed principally to prevent just this sort of embarrassing personal indiscretion rather than to maintain (for social, political, or economic reasons) the absolute secrecy of doctor-patient communications. In this regard, it is worth noting that Percival's Code of Medical Ethics (1803) includes the following admonition: "Patients should be interrogated concerning their complaint in a tone of voice which cannot be overheard." We in the medical profession frequently neglect these simple courtesies.

CONCLUSION

The principle of medical confidentiality described in medical codes of ethics and still believed in by patients no longer exists. In this respect, it is a decrepit concept. Rather than perpetuate the myth of confidentiality and invest energy vainly to preserve it, the public and the profession would be better served if they devoted their attention to determining which aspects of the original principle of confidentiality are worth retaining. Efforts could then be directed to salvaging those.

NO

Michael H. Kottow

MEDICAL CONFIDENTIALITY: AN INTRANSIGENT AND ABSOLUTE OBLIGATION

AUTHOR'S ABSTRACT

Clinicians' work depends on sincere and complete disclosures from their patients; they honour this candidness by confidentially safeguarding the information received. Breaching confidentiality causes harms that are not commensurable with the possible benefits gained. Limitations or exceptions put on confidentiality would destroy it, for the confider would become suspicious and un-co-operative, the confidant would become untrustworthy and the whole climate of the clinical encounter would suffer irreversible erosion. Excusing breaches of confidence on grounds of superior moral values introduces arbitrariness and ethical unreliability into the medical context. Physicians who breach the agreement of confidentiality are being unfair, thus opening the way for, and becoming vulnerable to, the morally obtuse conduct of others.

Confidentiality should not be seen as the cosy but dispensable atmosphere of clinical settings; rather, it constitutes a guarantee of fairness in medical actions. Possible perils that might accrue to society are no greater than those accepted when granting inviolable custody of information to priests, lawyers and bankers. To jeopardise the integrity of confidential medical relationships is too high a price to pay for the hypothetical benefits this might bring to the prevailing social order.

The contemporary expansion of ethics in general and medical ethics in particular harbours the danger of increasing scholasticism to the point where not even pressing practical problems are being offered workable solutions. People involved in health care may end up by distrusting the discipline of ethics, thus increasing the improbability of agreement between pragmatists and analysts (1). Even traditionally straightforward practices, such as confidentiality, have been subject to extensive review and analysis which have proved incapable of offering committed stances or unequivocal guidelines for

From Michael H. Kottow, "Medical Confidentiality: An Intransigent and Absolute Obligation," *Journal of Medical Ethics*, vol. 12 (1986). Copyright © 1986 by the *Journal of Medical Ethics*. Reprinted by permission.

action (2, 3). In an effort to illustrate that more stringency is desirable and possible, the status of confidentiality as an exceptionless or absolute commitment is here defended. It should be stated at the outset that I share general scepticism about absolute ethical propositions (4), and that confidentiality is here not defended as an inviolable moral value—a position that would be self-defeating—but as an interpersonal communications strategy that ceases to function unless strictly adhered to. Confidentiality is a brittle arrangement that disintegrates if misdirected in pursuance of other goals and, since it is a necessary component of medical practice, care should be taken to safeguard its integrity.

DEFINING CONFIDENTIALITY

The following definition of confidentiality is used: a situation is confidential when information revealing that harmful acts have been or possibly will be performed is consciously or voluntarily passed from one rationally competent person (confider) to another (confidant) in the understanding that this information shall not be further disclosed without the confider's explicit consent. The harm alluded to may be physical, but moral damage alone may also be the subject matter of a confidential exchange. When this sort of communication occurs in a medical setting it constitutes medical confidentiality.

WHAT IS AT ISSUE IN CONFIDENTIALITY CONFLICTS?

The main ethical controversy around confidentiality concerns the assessment of whether more harm is done by occasionally breaching confidentiality or by always respecting it regardless of the consequences. As long as the physician gathers private information, that is information that only concerns the confider and harbours no element of past or potential harm, confidentiality will concern exclusively the patient and any disclosure would be nothing but a malicious or at the very least gratuitous act of the physician, of little or no moral significance. It seems redundant to discuss other instances of confidentiality than those involving either the possibility of impending harm or testimonial of past injury, for these are the fundamental cases where dilemmas arise and a breach of confidence must seek justification.

Breaching is defended on the ground that the harm announced in the confidence is severe and can possibly only be averted by the confidant's disclosure (5, 6, 7). Exceptionless confidentiality, on the other hand, is upheld by the idea that breaching will relentlessly harm the confider, subjecting her or him to precautionary investigations and constraints of some sort, perhaps even with unavoidable defamatory consequences. The harm purportedly averted is merely potential and all the less likely to occur, the more exorbitant and preposterous the threatener's claims are. After all, excessively vicious menaces may well be uttered by psychotics who are rationally incompetent and therefore not protected by a pledge to confidentiality they can neither honour nor demand. Furthermore, the practice of confidentiality is in itself damaged by breaching because its trustworthiness is disqualified. Ultimately, degrees and probability of harm are so difficult to assess (8), that they will hardly deliver an intersubjectively acceptable argument for or against confidentiality, except for one: breaching confidentiality can not be a significant and enduring contribution against harmful actions, for these are no more than potential, whereas the damages caused to the confidant, to the practice of confidentiality and to the honesty of clinical relationships are unavoidable.

Perhaps less elusive is the conflict of rights—and their correlative obligations—which ensue in confidential situations. Confidentiality is an agreement bound by the principle of fairness (9); it gives the confider the right to expect discretion whereas the confidant has the right to hear the truth, but also the obligation to ensure guardianship of the information received. It could be argued against this right that past victims might be vindicated or potential ones helped by divulging confidential information that seems critical, and that these victims also have a right, namely to vindication or protection. In order for the victim's right to prevail, the confider must involuntarily forfeit her or his right to secrecy, which the confidant will forcefully violate by divulging information against the confider's will. This forfeiture of the confider's right can only occur subsequently to the confidence, for it is triggered by the contents of the confider's disclosure. To avoid the risk of losing the right to secrecy, confiders would have to confide falsely or not at all, a strategy that would erode their legitimate and initially granted right to be impunibly outspoken, distort or reduce confidentiality to lies and irrelevancies, and destroy both the confidant's right to hear the truth and the institution of confidentiality.

MEDICAL CONFIDENTIALITY

Physicians would appear to be under the *prima facie* obligation to respect the right to secrecy, but also to abide by the right of potential victims to be protected. In cases involving moral conflict they must necessarily override one of these rights. Infringing certain rights for the sake of other rights may be justifiable, but it leaves a sediment of negative feelings of regret, shame or guilt (10, 11). It is an unhealthy and paralysing notion to know that the relationship one enters into with patients may unexpectedly turn into a situation of conflict, infringement of rights, and guilt. This guilt may be compounded by the awareness that breaching relates to a family of dubious practices that misuse information obtained by resorting to deception or even duress. Of course, confidentiality is enacted in the unfettered environment of medical encounters, but its breaching infringes the rights of the confiders, harms them, and abrades confidentiality as an institution, all this in the name of elusive values and hard-to-specify protective and vindicative functions.

In the case where a physician believes the patient's exorbitant threats and alerts the police, a morally questionable principle becomes involved. The patient has sought the clinical encounter and proffered information on the understanding that this is necessary for an efficient therapy and also that the relationship with the physician is protected by a mantle of confidentiality. Confidence is offered and accepted in medical acts, and known to be an indispensable component of the clinical encounter, thus enticing the patient to deliver unbiased, unfiltered, uncensored and sincerely presented information (12).

Consequently, it appears contradictory and perverse first to offer confidentiality as an enticement to sincerity, only subsequently to breach it because the information elicited is so terrible it cannot remain unpublicised. Confidence is understood as an unconditional offer, otherwise it would not be accepted, and it appears profoundly unfair to disown the initial conditions once the act of confiding has occurred.

Should one decide to introduce exception clauses, it would only be fair to promulgate them beforehand, allowing every potential confider to know what to expect. But officially sanctioned exceptions would have the undesirable side-effect of creating a second-class kind of medicine for those cases where the patient considers it too risky to assume confidentiality. The communication between patient and physician would in these cases be hampered and would thus render the patient's medical care less than optimal.

GATHERING CONFIDENTIAL MATERIAL

The covenant of confidentiality only obtains if information is voluntarily and consciously given. No question of confidence arises unless the relationship involves rational, conscious and free individuals. But subtleties arise in the medical context when incriminating information reaches the physician unintentionally. Does this information fall within the confidence pact in virtue of being part of the clinical encounter? Or does it obey independent rules because it occurred marginally to the intended doctor/patient relationship?

During the clinical encounter a perspicacious physician may find tell-tale signs of matters the patient did not intend to disclose (skin blemishes perhaps caused by alcohol excess, suspiciously pin-point pupils, injection marks). This involuntary information transfer might not seem at first to fall under any confidentiality agreement according to the above presented definition. Nevertheless, it is the product of a conscious interaction between patient and physician. In consulting a doctor, a person implicitly accepts the risk of surrendering more information than intended but at the same time understands herself or himself to be under the protection of confidentiality. Information fortuitously gained within the freely chosen association of the clinical encounter is to be considered confidential and treated in the same way as information voluntarily disclosed by the patient. Everything that happens in the interpersonal relationship of a clinical encounter is confidential.

ARE THERE EXCEPTIONS TO CONFIDENTIALITY?

Exceptions to unrelenting confidentiality (6) have been invoked for the sake of the confider (paternalistic breaching in general and medical consultations as a special case thereof), in the name of potentially endangered innocent others, in the name of institutional or public interests, and less explicitly, in cases where the confidant is potentially in danger.

CONFIDENTIALITY THROUGHOUT TIME

Confidants may consider the potential harm of divulging information they have had in custody eventually to diffuse after the confider's death, so that a posthumous revelation will not be injurious. The contrary position that harm after death is possible is too weak to support obligations to the dead (13). A more convincing approach suggests that posthumous disclosures may be harmful to surviving persons. If the death of a famous politician should prompt a physician to uncover his knowledge about the deceased's homosexual inclination, still living patients of the same physician might register with distaste and fear the possibility that private information about them could eventually be disclosed after they died. This suspicion may well be unsettling and therefore harmful to them, especially if they happen to believe in some form of 'after-life', the quality of which would be polluted by indiscretions occurring after their biological death. Also to be considered are the negative effects a disparaging disclosure might have upon surviving family members as well as groups of individuals with whom the deceased had a commonality of interests. Death does not cancel the obligation of confidentiality which remains of import to all survivors within the radius of interests of the deceased.

PATERNALISTIC BREACHING

A commonly suggested exemption to confidentiality is that some patients' interests might be better served by physicians' indiscretion (14). Harming confiders for their own purported good is like forcing therapeutic decisions on patients for the sake of their health care. Such stern paternalism has nothing to recommend it, for it is generally agreed that autonomous individuals are not to be compelled into undergoing medical procedures they have explicitly rejected. If rationally competent patients refuse a medical procedure that would do them good, the physician is not authorised to insist, let alone proceed. Rationally competent individuals are allowed to take decisions against their own interests and this does not make them irrational, as

some have misleadingly suggested (15). Why, then, should confidentiality function differently? If patients wish certain knowledge to be kept confidential even if this course of action injures their own interests, they are entitled to do so and no one, not even the physician, has the right to breach confidentiality in the name of patients' welfare.

MEDICAL CONSULTATIONS

Multi-professional care seems to offer plausible alibis to breach confidentiality for the sake of the confider (16). It has been argued that patients negotiate confidentiality with their primary-care physician and that if additional professionals are involved in the patient's care they are to report to the confidant physician. This position is discarded by those who believe that patients, in as much as their autonomy is respected, are to re-negotiate—or count upon—confidentiality with every physician involved. Such a line of thought has much to recommend it since every physician/patient encounter may unveil unedited information which the patient is willing to discuss in a certain setting but is reluctant to have brought to the attention of the primary-care physician. Consultations and other expansions of a medical care programme do not serve as an excuse to exchange information about patients against their will. If they did, they would be supporting double morality and possibly double-quality medicine, where primary health-care would have a paternalistic format embedded in trust and confidence whilst secondary and tertiary services would operate in a contractual setting. This would not be acceptable, it being preferable that each act of confidence be

equally and non-transmittably entrenched in all medical encounters.

HARM TO INNOCENT OTHERS

Another major exception invoked against
absolute confidentiality concerns the
aversion of damage to uninvolved and
innocent third parties. These are the oft-
quoted cases of the doctor telling the
bride that her fiancé is homosexual, or
calling the wife because he is treating the
husband for venereal disease. Escalating
examples include informing authorities
about a confider's intention to kill someone, as well as encounters with terrorists
at large.

This postulated exemption to confidentiality is self-defeating. Firstly, if
physicians become known as confidence-
violators, problem-ridden patients will
try to lie, accommodate facts to their
advantage or, if this does not work,
avoid physicians altogether (17). Physicians would then be unable to give optimal advice or treatment to the detriment
of both the reluctant patients and their
threatened environment. It is better to
treat and advise the syphilitic husband
without informing the wife than not
have him come at all for fear of undesired
revelations.

Physicians who believe themselves in
possession of information that must be
disclosed in order to safeguard public
interests are contemplating preventive
action against the putative malefactor.
Like all preventive policies, breaching
confidentiality is difficult to analyse in
terms of costs/benefits: is the danger
real, potential or fictitious? what preventive measure will appear justified? how
much harm may these measures cause
before they lose justification? Since physicians will rarely be instrumental in deciding or carrying out preventive actions,
they have no way of knowing in advance
whether taking the risk of honouring
confidentiality will eventually prove
more or less harmful than breaching it.

If physicians play it safe and commit
frequent breaches of confidentiality they
will unleash overreacting preventive programmes, at the same time progressively
losing credibility as reliable informers.
On the other hand, should they remain
critical and carefully decide each case on
its own merits, they will be equally suspect and unreliable informers, for their
conscientiousness and judgement might
well deviate from what other authorities,
notably the police, consider adequate.

In apparently more delicate cases it
could be argued that physicians might
subject their co-operation with the authorities to some conditions in order to
defuse the dramatic moment. They may
suggest that violence be refrained from,
that their own intervention be kept secret, that the preventive action be dis-
creet. But certainly, if physicians accept
that their confidential relationship with
patients is conditional, they must consequently expect authorities to handle their
own role as informants in a similarly
unpredictable and contingent way. Physicians who breach confidentiality cannot expect to be protected by it just
because they have exchanged the confidant for the confider role. Physicians
who are known to take confidentiality as
a *prima facie* value cannot demand that
the authorities they are serving by disclosing information should honour their
request for discretion. For similar reasons they must expect some patients to
become increasingly inconsiderate or
even vicious. By breaking confidentiality,
physicians are helping sustain a language of dishonesty and they cannot

expect violence-prone patients to refrain from blackmailing, threatening or otherwise molesting them. As a physician, I would be most unsettled if it became a matter of policy that my colleagues violated confidentiality for the public good, for it would leave me defenceless when confronted with a public offender. No amount of promising would help, since physicians would already have a reputation as unpredictable violators of agreements.

Who should control the policy of confidentiality in medicine anyhow? If public interest demands a catalogue of situations where the physician would be under obligation to inform, medicine becomes subaltern to political design and starts down a treacherous path. Should one prefer to leave the management of confidentiality to the physician's conscience and moral judgement, public interest would not be relying on a consistent and trustworthy source of information. Fear of either political misuse or personal arbitrariness should make us wary of opening the doors of confidentiality for the sake of public interest.

What about possible conflicts between the frailties of public figures and the purported interests of society? National leaders from time to time suffer from disabilities due to old age and the question is raised whether the attending medical team are under an obligation to publish full-fledged clinical reports. It must again be brought to mind that the medical team have been commissioned not to safeguard the public interest but to care for the health of this individual who happens to be influential. Consequently, the medical team's duties remain in the clinical realm, not in the political arena. Furthermore, if the leader in question were in such a precarious situation as to

constitute a public danger, his political mismanagement would become obvious to other individuals more qualified to take public decisions and would not require the physicians to play the role of enlightening figures. Observers of the political scene have preferred to suggest constitutional amendments and political measures to cope with this problem, being aware that cajoling physicians out of their commitment to confidentiality is no solution (18).

COMPETING CLAIMS TO CONFIDENTIAL MATERIAL

This issue refers to conflicts arising from individual interests colliding with those of groups or institutions. It differs from those previously discussed in that here physicians do not necessarily engage in active disclosure but restrict themselves to a one-sided co-operation. The emphasis here is not so much on harm being prevented—although this also plays a major role—but on conflicting parties claiming the physician's loyalty.

Company doctors doing routine examinations of employees are under obligation to report even disparaging findings, for their duty is to the commissioning company. By failing to report an epileptic bus driver or a hypertensive pilot, the doctor is deceiving the company and hindering its efforts to secure safe transportation. If, on the contrary, the same bus driver or pilot goes to the private office of a doctor unconnected with his employer, there would be no excuse for unauthorisedly reporting any findings to the company, for the physician is now being commissioned by the individual, not by the institution, to perform a medical act under the mantle of confidentiality. If this results in the bus driver continuing to work under precarious conditions it means that the company has not established an efficient medical service to check its drivers and is negligent. Physicians are to declare themselves explicitly and unmistakably loyal to those who engage their services, for, again, the legitimate claim to confidentiality is in the act of entering an agreement, not in the contents of the confided material.

Not even these competing claims of loyalty can be settled unless a robust and relentless position in favour of exceptionless confidentiality is upheld. If a physician owes loyalty to an institution, he has no right to misuse the confidence of his employer in order to honour any personal desire for confidentiality. Conversely, when physicians are committed to the confidential situations that arise in their consulting rooms, they lack the right to infringe this agreement to the benefit of other interests.

DOES RISK TO THE CONFIDANT JUSTIFY BREACHING?

The situation could arise where the patient's revelations contain threats of harm or disclosure of damage already done directly to the confidant physician, his or her family members or their interests. Can the physician disclaim the obligation to confidentiality in the name of self-defence? If physicians were morally allowed to breach confidentiality in defence of their own interests, it would mean accepting the principle that one can inflict harm upon others for self-interested reasons. It has already been stated that in disclosing confidential information there is no adequate way of comparing amounts of harm inflicted with harm prevented, so it might well occur that a person brought about severe harm to others in an effort to avert a fairly trivial or improbable harm to her or his own interests, comparable to killing a burglar who is running away with some property—perhaps no more than a loaf of bread. Since an unbiased view can hardly be expected from someone who believes his interests to be in jeopardy, legal systems do not tolerate self-administered justice and condemn, albeit with leniency, injuring others in the face of putative menace to self-interests. Physicians may not safeguard their own interests by mishandling patients, so why should they be allowed to cause harm by breaching confidentiality only because they believe or fear their interests to be imperilled?

Although imaginary situations can be concocted that make it awkward to insist on not breaching, the basic attitude should still be to respect confidentiality to the utmost. Admittedly, if the patient's disclosure implies impending harm to the confidant, the moral obligation to the confidential relationship is weakened in its core, but this admission requires a double qualification: firstly, such situations are highly improbable and therefore of little paradigmatic interest; secondly, even if they should obtain, breaching confidentiality should be used as a last, certainly not first, resort to resolve the conflict, precisely because there is no suasive justification for employing confidentiality as a weapon to avert harm.

CONCLUDING REMARKS

Confidentiality is a widely recognised implicit warranty of fairness in clinical situations and thus constitutes a technically and morally essential element of efficient medical care. If breaches of confidentiality occur, they do so necessarily after the communication and therefore retroactively introduce unfairness into the clinical encounter. A situation that is potentially, even if only occasionally, unfair can no longer be described as fair, especially if breaching occurs unpredictably. All possible exceptions to an attitude of unrelenting confidentiality lead to morally untenable situations where harm avoided v harm inflicted is incommensurable, and rights preserved are less convincing than rights eroded. Confidentiality collapses unless strictly adhered to, for even occasional, exceptional or otherwise limited leaks are sufficient to discredit confidentiality into inefficiency.

The clinical encounter is consistently described as a confidential relationship. If this statement is adhered to, there can be no room for violation without making the initial statement untrue. Nor can the description be qualified—'usually confidential'—or made into a conditional—'confidential unless'—statement, for these half-hearted commitments are, from the confider's point of view, as worthless as no guarantee of confidentiality at all. Confidentiality cannot but be, factually and morally, an all or none proposition. It might perhaps be easier to present a plausible defence of conditional confidentiality, but the ethical atmosphere of the clinical encounter, the autonomy of patients and the sovereignty of the medical profession are all better served by making confidentiality an unexceptionable element of medicine.

REFERENCES

1. MacIntyre A. Moral philosophy: what next? In: Hauerwas S, MacIntyre A, eds. *Revisions: changing perspectives in moral philosophy.* Notre Dame/London: University of Notre Dame Press, 1983: 1–15.

2. Thompson I E. The nature of confidentiality. *Journal of medical ethics* 1979; 5: 57–64.

3. Pheby D F H. Changing practice on confidentiality: a cause for concern. *Journal of medical ethics* 1982; 8: 12–18.

4. Anscombe G E M. Modern moral philosophy. In: Anscombe G E M. *Ethics, religion and politics.* Oxford: Blackwell, 1981: 26–42.

5. Walters L. Confidentiality. In: Beauchamp T L, Walters L, eds. *Contemporary issues in bioethics.* Encino/Belmont: Dickenson, 1978: 169–175.

6. *Handbook of medical ethics.* London: British Medical Association 1981.

7. Anonymous. Medical confidentiality [editorial]. *Journal of medical ethics* 1984; 10: 3–4.

8. Carli T. Confidentiality and privileged communication: a psychiatrist's perspective. In: Basson M D, ed. *Ethics, humanism, and medicine.* New York: Liss, 1980: 245–251.

9. Rawls J. *A theory of justice.* Cambridge, Mass: Belknap Press, 1971: 342–350.

10. Melden A I. *Rights and persons.* Oxford: Blackwell, 1977: 47–48.

11. Morris H. The status of rights. *Ethics* 1981; 92: 40–56.

12. Veatch R M. *A theory of medical ethics.* New York: Basic Books, 1981: 184–189.

13. Levenbook B B. Harming someone after his death. *Ethics* 1984; 94: 407–419.

14. Veatch R M. *Case studies in medical ethics.* Cambridge/London: Harvard University Press, 1977: 131–135.

15. Culver C M, Gert B. *Philosophy in medicine.* New York: Oxford, 1983: 26–28.

16. Siegler M. Medical consultations in the context of the physician-patient relationship. In: Agich G J, ed. *Responsibility in health care.* Dordrecht: Reidel, 1982: 141–162.

17. Havard J. Medical confidence. *Journal of medical ethics* 1985; 11: 8–11.

18. Robins R S, Rothschild H. Hidden health disabilities and the presidency: medical management and political consideration. *Perspectives in biology and medicine* 1981; 24: 240–253.

POSTSCRIPT

Are There Limits to Confidentiality?

The decision in *Tarasoff* was widely criticized by lawyers and mental health professionals. Nevertheless, the doctrine that therapists have a duty to protect potential victims has been endorsed by several other state and federal courts, for example, in New Jersey, Nebraska, Indiana, Georgia, Michigan, Washington, and Kansas. In one New Jersey case, a court held a psychiatrist liable for failing to protect a patient's former girlfriend who was killed by the adolescent patient—even though the patient had never expressed any intent to harm her and had only talked about his jealous feelings. However, some courts have limited the duty to protect to known, identifiable victims. A 1986 decision of the Vermont Supreme Court, on the other hand, in a case involving a barn burning, creates liability for property damage as well as for personal injury.

Prosenjit Poddar, the man who killed Tatiana Tarasoff, was convicted of second-degree murder, but the conviction was overturned on appeal because the jury had been incorrectly instructed. Since more than five years had elapsed since the crime, the state decided not to retry Poddar but to release him if he would promise to return to India, which he did. For the aftermath of the decision, see "Protecting Third Parties: A Decade After *Tarasoff*," by Mark J. Mills, Greer Sullivan, and Spencer Eth, *American Journal of Psychiatry* (January 1987); Vanessa Merton, "Confidentiality and the 'Dangerous' Patient: Implications of *Tarasoff* for Psychiatrists and Lawyers," *Emory Law Journal* (vol. 31, 1982); Paul S. Appelbaum, "Tarasoff and the Clinician: Problems in Fulfilling the Duty to Protect," *American Journal of Psychiatry* (April 1985); and Alan A. Stone, "Vermont Adopts Tarasoff: A Real Barn-Burner," *American Journal of Psychiatry* (March 1986). See also Alan R. Felthous, *The Psychotherapist's Duty to Warn or Protect* (Charles C. Thomas, 1989).

A consensus is developing concerning appropriate exceptions to confidentiality in the case of an HIV-infected person who refuses to notify a third party at risk because of sexual contact. In July 1988 the American Medical Association stated that "Ideally, a physician should attempt to persuade the infected party to cease endangering the third party; if persuasion fails, the authorities should be notified; and if the authorities take no action, the physician should notify and counsel the endangered third party." New York State has passed AIDS confidentiality protection legislation that allows for this sort of exception. Two articles addressing this issue are Kenneth E. Labowitz, "Beyond *Tarasoff*: AIDS and the Obligation to Breach Confidentiality," *Saint Louis University Public Law Review* (1990), and Bernard M. Dickens, "Confidentiality and the Duty to Warn," in Lawrence O. Gostin, editor, *AIDS and the Health Care System* (Yale University Press, 1990).

On confidentiality in general, see *Secrets* by Sissela Bok (Pantheon, 1982). See also Robert M. Veatch, *Case Studies in Medical Ethics* (Harvard, 1977), chapter 5; and Louis Everstine et al., "Threats to Confidentiality," *American Psychologist* (September 1980).

ISSUE 9

Is Involuntary Commitment Wrong?

YES: Thomas S. Szasz, from *Ideology and Insanity* (Doubleday, 1970)

NO: Paul Chodoff, from "The Case for Involuntary Hospitalization of the Mentally Ill," *American Journal of Psychiatry* (May 1976)

ISSUE SUMMARY

YES: Psychiatrist Thomas S. Szasz maintains that the detention of persons in mental institutions against their will is a crime against humanity. People are committed not because they are "mentally ill" or "dangerous" but because society wants to control their behavior.

NO: Psychiatrist Paul Chodoff believes that the rights of the mentally ill to be treated are being set aside in the rush to give them their freedom. He favors a return to the use of medical criteria by psychiatrists, albeit with legal safeguards.

In every society, some people behave in odd and nonconforming ways, though what is considered abnormal may vary considerably. Throughout history explanations of why some people are "crazy" or "mad" have varied. The moon was the cause (hence *lunatic*), thought some early people; the devil or spirits did it, thought others. Some of these deviant people were kept in chains and displayed publicly for the amusement of the crowds; others were loaded onto "ships of fools" and set free to wander. Still others were tolerated within their community or even respected because they were thought to have special powers. As early as 1400, in England, a special institution designed to house the outcasts—Bethlehem Royal Hospital, or "Bedlam"—was established. One can only imagine what it was like, since *bedlam* came to mean a place of great confusion and disorder.

In our own times, the most prevalent view is that people whose behavior is strange and often self-destructive are "sick" and need treatment. They are, it is said, "mentally ill." The medical model of deviant behavior developed in the nineteenth century as part of the growth of scientific knowledge, the belief in rationality, and a sense of social responsibility about the helpless. Laws permitting people to be hospitalized in mental institutions against their will are based on the assumption, inherent in the medical model, that the state has a right—even an obligation—to provide treatment for those whose condition has impaired their capacity for rational thought.

The philosophy of an influential group of antipsychiatrists goes against the conventional view. Two of the most prominent— R. D. Laing of Scotland and Thomas S. Szasz of the United States—were themselves trained as psychiatrists. But they reject the notion that there is such a thing as "mental illness"; it is, they say, only a label that society has placed on those whose behavior it rejects, for social, ethical, political, aesthetic, or other reasons.

In the United States, the pendulum has swung back and forth between periods in which involuntary commitment has been relatively easy to accomplish and periods in which its use has been restricted. As psychiatrist Paul S. Appelbaum has put it, "When concern with rapid treatment has been paramount (as in the Progressive Era at the turn of the century), procedures have been streamlined to permit greater physician and family discretion. On the other hand, when concern with civil liberties has been on the ascendance, as in the 1970s, procedures have come more closely to resemble the criminal model." In this model patients have rights of due process, including the right to an attorney and limited duration of stay.

An important limitation on the state's right to commit people to mental institutions was set forth in the 1975 Supreme Court Decision of *Donaldson v. O'Connor*. That case involved Kenneth Donaldson, a forty-five-year-old man whose parents had committed him to a Florida mental hospital fifteen years earlier because they believed he had a "persecution complex." The court ruled that the state cannot constitutionally confine a "nondangerous individual who is capable of surviving safely in freedom by himself or with the help of willing and responsible family members or friends."

The following selections represent two opposing views in this long-standing debate. Thomas S. Szasz cites medical, moral, historical, and literary evidence to show that commitment does not serve the purpose of helping or treating people whose behavior deviates from or threatens prevailing social norms or moral standards. Nor does it protect the rest of society from harm. Paul Chodoff insists that mental illness is not a myth and that those who suffer from it need care and treatment. With appropriate legal safeguards, involuntary commitment can be an effective and moral practice.

YES
Thomas S. Szasz

INVOLUNTARY
MENTAL HOSPITALIZATION:
A CRIME AGAINST HUMANITY

I

For some time now I have maintained that commitment—that is, the detention of persons in mental institutions against their will—is a form of imprisonment;[1] that such deprivation of liberty is contrary to the moral principles embodied in the Declaration of Independence and the Constitution of the United States;[2] and that it is a crass violation of contemporary concepts of fundamental rights.[3] The practice of "sane" men incarcerating their "insane" fellow men in "mental hospitals" can be compared to that of white men enslaving black men. In short, I consider commitment a crime against humanity.

Existing social institutions and practices, especially if honored by prolonged usage, are generally experienced and accepted as good and valuable. For thousands of years slavery was considered a "natural" social arrangement for the securing of human labor; it was sanctioned by public opinion, religious dogma, church, and state;[4] it was abolished a mere one hundred years ago in the United States; and it is still a prevalent social practice in some parts of the world, notably in Africa.[5] Since its origin, approximately three centuries ago, commitment of the insane has enjoyed equally widespread support; physicians, lawyers, and the laity have asserted, as if with a single voice, the therapeutic desirability and social necessity of institutional psychiatry. My claim that commitment is a crime against humanity may thus be countered—as indeed it has been—by maintaining, first, that the practice is beneficial for the mentally ill, and second, that it is necessary for the protection of the mentally healthy members of society.

Illustrative of the first argument is Slovenko's assertion that "Reliance solely on voluntary hospital admission procedures ignores the fact that some persons may desire care and custody but cannot communicate their desire directly."[6] Imprisonment in mental hospitals is here portrayed—by a professor of law!—as a service provided to persons by the state because they "desire" it but do not know how to ask for it. Felix defends involuntary mental hospitalization by asserting simply, "We *do* [his italics] deal with illnesses of the mind."[7]

Illustrative of the second argument is Guttmacher's characterization of my book *Law, Liberty, and Psychiatry* as " . . . a pernicious book . . . certain to produce intolerable and unwarranted anxiety in the families of psychiatric patients."[8] This is an admission of the fact that the families of "psychiatric patients" frequently resort to the use of force in order to control their "loved ones," and that when attention is directed to this practice it creates embarrassment and guilt. On the other hand, Felix simply defines the psychiatrist's duty as the protection of society: "Tomorrow's psychiatrist will be, as is his counterpart today, one of the gatekeepers of his community."[9]

These conventional explanations of the nature and uses of commitment are, however, but culturally accepted justifications for certain quasi-medical forms of social control, exercised especially against individuals and groups whose behavior does not violate criminal laws but threatens established social values.

II

What is the evidence that commitment does not serve the purpose of helping or treating people whose behavior deviates from or threatens prevailing social norms or moral standards; and who, because they inconvenience their families, neighbors, or superiors, may be incriminated as "mentally ill"?

1. *The medical evidence.* Mental illness is a metaphor. If by "disease" we mean a disorder of the physiochemical machinery of the human body, then we can assert that what we call functional mental diseases are not diseases at all.[10] Persons said to be suffering from such disorders are socially deviant or inept, or in conflict with individuals, groups, or institutions. Since they do not suffer from disease, it is impossible to "treat" them for any sickness.

Although the term "mentally ill" is usually applied to persons who do not suffer from bodily disease, it is sometimes applied also to persons who do (for example, to individuals intoxicated with alcohol or other drugs, or to elderly people suffering from degenerative disease of the brain). However, when patients with demonstrable diseases of the brain are involuntarily hospitalized, the primary purpose is to exercise social control over their behavior;[11] treatment of the disease is, at best, a secondary consideration. Frequently, therapy is non-existent, and custodial care is dubbed "treatment."

In short, the commitment of persons suffering from "functional psychoses" serves moral and social, rather than medical and therapeutic, purposes. Hence, even if, as a result of future research, certain conditions now believed to be "functional" mental illnesses were to be shown to be "organic," my argument against involuntary mental hospitalization would remain unaffected.

2. *The moral evidence.* In free societies, the relationship between physician and patient is predicated on the legal presumption that the individual "owns" his body and his personality.[12] The physi-

cian can examine and treat a patient only with his consent; the latter is free to reject treatment (for example, an operation for cancer).[13] After death, "ownership" of the person's body is transferred to his heirs; the physician must obtain permission from the patient's relatives for a postmortem examination. John Stuart Mill explicitly affirmed that " . . . each person is the proper guardian of his own health, whether bodily, or mental and spiritual."[14] Commitment is incompatible with this moral principle.

3. *The historical evidence.* Commitment practices flourished long before there were any mental or psychiatric "treatments" of "mental diseases." Indeed, madness or mental illness was not always a necessary condition for commitment. For example, in the seventeenth century, "children of artisans and other poor inhabitants of Paris up to the age of 25, . . . girls who were debauched or in evident danger of being debauched, . . ." and other "miseqrables" of the community, such as epileptics, people with venereal diseases, and poor people with chronic diseases of all sorts, were all considered fit subjects for confinement in the Hoepital Geqneqral.[15] And, in 1860, when Mrs. Packard was incarcerated for disagreeing with her minister-husband,[16] the commitment laws of the State of Illinois explicitly proclaimed that " . . . married women . . . may be entered or detained in the hospital at the request of the husband of the woman or the guardian. . . . , without the evidence of insanity required in other cases."[17] It is surely no coincidence that this piece of legislation was enacted and enforced at about the same time that Mill published his essay *The Subjection of Women.*[18]

4. *The literary evidence.* Involuntary mental hospitalization plays a significant part in numerous short stories and novels from many countries. In none that I have encountered is commitment portrayed as helpful to the hospitalized person; instead, it is always depicted as an arrangement serving interests antagonistic of those of the so-called patient.[19]

III

The claim that commitment of the "mentally ill" is necessary for the protection of the "mentally healthy" is more difficult to refute, not because it is valid, but because the danger that "mental patients" supposedly pose is of such an extremely vague nature.

1. *The medical evidence.* The same reasoning applies as earlier: If "mental illness" is not a disease, there is no medical justification for protection from disease. Hence, the analogy between mental illness and contagious disease falls to the ground: The justification for isolating or otherwise constraining patients with tuberculosis or typhoid fever cannot be extended to patients with "mental illness."

Moreover, because the accepted contemporary psychiatric view of mental illness fails to distinguish between illness as a biological condition and as a social role,[20] it is not only false, but also dangerously misleading, especially if used to justify social action. In this view, regardless of its "causes"—anatomical, genetic, chemical, psychological, or social—mental illness has "objective existence." A person either has or has not a mental illness; he is either mentally sick or mentally healthy. Even if a person is cast in the role of mental patient against his will, his "mental illness" exists "objectively"; and even if, as in the cases of the Very

Important Person, he is never treated as a mental patient, his "mental illness" still exists "objectively"—apart from the activities of the psychiatrist.[21]

The upshot is that the term "mental illness" is perfectly suited for mystification: It disregards the crucial question of whether the individual assumes the role of mental patient voluntarily, and hence wishes to engage in some sort of interaction with the psychiatrist; or whether he is cast in that role against his will, and hence is opposed to such a relationship. This obscurity is then usually employed strategically, either by the subject himself to advance *his* interests, or by the subject's adversaries to advance *their* interests.

In contrast to this view, I maintain, first, that the involuntarily hospitalized mental patient is, by definition, the occupant of an ascribed role; and, second, that the "mental disease" of such a person—unless the use of this term is restricted to demonstrable lesions or malfunctions of the brain—is always the product of interaction between psychiatrist and patient.

2. *The moral evidence.* The crucial ingredient in involuntary mental hospitalization is coercion. Since coercion is the exercise of power, it is always a moral and political act. Accordingly, regardless of its medical justification, commitment is primarily a moral and political phenomenon—just as, regardless of its anthropological and economic justifications, slavery was primarily a moral and political phenomenon.

Although psychiatric methods of coercion are indisputably useful for those who enjoy them, they are clearly not indispensable for dealing with the problems that so-called mental patients pose for those about them. If an individual threatens others by virtue of his beliefs or actions, he could be dealt with by methods other than "medical"; if his conduct is ethically offensive, moral sanctions against him might be appropriate; if forbidden by law, legal sanctions might be appropriate. In my opinion, both informal, moral sanctions, such as social ostracism or divorce, and formal, judicial sanctions, such as fine and imprisonment, are more dignified and less injurious to the human spirit than the quasi-medical psychiatric sanction of involuntary mental hospitalization.[22]

3. *The historical evidence.* To be sure, confinement of so-called mentally ill persons does protect the community from certain problems. If it didn't, the arrangement would not have come into being and would not have persisted. However, the question we ought to ask is not *whether* commitment protects the community from "dangerous mental patients," but rather from precisely *what danger* it protects and by *what means*? In what way were prostitutes or vagrants dangerous in seventeenth-century Paris? Or married women in nineteenth-century Illinois?

It is significant, moreover, that there is hardly a prominent person who, during the past fifty years or so, has not been diagnosed by a psychiatrist as suffering from some type of "mental illness." Barry Goldwater was called a "paranoid schizophrenic";[23] Whittaker Chambers, a "psychopathic personality";[24] Woodrow Wilson, a "neurotic" frequently "very close to psychosis";[25] and Jesus, "a born degenerate" with a "fixed delusional system," and a "paranoid" with a "clinical picture [so typical] that it is hardly conceivable that people can even question the accuracy of the diagnosis."[26] The list is endless.

Sometimes, psychiatrists declare the same person sane *and* insane, depending on the political dictates of their superiors and the social demand of the moment. Before his trial and execution, Adolph Eichmann was examined by several psychiatrists, all of whom declared him to be normal; after he was put to death, "medical evidence" of his insanity was released and widely circulated.

According to Hannah Arendt, "Half a dozen psychiatrists had certified him [Eichmann] as 'normal.' " One psychiatrist asserted, " . . . his whole psychological outlook, his attitude toward his wife and children, mother and father, sisters and friends, was 'not only normal but most desirable.' . . ." And the minister who regularly visited him in prison declared that Eichmann was "a man with very positive ideas."[27] After Eichmann was executed, Gideon Hausner, the Attorney General of Israel, who had prosecuted him, disclosed in an article in *The Saturday Evening Post* that psychiatrists diagnosed Eichmann as " 'a man obsessed with a dangerous and insatiable urge to kill,' 'a perverted, sadistic personality.' "[28]

Whether or not men like those mentioned above are considered "dangerous" depends on the observer's religious beliefs, political convictions, and social situation. Furthermore, the "dangerousness" of such persons—whatever we may think of them—is not analogous to that of a person with tuberculosis or typhoid fever; nor would rendering such a person "non-dangerous" be comparable to rendering a patient with a contagious disease noninfectious.

In short, I hold—and I submit that the historical evidence bears me out—that people are committed to mental hospitals neither because they are "dangerous," nor because they are "mentally ill," but rather because they are society's scapegoats, whose persecution is justified by psychiatric propaganda and rhetoric.[29]

4. *The literary evidence.* No one contests that involuntary mental hospitalization of the so-called dangerously insane "protects" the community. Disagreement centers on the nature of the threat facing society, and on the methods of legitimacy of the protection it employs. In this connection, we may recall that slavery, too, "protected" the community: it freed the slaveowners from manual labor. Commitment likewise shields the non-hospitalized members of society: first, from having to accommodate themselves to the annoying or idiosyncratic demands of certain members of the community who have not violated any criminal statutes; and, second, from having to prosecute, try, convict, and punish members of the community who have broken the law but who either might not be convicted in court, or, if they would be, might not be restrained as effectively or as long in prison as in a mental hospital. The literary evidence cited earlier fully supports this interpretation of the function of involuntary mental hospitalization.

IV

I have suggested that commitment constitutes a social arrangement whereby one part of society secures certain advantages for itself at the expense of another part. To do so, the oppressors must possess an ideology to justify their aims and actions; and they must be able to enlist the police power of the state to impose their will on the oppressed members. What makes such an arrangement a "crime against humanity"? It may be argued that the use of state power is legitimate when law-abiding citizens punish lawbreakers. What is the difference between this use of state power and its use in commitment?

In the first place, the difference between committing the "insane" and imprisoning the "criminal" is the same as that between the rule of man and the rule of law:[30] whereas the "insane" are subjected to the coercive controls of the state because persons more powerful than they have labeled them as "psychotic," "criminals" are subjected to such controls because they have violated legal rules applicable equally to all.

The second difference between these two proceedings lies in their professed aims. The principal purpose of imprisoning criminals is to protect the liberties of the law-abiding members of society.[31] Since the individual subject to commitment is not considered a threat to liberty in the same way as the accused criminal is (if he were, he would be prosecuted), his removal from society cannot be justified on the same grounds. Justification for commitment must thus rest on its therapeutic promise and potential: it will help restore the "patient" to "mental health." But if this can be accomplished only at the cost of robbing the individual of liberty, "involuntary mental hospitalization" becomes only a verbal camouflage for what is, in effect, punishment. This "therapeutic" punishment differs, however, from traditional judicial punishment, in that the accused criminal enjoys a rich panoply of constitutional protections against false accusation and oppressive prosecution, whereas the accused mental patient is deprived of these protections.[32]

NOTES

1. Szasz, T.S.: "Commitment of the mentally ill: Treatment or social restraint?" *J. Nerv. & Ment. Dis.* 125:293-307 (Apr.-June) 1957.

2. Szasz, T.S.: *Law, Liberty, and Psychiatry: An Inquiry into the Social Uses of Mental Health Practices* (New York: Macmillan, 1963), pp. 149-90.

3. *Ibid.*, pp. 223-55.

4. Davis, D.B.: *The Problem of Slavery in Western Culture* (Ithaca, N.Y.: Cornell University Press, 1966).

5. See Cohen, R.: "Slavery in Africa." *Trans-Action* 4:44-56 (Jan.-Feb.), 1967; Tobin, R.L.: "Slavery still plagues the earth." *Saturday Review,* May 6, 1967, pp. 24-25.

6. Slovenko, R.: "The psychiatric patient, liberty, and the law." *Amer. J. Psychiatry,* 121:534-39 (Dec.), 1964, p. 536.

7. Felix, R.H.: "The image of the psychiatrist: Past, present, and future." *Amer. J. Psychiatry,* 121:318-22 (Oct.), 1964, p. 320.

8. Guttmacher, M.S.: "Critique of views of Thomas Szasz on legal psychiatry." *AMA Arch. Gen. Psychiatry,* 10:238-45 (March), 1964, p. 244.

9. Felix, op. cit., p. 231.

10. See Szasz, T.S.: "The myth of mental illness." This volume [original source] pp. 12-24; *The Myth of Mental Illness: Foundations of a Theory of Personal Conduct* (New York: Hoeber-Harper, 1961); "Mental illness is a myth." *The New York Times Magazine,* June 12, 1966, pp. 30 and 90-92.

11. See, for example, Noyes, A.P.: *Modern Clinical Psychiatry,* 4th ed. (Philadelphia: Saunders, 1956), p. 278.

12. Szasz, T.S.: "The ethics of birth control; or, who owns your body?" *The Humanist,* 20:332-36 (Nov.-Dec.) 1960.

13. Hirsch, B.D.: "Informed consent to treatment," in Averbach, A. and Belli, M.M., eds., *Tort and Medical Yearbook* (Indianapolis: Bobbs-Merrill, 1961), Vol. I, pp. 631-38.

14. Mill, J.S.: *On Liberty* [1859] (Chicago: Regnery, 1955), p. 18.

15. Rosen, G.: "Social attitudes to irrationality and madness in 17th and 18th century Europe." *J. Hist. Med. & Allied Sciences,* 18:220-40 (1963), p. 223.

16. Packard, E.W.P.: *Modern Persecution, or Insane Asylums Unveiled,* 2 Vols. (Hartford: Case, Lockwood, and Brainard, 1873).

17. Illinois Statute Book, Sessions Laws 15, Section 10, 1851. Quoted in Packard, E.P.W.: *The Prisoner's Hidden Life* (Chicago: published by the author, 1868), p. 37.

18. Mill, J.S.: *The Subjection of Women* [1869] (London: Dent, 1965).

19. See, for example, Chekhov, A.P.: *Ward No. 6,* [1892], in *Seven Short Novels by Chekhov* (New

York: Bantam Books, 1963), pp. 106-57; De Assis, M.: *The Psychiatrist* [1881-82], in De Assis, M., *The Psychiatrist and Other Stories* (Berkeley and Los Angeles: University of California Press, 1963), pp. 1-45; London, J.: *The Iron Heel* [1907] (New York: Sagamore Press, 1957); Porter, K.A.: *Noon Wine* [1937], in Porter, K.A., *Pale Horse, Pale Rider: Three Short Novels* (New York: Signet, 1965), pp. 62-112; Kesey, K.: *One Flew Over the Cuckoo's Nest* (New York: Viking, 1962); Tarsis, V.: *Ward 7: An Autobiographical Novel* (London and Glasgow: Collins and Harvill, 1965).

20. See Szasz, T.S.: "Alcoholism: A socio-ethical perspective." *Western Medicine*, 7:15-21 (Dec.) 1966.

21. See, for example, Rogow, A.A.: *James Forrestal: A Study of Personality, Politics, and Policy* (New York: Macmillan, 1964); for a detailed criticism of this view, see Szasz, T.S.: "Psychiatric classification as a strategy of personal constraint." This volume [original source] pp. 190-217.

22. Szasz, T.S.: *Psychiatric Justice* (New York: Macmillan, 1965).

23. "The Unconscious of a Conservative: A Special Issue on the Mind of Barry Goldwater." *Fact*, Sept.-Oct. 1964.

24. Zeligs, M.A.: *Friendship and Fratricide: An Analysis of Whittaker Chambers and Alger Hiss* (New York: Viking, 1967).

25. Freud, S., and Bullitt, W.C.: *Thomas Woodrow Wilson: A Psychological Study* (Boston: Houghton Mifflin, 1967).

26. Quoted in Schweitzer, A.: *The Psychiatric Study of Jesus* [1913] transl. by Charles R. Joy (Boston: Beacon Press, 1956), pp. 37, 40-41.

27. Arendt, H.: *Eichmann in Jerusalem: A Report on the Banality of Evil* (New York: Viking, 1963), p. 22.

28. *Ibid.*, pp. 22-23.

29. For a full articulation and documentation of this thesis, see Szasz, T.S.: *The Manufacture of Madness: A Comparative Study of the Inquisition and the Mental Health Movement* (New York: Harper & Row, 1970).

30. Hayek, F.A.: *The Constitution of Liberty* (Chicago: University of Chicago Press, 1960), especially pp. 162-92.

31. Mabbott, J.D.: "Punishment" [1939], in Olafson, F.A., ed., *Justice and Social Policy: A Collection of Essays* (Englewood Cliffs, N.J.: Prentice-Hall, 1961), pp. 39-54.

32. For documentation, see Szasz, T.S.: *Law, Liberty, and Psychiatry: An Inquiry into the Social Uses of Mental Health Practices* (New York: Macmillan, 1963); *Psychiatric Justice* (New York: Macmillan, 1965).

NO

Paul Chodoff

THE CASE FOR INVOLUNTARY
HOSPITALIZATION
OF THE MENTALLY ILL

I will begin this paper with a series of vignettes designed to illustrate graphically the question that is my focus: under what conditions, if any, does society have the right to apply coercion to an individual to hospitalize him against his will, by reason of mental illness?

Case 1. A woman in her mid 50s, with no previous overt behavioral difficulties, comes to believe that she is worthless and insignificant. She is completely preoccupied with her guilt and is increasingly unavailable for the ordinary demands of life. She eats very little because of her conviction that the food should go to others whose need is greater than hers, and her physical condition progressively deteriorates. Although she will talk to others about herself, she insists that she is not sick, only bad. She refuses medication, and when hospitalization is suggested she also refuses that on the grounds that she would be taking up space that otherwise could be occupied by those who merit treatment more than she.

Case 2. For the past 6 years the behavior of a 42-year-old woman has been disturbed for periods of 3 months or longer. After recovery from her most recent episode she has been at home, functioning at a borderline level. A month ago she again started to withdraw from her environment. She pays increasingly less attention to her bodily needs, talks very little, and does not respond to questions or attention from those about her. She lapses into a mute state and lies in her bed in a totally passive fashion. She does not respond to other people, does not eat, and does not void. When her arm is raised from the bed it remains for several minutes in the position in which it is left. Her medical history and a physical examination reveal no evidence of primary physical illness.

Case 3. A man with a history of alcoholism has been on a binge for several weeks. He remains at home doing little else than drinking. He eats very little. He becomes tremulous and misinterprets spots on the wall as animals about to

From Paul Chodoff, "The Case for Involuntary Hospitalization of the Mentally Ill," *American Journal of Psychiatry,* vol. 133, no. 5 (May 1976). Copyright © 1976 by the American Psychiatric Association. Reprinted by permission.

attack him, and he complains of "creeping" sensations in his body, which he attributes to infestation by insects. He does not seek help voluntarily, insists there is nothing wrong with him, and despite his wife's entreaties he continues to drink.

Case 4. Passersby and station personnel observe that a young woman has been spending several days at Union Station in Washington, D.C. Her behavior appears strange to others. She is finally befriended by a newspaper reporter who becomes aware that her perception of her situation is profoundly unrealistic and that she is, in fact, delusional. He persuades her to accompany him to St. Elizabeth's Hospital, where she is examined by a psychiatrist who recommends admission. She refuses hospitalization and the psychiatrist allows her to leave. She returns to Union Station. A few days later she is found dead, murdered, on one of the surrounding streets.

Case 5. A government attorney in his late 30s begins to display pressured speech and hyperactivity. He is too busy to sleep and eats very little. He talks rapidly, becomes irritable when interrupted, and makes phone calls all over the country in furtherance of his political ambitions, which are to begin a campaign for the Presidency of the United States. He makes many purchases, some very expensive, thus running through a great deal of money. He is rude and tactless to his friends, who are offended by his behavior, and his job is in jeopardy. In spite of his wife's pleas he insists that he does not have the time to seek or accept treatment, and he refuses hospitalization. This is not the first such disturbance for this individual; in fact, very similar episodes have been occurring at roughly 2-year intervals since he was 18 years old.

Case 6. Passersby in a campus area observe two young women standing together, staring at each other, for over an hour. Their behavior attracts attention, and eventually the police take the pair to a nearby precinct station for questioning. They refuse to answer questions and sit mutely, staring into space. The police request some type of psychiatric examination but are informed by the city attorney's office that state law (Michigan) allows persons to be held for observation only if they appear obviously dangerous to themselves or others. In this case, since the women do not seem homicidal or suicidal, they do not qualify for observation and are released.

Less than 30 hours later the two women are found on the floor of their campus apartment, screaming and writhing in pain with their clothes ablaze from a self-made pyre. One woman recovers; the other dies. There is no conclusive evidence that drugs were involved (1).

Most, if not all, people would agree that the behavior described in these vignettes deviates significantly from even elastic definitions of normality. However, it is clear that there would not be a similar consensus on how to react to this kind of behavior and that there is a considerable and increasing ferment about what attitude the organized elements of our society should take toward such individuals. Everyone has a stake in this important issue, but the debate about it takes place principally among psychiatrists, lawyers, the courts, and law enforcement agencies.

Points of view about the question of involuntary hospitalization fall into the following three principal groups: the "abolitionists," medical model psychiatrists, and civil liberties lawyers.

THE ABOLITIONISTS

Those holding this position would assert that in none of the cases I have described should involuntary hospitalization be a viable option because, quite simply, it should never be resorted to under any circumstances. As Szasz (2) has put it, "we should value liberty more highly than mental health no matter how defined" and "no one should be deprived of his freedom for the sake of his mental health." Ennis (3) has said that the goal "is nothing less than the abolition of involuntary hospitalization."

Prominent among the abolitionists are the "anti-psychiatrists," who, somewhat surprisingly, count in their ranks a number of well-known psychiatrists. For them mental illness simply does not exist in the field of psychiatry (4). They reject entirely the medical model of mental illness and insist that acceptance of it relies on a fiction accepted jointly by the state and by psychiatrists as a device for exerting social control over annoying or unconventional people. The anti-psychiatrists hold that these people ought to be afforded the dignity of being held responsible for their behavior and required to accept its consequences. In addition, some members of this group believe that the phenomena of "mental illness" often represent essentially a tortured protest against the insanities of an irrational society (5). They maintain that society should not be encouraged in its oppressive course by affixing a pejorative label to its victims.

Among the abolitionists are some civil liberties lawyers who both assert their passionate support of the magisterial importance of individual liberty and react with repugnance and impatience to what they see as the abuses of psychiatric practice in this field—the commitment of some individuals for flimsy and possibly self-serving reasons and their inhuman warehousing in penal institutions wrongly called "hospitals."

The abolitionists do not oppose psychiatric treatment when it is conducted with the agreement of those being treated. I have no doubt that they would try to gain the consent of the individuals described earlier to undergo treatment, including hospitalization. The psychiatrists in this group would be very likely to confine their treatment methods to psychotherapeutic efforts to influence the aberrant behavior. They would be unlikely to use drugs and would certainly eschew such somatic therapies as ECT. If efforts to enlist voluntary compliance with treatment failed, the abolitionists would not employ any means of coercion. Instead, they would step aside and allow social, legal, and community sanctions to take their course. If a human being should be jailed or a human life lost as a result of this attitude, they would accept it as a necessary evil to be tolerated in order to avoid the greater evil of unjustified loss of liberty for others (6).

THE MEDICAL MODEL PSYCHIATRISTS

I use this admittedly awkward and not entirely accurate label to designate the position of a substantial number of psychiatrists. They believe that mental illness is a meaningful concept and that under certain conditions its existence justifies the state's exercise, under the doctrine of parens patriae, of its right and obligation to arrange for the hospitalization of the sick individual even though coercion is involved and he is deprived of his liberty. I believe that these psychiatrists would recommend involuntary hospitalization for all six of the patients described earlier.

The Medical Model

There was a time, before they were considered to be ill, when individuals who displayed the kind of behavior I described earlier were put in "ships of fools" to wander the seas or were left to the mercies, sometimes tender but often savage, of uncomprehending communities that regarded them as either possessed or bad. During the Enlightenment and the early nineteenth century, however, these individuals gradually came to be regarded as sick people to be included under the humane and caring umbrella of the Judeo-Christian attitude toward illness. This attitude, which may have reached its height during the era of moral treatment in the early nineteenth century, has had unexpected and ambiguous consequences. It became overextended and partially perverted, and these excesses led to the reaction that is so strong a current in today's attitude toward mental illness.

However, reaction itself can go too far, and I believe that this is already happening. Witness the disastrous consequences of the precipitate dehospitalization that is occurring all over the country. To remove the protective mantle of illness from these disturbed people is to expose them, their families, and their communities to consequences that are certainly maladaptive and possibly irreparable. Are we really acting in accordance with their best interests when we allow them to "die with their rights on" (1) or when we condemn them to a "preservation of liberty which is actually so destructive as to constitute another form of imprisonment" (7)? Will they not suffer "if [a] liberty they cannot enjoy is made superior to a health that must sometimes be forced on them" (8)?

Many of those who reject the medical model out of hand as inapplicable to so-called "mental illness" have tended to oversimplify its meaning and have, in fact, equated it almost entirely with organic disease. It is necessary to recognize that it is a complex concept and that there is a lack of agreement about its meaning. Sophisticated definitions of the medical model do not require only the demonstration of unequivocal organic pathology. A broader formulation, put forward by sociologists and deriving largely from Talcott Parsons' description of the sick role (9), extends the domain of illness to encompass certain forms of social deviance as well as biological disorders. According to this definition, the medical model is characterized not only by organicity but also by being negatively valued by society, by "nonvoluntariness," thus exempting its exemplars from blame, and by the understanding that physicians are the technically competent experts to deal with its effects (10).

Except for the question of organic disease, the patients I described earlier conform well to this broader conception of the medical model. They are all suffering both emotionally and physically, they are incapable by an effort of will of stopping or changing their destructive behavior, and those around them consider them to be in an undesirable sick state and to require medical attention.

Categorizing the behavior of these patients as involuntary may be criticized as evidence of an intolerably paternalistic and antitherapeutic attitude that fosters the very failure to take responsibility for their lives and behavior that the therapist should uncover rather than encourage.

However, it must also be acknowledged that these severely ill people are not capable at a conscious level of deciding what is best for themselves and that in order to help them examine their behavior and motivation, it is necessary that they be alive and available for treatment. Their verbal message that they will not accept treatment may at the same time be conveying other more covert messages—that they are desperate and want help even though they cannot ask for it (11).

Although organic pathology may not be the only determinant of the medical model, it is of course an important one and it should not be avoided in any discussion of mental illness. There would be no question that the previously described patient with delirium tremens is suffering from a toxic form of brain disease. There are a significant number of other patients who require involuntary hospitalization because of organic brain syndrome due to various causes. Among those who are not overtly organically ill, most of the candidates for involuntary hospitalization suffer from schizophrenia or one of the major affective disorders. A growing and increasingly impressive body of evidence points to the presence of an important genetic-biological factor in these conditions; thus, many of them qualify on these grounds as illnesses.

Despite the revisionist efforts of the anti-psychiatrists, mental illness *does* exist. It does not by any means include all of the people being treated by psychiatrists (or by nonpsychiatrist physicians), but it does encompass those few desperately sick people for whom involuntary commitment must be considered. In the words of a recent article, "The problem is that mental illness is not a myth. It is not some palpable falsehood propagated among the populace by power-mad psy-chiatrists, but a cruel and bitter reality that has been with the human race since antiquity" (12, p. 1483).

Criteria for Involuntary Hospitalization

Procedures for involuntary hospitalization should be instituted for individuals who require care and treatment because of diagnosable mental illness that produces symptoms, including marked impairment in judgment, that disrupt their intrapsychic and interpersonal functioning. All three of these criteria must be met before involuntary hospitalization can be instituted.

1. *Mental illness.* This concept has already been discussed, but it should be repeated that only a belief in the existence of illness justifies involuntary commitment. It is a fundamental assumption that makes aberrant behavior a medical matter and its care the concern of physicians.

2. *Disruption of functioning.* This involves combinations of serious and often obvious disturbances that are both intrapsychic (for example, the suffering of severe depression) and interpersonal (for example, withdrawal from others because of depression). It does not include minor peccadilloes or eccentricities. Furthermore, the behavior in question must represent symptoms of the mental illness from which the patient is suffering. Among these symptoms are actions that are imminently or potentially dangerous in a physical sense to self or others, as well as other manifestations of mental illness such as those in the cases I have described. This is not to ignore dangerousness as a criterion for commitment but rather to put it in its proper place as one of a number of symptoms of the illness. A further manifestation of the illness, and indeed, the one that makes

involuntary rather than voluntary hospitalization necessary, is impairment of the patient's judgment to such a degree that he is unable to consider his condition and make decisions about it in his own interests.

3. *Need for care and treatment.* The goal of physicians is to treat and cure their patients; however, sometimes they can only ameliorate the suffering of their patients and sometimes all they can offer is care. It is not possible to predict whether someone will respond to treatment; nevertheless, the need for treatment and the availability of facilities to carry it out constitute essential preconditions that must be met to justify requiring anyone to give up his freedom. If mental hospital patients have a right to treatment, then psychiatrists have a right to ask for treatability as a front-door as well as a backdoor criterion for commitment (7). All of the six individuals I described earlier could have been treated with a reasonable expectation of returning to a more normal state of functioning.

I believe that the objections to this formulation can be summarized as follows.

1. The whole structure founders for those who maintain that mental illness is a fiction.

2. These criteria are also untenable to those who hold liberty to be such a supreme value that the presence of mental illness per se does not constitute justification for depriving an individual of his freedom; only when such illness is manifested by clearly dangerous behavior may commitment be considered. For reasons to be discussed later, I agree with those psychiatrists (13, 14) who do not believe that dangerousness should be elevated to primacy above other manifestations of mental illness as a sine qua non for involuntary hospitalization.

3. The medical model criteria are "soft" and subjective and depend on the fallible judgment of psychiatrists. This is a valid objection. There is no reliable blood test for schizophrenia and no method for injecting grey cells into psychiatrists. A relatively small number of cases will always fall within a grey area that will be difficult to judge. In those extreme cases in which the question of commitment arises, competent and ethical psychiatrists should be able to use these criteria without doing violence to individual liberties and with the expectation of good results. Furthermore, the possible "fuzziness" of some aspects of the medical model approach is certainly no greater than that of the supposedly "objective" criteria for dangerousness, and there is little reason to believe that lawyers and judges are any less fallible than psychiatrists.

4. Commitment procedures in the hands of psychiatrists are subject to intolerable abuses. Here, as Peszke said, "It is imperative that we differentiate between the principle of the process of civil commitment and the practice itself" (13, p. 825). Abuses can contaminate both the medical and the dangerousness approaches, and I believe that the abuses stemming from the abolitionist view of no commitment at all are even greater. Measures to abate abuses of the medical approach include judicial review and the abandonment of indeterminate commitment. In the course of commitment proceedings and thereafter, patients should have access to competent and compassionate legal counsel. However, this latter safeguard may itself be subject to abuse if the legal counsel acts solely in the adversary tradition and undertakes

to carry out the patient's wishes even when they may be destructive.

Comment

The criteria and procedures outlined will apply most appropriately to initial episodes and recurrent attacks of mental illness. To put it simply, it is necessary to find a way to satisfy legal and humanitarian considerations and yet allow psychiatrists access to initially or acutely ill patients in order to do the best they can for them. However, there are some involuntary patients who have received adequate and active treatment but have not responded satisfactorily. An irreducible minimum of such cases, principally among those with brain disorders and process schizophrenia, will not improve sufficiently to be able to adapt to even a tolerant society.

The decision of what to do at this point is not an easy one, and it should certainly not be in the hands of psychiatrists alone. With some justification they can state that they have been given the thankless job of caring, often with inadequate facilities, for badly damaged people and that they are now being subjected to criticism for keeping these patients locked up. No one really knows what to do with these patients. It may be that when treatment has failed they exchange their sick role for what has been called the impaired role (15), which implies a permanent negative evaluation of them coupled with a somewhat less benign societal attitude. At this point, perhaps a case can be made for giving greater importance to the criteria for dangerousness and releasing such patients if they do not pose a threat to others. However, I do not believe that the release into the community of these severely malfunctioning individuals will serve their inter-

ests even though it may satisfy formal notions of right and wrong.

It should be emphasized that the number of individuals for whom involuntary commitment must be considered is small (although, under the influence of current pressures, it may be smaller than it should be). Even severe mental illness can often be handled by securing the cooperation of the patient, and certainly one of the favorable effects of the current ferment has been to encourage such efforts. However, the distinction between voluntary and involuntary hospitalization is sometimes more formal than meaningful. How "voluntary" are the actions of an individual who is being buffeted by the threats, entreaties, and tears of his family?

I believe, however, that we are at a point (at least in some jurisdictions) where, having rebounded from an era in which involuntary commitment was too easy and employed too often, we are now entering one in which it is becoming very difficult to commit anyone, even in urgent cases. Faced with the moral obloquy that has come to pervade the atmosphere in which the decision to involuntarily hospitalize is considered, some psychiatrists, especially younger ones, have become, as Stone (16) put it, "soft as grapes," when faced with the prospect of committing anyone under any circumstances. . . .

DISCUSSION

It is obvious that it is good to be at liberty and that it is good to be free from the consequences of disabling and dehumanizing illness. Sometimes these two values are incompatible, and in the heat of the passions that are often aroused by opposing views of right and wrong, the partisans of each view may tend to minimize the importance of the other. Both sides can present their horror stories—the psychiatrists, their dead victims of the failure of the involuntary hospitalization process, and the lawyers, their Donaldsons. There is a real danger that instead of acknowledging the difficulty of the problem, the two camps will become polarized, with a consequent rush toward extreme and untenable solutions rather than working toward reasonable ones.

The path taken by those whom I have labeled the abolitionists is an example of the barren results that ensue when an absolute solution is imposed on a complex problem. There are human beings who will suffer greatly if the abolitionists succeed in elevating an abstract principle into an unbreakable law with no exceptions. I find myself oppressed and repelled by their position, which seems to stem from an ideological rigidity which ignores that element of the contingent immanent in the structure of human existence. It is devoid of compassion.

The positions of those who espouse the medical model and the dangerousness approaches to commitment are, one hopes, not completely irreconcilable. To some extent these differences are a result of the vantage points from which lawyers and psychiatrists view mental illness and commitment. The lawyers see and are concerned with the failures and abuses of the process. Furthermore, as a result of their training, they tend to apply principles to classes of people rather than to take each instance as unique. The psychiatrists, on the other hand, are required to deal practically with the singular needs of individuals. They approach the problem from a clinical rather than a deductive stance. As physicians, they want to be in a position to take care of and to help suffering people whom they regard as sick patients. They sometimes become impatient with the rules that prevent them from doing this.

I believe we are now witnessing a pendular swing in which the rights of the mentally ill to be treated and protected are being set aside in the rush to give them their freedom at whatever cost. But is freedom defined only by the absence of external constraints? Internal physiological or psychological processes can contribute to a throttling of the spirit that is as painful as any applied from the outside. The "wild" manic individual without his lithium, the panicky hallucinator without his injection of fluphenazine hydrochloride and the understanding support of a concerned staff, the sodden alcoholic—are they free? Sometimes, as Woody Guthrie said, "Freedom means no place to go."

Today the civil liberties lawyers are in the ascendancy and the psychiatrists on the defensive to a degree that is harmful to individual needs and the public welfare. Redress and a more balanced position will not come from further extension of the dangerousness doctrine. I favor a return to the use of medical criteria by psychiatrists—psychiatrists, however, who have been chastened by the buffeting they have received and are quite willing to go along with even strict legal safeguards as long as they are constructive and not tyrannical.

REFERENCES

1. Treffert DA: The practical limits of patients' rights. Psychiatric Annals 5(4):91-96, 1971
2. Szasz, T: Law, Liberty and Psychiatry. New York, Macmillan Co, 1963
3. Ennis B: Prisoners of Psychiatry. New York, Harcourt, Brace, Jovanovich, 1972

4. Szasz T: The Myth of Mental Illness. New York, Harper & Row, 1961

5. Laing R: The Politics of Experience. New York, Ballantine Books, 1967

6. Ennis B: Ennis on 'Donaldson.' Psychiatric News, Dec 3, 1975, pp 4, 19, 37

7. Peele R, Chodoff P, Taub N: Involuntary hospitalization and treatability. Observations from the DC experience. Catholic University Law Review 23:744-753, 1974

8. Michels R: The Right to Refuse Psychotropic Drugs, Hastings Center Report. Hastings-on-Hudson, NY, Hastings Institute of Health and Human Values, 1973

9. Parsons T: The Social System. New York, Free Press, 1951

10. Veatch RM: The medical model: its nature and problems. Hastings Center Studies 1(3): 59-76, 1973

11. Katz J: The right to treatment—an enchanting legal fiction? University of Chicago Law Review 36:755-783, 1969

12. Moore MS: Some myths about "mental illness." Arch Gen Psychiatry 32:1483-1497, 1975

13. Peszke MA: Is dangerousness an issue for physicians in emergency commitment? Am J Psychiatry 132:825-828, 1975

14. Stone AA: Comment on Peszke MA: Is dangerousness an issue for physicians in emergency commitment? Ibid, 829-831

15. Siegler M, Osmond H: Models of Madness, Models of Medicine. New York, Macmillan Co, 1974

16. Stone A: Lecture for course on The Law, Litigation, and Mental Health Services. Adelphi, Md, Mental Health Study Center, September 1974.

POSTSCRIPT

Is Involuntary Commitment Wrong?

As a result of the ideological power of the antipsychiatrists, the dreadful condition of many large state mental institutions in which patients had been warehoused for years, the development of antipsychotic medications to control overtly disruptive behavior, and the reduction of mental health budgets, a mass exodus of patients from institutions began in the 1970s. The promise of deinstitutionalization, as this process is called, has not been fulfilled, and the streets of all major American cities are filled with homeless former mental patients who are both potential victims and potential victimizers. See E. Fuller Torrey, *Nowhere to Go: The Tragic Odyssey of the Homeless Mentally Ill* (Harper & Row, 1988). The debate over involuntary hospitalization that began two decades ago must now go on in a somewhat different context, for there are not as many institutions to which people can be confined, there is less optimism about patients' eventual restoration to normality, and there is, perhaps most important, less public money to support treatment.

As incidents in which released mental patients have committed violent crimes become publicized, and as the growing problem of mental illness among homeless people becomes more visible, the pendulum is swinging back toward involuntary commitment.

In New York City the case of Billie Boggs, a homeless woman who resisted the city's efforts to hospitalize her, exemplified the dilemma. The mayor personally became involved in the case, urging involuntary treatment. She was eventually released by the courts. In August 1990 an agreement was signed by the mayor and the governor of New York to provide permanent housing and social services for 5,225 homeless mentally ill people in New York City by 1992.

In 1985 the American Psychiatric Association proposed a model law that would reduce the emphasis on potential dangerousness as a criterion and would focus instead on *significant deterioration*, a version of the *need for treatment* standard.

In February 1990 the Supreme Court ruled that prison officials can treat mentally ill prisoners with antipsychotic drugs against their will without first receiving permission. The majority decision said that "the due process clause permits the state to treat a prison inmate who has a serious mental illness with antipsychotic drugs against his will, if the inmate is dangerous to himself or others and the treatment is in the inmate's medical interest."

Thomas S. Szasz's views are amplified in several books, among them *The Myth of Mental Illness*, revised edition (Harper & Row, 1974). A supporting view is found in Nicholas Kittrie, *The Right to Be Different: Deviance and Enforced Therapy* (Johns Hopkins, 1971). The justifications for involuntary hospitalization are found in Charles M. Culver and Bernard Gert, "The Morality of Involuntary Hospitalization," in *The Law-Medicine Relation: A Philosophical Critique*, edited by H. T. Engelhardt, Jr., and Stuart Spicker (Reidel, 1981). See George J. Annas, "*Donaldson v. O'Connor*: Insanity Inside Out," *Hastings Center Report* (August 1976), and Michael A. Peszke, *Involuntary Treatment of the Mentally Ill: The Problem of Autonomy* (Thomas, 1975); also Richard Van Duizend, Bradley D. McGraw, and Ingo Keilitz, "An Overview of State Involuntary Civil Commitment Statutes," *Mental and Physical Disability Law Reporter* (May-June 1984). Also see Rebecca Dresser, "Involuntary Confinement: Legal and Psychiatric Perspectives," *Journal of Medicine and Philosophy* (August 1984).

ISSUE 10

Should Surgical Patients Be Screened for HIV?

YES: Robert W. M. Frater and Douglas Condit, from "Preoperative HIV Screening," *Infections in Surgery* (July 1988)

NO: Lynn M. Peterson, from "AIDS: The Ethical Dilemma for Surgeons," *Law, Medicine & Health Care* (Summer 1989)

ISSUE SUMMARY

YES: Surgeon Robert W. M. Frater and physician assistant Douglas Condit of the division of cardiothoracic surgery at Montefiore Medical Center in New York City argue that preoperative HIV screening is in the best interests of patients, health care workers, and employers as long as it is performed in an atmosphere of confidentiality and mandatory supportive counseling.

NO: Surgeon Lynn M. Peterson believes that from both a practical and ethical point of view, physicians should not rely on preoperative HIV screening for their own protection but should instead follow universal infection control procedures.

Throughout history, epidemics of infectious disease have created social and political havoc. The discovery of antibiotics and the development of vaccines in the 1940s led to a sense of security that infectious diseases were no longer a major threat in the United States. In 1981 that sense of security turned out to be false. In Los Angeles, then in New York and San Francisco, physicians reported to the Centers for Disease Control (CDC), the federal agency concerned with monitoring health problems in this country, a mysterious series of rare infections and cancers in previously health homosexual young men. As the cases increased, the name acquired immunodeficiency syndrome—AIDS—was given to this disease. Now it is one of the most feared, most misunderstood, and most complex diseases to confront our society.

AIDS is the end stage of a spectrum of illness caused by the human immunodeficiency virus (HIV). The presence of the virus appears to be necessary for infection to occur, but other, unknown factors may determine which infected people develop symptoms of illness and how rapidly. HIV cannot be transmitted by casual contact—that is, the kinds of contact people ordinarily have in the workplace, public places, or at home. It can only be transmitted through intimate sexual contact, blood, and from infected mother to fetus.

The most common risk behaviors are thus sexual intercourse (homosexual or heterosexual) and drug use (especially the use of shared needles and syringes, which may be contaminated with infected blood). Screening blood donations for antibodies to the virus—evidence of infection—greatly reduces the risk of transmission through blood transfusions or blood products. (In other parts of the world, however, where this technology is not readily available, transmission in the health care setting is a serious problem.)

While screening blood and organ donations is not controversial, other possible mandatory or "routine" uses have been challenged because of the potential for discrimination in employment, housing, and insurance, and for stigmatization and rejection by friends and family. As the benefits of early intervention in the disease process become clearer, more individuals are voluntarily choosing to be tested on an anonymous or confidential basis.

The debate about whether testing should be required, not just encouraged, is now centered around the risks of occupational exposure. Some health care workers have become infected through accidental needle-sticks or blood spills. Many feel that they have the right to know whether the patients they care for are HIV-infected; if they had that knowledge, they believe, they would be better able to protect themselves. Others, including the CDC, call for stringent infection control procedures for all patients. Underlying the discussion about risk is the growing prevalence of outright discrimination or avoidance of HIV-infected patients (see the issue on treating AIDS patients).

The following two selections explore the testing issue from the surgeon's perspective. Surgeons and members of their operating teams have the most obvious risk, although to date most occupational exposures have occurred in routine blood drawing and nursing care. Robert W. M. Frater and Douglas Condit call for universal preoperative HIV screening to protect health care personnel. Lynn M. Peterson sees universal screening as technologically and ethically flawed, and reiterates the importance of universal infection control procedures.

YES

**Robert W. M. Frater
and Douglas Condit**

PREOPERATIVE HIV SCREENING

Grethe Rask, M.D., was bred of stoic Scandinavian stock in Twisted, Denmark. A talented, fiercely independent surgeon, she devoted her career to serving the medically deprived in Africa rather than enjoying a lucrative, comfortable practice in the style of her peers in bureaucratic Copenhagen. In a primitive hospital in Abumombazi, Zaire, she practiced under conditions unimaginable in even the poorest sections of the U.S. Faced with a severe shortage of supplies, she had no choice but to reuse "disposable" syringes, discarding them only after they had broken. She also reused the few gloves she could find, discarding them only after they had too many holes to be useful. It was not unusual for her to perform surgery with her hands bare.

Despite the peculiar brand of surgery she practiced, she remained remarkably healthy until 1974, when she was stricken with unrelenting diarrhea and fatigue. Her symptoms abated with medication in 1975, but in 1976 she developed increasing fatigability, generalized lymphadenopathy, and progressive weight loss. She returned to Denmark where she was examined and treated by some of the best and brightest clinicians, with all the implements of modern medicine at their disposal.

Dr. Rask's learned colleagues discovered that there was something terribly wrong with her immune system: for unknown reasons, she lacked T cells. This deficiency rendered her body defenseless against the fungus growing in her mouth and the *Staphylococcus* inhabiting her blood. At the age of 47, on December 12, 1977, Dr. Rask finally succumbed to *Pneumocystis carinii* pneumonia, the first Westerner in the current epidemic to die of what is now known as AIDS, which she apparently acquired through occupational exposure.

Since Dr. Rask's untimely death, medicine has come a long way in its understanding of this illness, now formally known as the acquired immune deficiency syndrome. The causative agent, human immunodeficiency virus (HIV), has been identified and a test is now commercially available to identify antibodies in the majority of infected individuals.

In many states health care workers are not permitted to order an HIV test without the patient's written consent and submission of the blood specimen to a health department laboratory—cumbersome and time-consuming stipulations. For the first time, clinicians are faced with legal restrictions on obtaining full knowledge of the health status of their patients. The justification for these laws is that the diagnosis of HIV infection causes stigma and social disadvantage far greater than that associated with the result of any other routine test ordered without special consent.

Despite such restrictions on testing, a case can be made for universal preoperative screening for HIV to benefit patients, health care workers, and medical institutions.

Benefits to patients. The primary rationale for any medical test is to benefit the patient. The reason for concern about HIV testing has been the fear that test results could be used to the detriment of the patient—for example, that a positive screening result could lead to a refusal to perform elective surgery on the grounds that the patient had a terminal illness. By the laws of New York City, refusal to provide care constitutes discrimination if based solely on a positive HIV result.

The facts currently available are that it takes a period of weeks to months before individuals who become infected with HIV seroconvert to a positive test result. Following seroconversion, 36% of those with HIV infection develop AIDS within 7 years.[1] However, as 64% do not develop AIDS within that interval, a positive HIV test should not of itself be used to discriminate against an HIV-positive patient facing elective surgery. Indeed, the patient will benefit from testing in several ways.

First, knowing the HIV status of a patient allows the surgeon to avoid treatments that are contraindicated in HIV infection. Reports are currently entering the literature regarding individuals with quiescent HIV infection who convert to the overt deficiency syndrome following surgical intervention.[2,3] Whether this conversion is coincidental or related to the surgical procedure can only be determined by large-scale, prospective studies. Therefore, knowing a patient's HIV status is indeed an important consideration, especially for patients facing elective surgical procedures.

Second, HIV screening makes it possible for a patient who is HIV-positive to be seen preoperatively by an infectious disease specialist and thus to have the benefit of counseling, specialized laboratory tests (e.g., T-cell counts), and any treatments that may reduce the chance of exacerbating a quiescent state of infection. Furthermore, the patient may be followed postoperatively by the AIDS specialist.

Third, knowing a patient's HIV status allows judicious use of pharmacologic agents. Certain antibiotics are known to depress immune response, including tetracycline, chloramphenicol, oxytetracycline, streptomycin, gentamicin, kanamycin, and neomycin. Furthermore, B- and T-cell mitogenic capabilities are inhibited by some anesthetic agents, including halothane, cyclopropane, ether, and nitrous oxide.[4] Such agents could theoretically have detrimental effects in the HIV-positive patient.

Knowledge of HIV status is of particular importance to patients facing surgery that leads to immune compromise, such as organ transplantation and open heart surgery. Immunosuppression is chemically induced in patients undergoing organ transplantation to prevent organ rejection. Patients having open heart surgery are placed on extracorporeal circulation, which depresses the function of all components of the immune system, resulting in a temporary immunosuppressed state.[4] Consequently, both organ transplantation and open heart surgery pose a theoretical risk to HIV-positive patients. Some hospitals are hesitant to transplant an organ into an HIV-positive recipient, but the only way to ascertain the risk-benefit ratio of such procedures is through prospective studies in which the HIV status of every patient is known.

Other benefits of screening include the possibility that the HIV-infected patient will receive counseling regarding measures to prevent further transmission of the virus. Studies have suggested that most individuals who are HIV-positive curtail unsafe sexual practices when they are aware of their status.[5] Furthermore, individuals of childbearing age may also receive counseling regarding HIV infection and procreation.[6]

Benefits to health care personnel. Currently there are very few documented cases of occupationally related HIV transmission to health care workers. With widespread implementation of HIV screening in surgical patients, it is hoped that the number of health care workers who become infected with HVI in the future will be further reduced. If they know the HIV status of surgical patients, health care workers are alerted to take special precautions with body fluids. For years, patients infected with hepatitis antigen have been identified so medical personnel can be extremely cautious when handling the patients' body fluids.

Health care workers with open sores, chapped lips, dermatitis, or other compromise of barrier defenses should *not* be permitted to participate in invasive procedures on HIV-infected patients. When invasive procedures are performed, health care workers who have direct contact with the patient should use protective clothing, including eye shields, to further reduce the potential for HIV transmission.

It is often stated that all health care workers should use all the precautions against HIV infection in the care of every patient, making knowledge of HIV status irrelevant. If this is a valid argument, why has it been routine and longstanding practice to alert health care workers to use special precautions for handling body fluids of patients infected with hepatitis B?

As accidents leading to inoculation with HIV are more likely to occur when an inexperienced health care provider is learning a new procedure, a patient who is identified as being HIV-positive should not be utilized as a teaching case, but rather should be treated by the most experienced personnel available. The adage "See one, do one, teach one" should *not* be applied to HIV-positive patients.

In the event of an accident involving the transmission of body fluids, it obviously makes an enormous difference to the health care worker if it is known whether the patient is HIV-infected. With a patient known to be HIV-negative, the degree of anxiety and inconvenience to the health care worker is considerably lessened. In contrast, if the patient is known to be infected with HIV, the health care worker *must* undergo serial HIV testing and may need to modify sexual behavior (even with his or her spouse) for an indefinite period. . . .

Benefits to health care employers. Currently, the threat of liability for health care workers who have allegedly acquired HIV from their employment is a major concern of medical employers. By implementing a comprehensive program of screening and prevention, as outlined above, these businesses should benefit from a reduction in the number of accidents related to HIV-positive patients and an even greater reduction in their potential liability.

Issues of confidentiality. . . . AIDS is now known to extend far beyond the homosexual population; HIV does not discriminate based on race, sex, or sexual orientation. The medical community must therefore incorporate measures to ensure strict confidentiality of screening procedures and medical records. Furthermore, whenever and wherever HIV testing is performed, it is mandatory that qualified counseling be made available to assist the patient in understanding the significance of test results. A positive result of HIV screening may have a greater psychosocial impact than any other test in medical history. Some individuals have committed suicide after receiving a positive result. Other individuals have severed their employment and made preparations for a fatal illness, only to learn that the test had been falsely positive[7] or that they had, for unknown reasons, subsequently seroconverted from positive to negative.

These problems must be anticipated until the prognosis for this infection improves. Knowledgeable, reliable, competent counseling must be mandatory for all individuals subjected to HIV screening tests. . . .

Summary. Preoperative testing of all surgical patients would benefit surgical patients, health care workers, and medical employers. Although numerous obstacles must be overcome before such a policy can be implemented, health care workers should work to make routine preoperative HIV screening a reality.

REFERENCES

1. Hessol NA, Rutherford GW, O'Malley PM, et al: The natural history of human immunodeficiency virus infection in a cohort of homosexual and bisexual men: A 7-year prospective study. Read before the Third International Conference on AIDS, Washington, DC, 1–5 June 1987.

2. Barbui T, Cortelazzo S, Minetti B, et al: Does splenectomy enhance risk of AIDS in HIV-positive patients with chronic thrombocytopenia? *Lancet* 2:342–343, 1987.

3. Konotek-Ahulu FID: Surgery and risk of AIDS in HIV-positive patients. *Lancet* 2:1146, 1987.

4. Utley JR: The immune response, in Utley JR (ed): *Pathophysiology and Techniques of Cardiopulmonary Bypass*, vol 1. Baltimore, Williams & Wilkins, 1982, pp. 132–144.

5. Centers for Disease Control: Self-reported changes in sexual behavior among homosexual men from the San Francisco City Clinic cohort. *MMWR*, 3 Apr 1987.

6. Minkoff HL: Care of pregnant women infected with human immunodeficiency virus. *JAMA* 258:2714–2717, 1987.

7. Vernon A, Hoagland MH, Perlman EJ: AIDS wrongly diagnosed. *JAMA* 258:2063–2064, 1987.

NO
Lynn M. Peterson

AIDS: THE ETHICAL DILEMMA
FOR SURGEONS

Some surgeons have refused to operate on patients infected with human immunodeficiency virus (HIV)[1] and more than 90 percent of 1000 surgeons responding to a survey supported the refusals.[2] The refusing surgeons based their action on the danger of AIDS to themselves and their families and the threat of transmission to other patients, thereby fueling the epidemic. Having operated on AIDS patients over the past eight years, I can attest to the reality of their fear. In addition to overt refusals, physicians treat HIV patients differently[3] in order to reduce the risk of transmission and it may be entirely appropriate, at times, to use a less risky but *equally effective* treatment. The refusing surgeons are not ignorant or malicious. The danger is real and its perception should not be denied. Awareness of the risk should even be reinforced in order to reduce transmission.

Despite the danger, and even though the disease is incurable, AIDS patients can be 'aided' significantly by medical care, their lives can be prolonged and their suffering relieved. At present, HIV has infected over one million Americans, produced AIDS in 50,000 and claimed over 20,000 lives. By 1991 more than 300,000 people will have contracted AIDS.[4] Most importantly, AIDS patients may require care unexpectedly in emergencies, or when hospitalized they may need urgent tracheal intubation or vascular access. The potential for significant benefit, the rising incidence and the unpredictability underscore the need for a dependable health care system capable of dealing with an epidemic. Such a need seems incompatible with individual surgeons refusing to treat patients because they are infected with HIV.

Must all surgeons accept the danger and provide needed care? If so, why? Are there no limits on the level of danger? What can surgeons do to protect themselves? . . . Physicians who sacrifice their lives for a noble cause perform supererogatory acts, going beyond the reach of culpability or medical duty. We praise such physician acts as superhuman efforts but refrain from blaming those who fail to make such extreme sacrifices. In

From Lynn M. Peterson, "AIDS: The Ethical Dilemma for Surgeons," *Law, Medicine & Health Care*, vol. 17, no. 2 (Summer 1989). Copyright © 1989 by the American Society of Law & Medicine. Reprinted by permission.

addition, a fine line separates the virtue of courage from the vice of foolhardiness; we condone courage but not self-destruction. Bad Samaritan laws in European countries, Vermont and Minnesota make danger to self the limit of responsibility to help others.[5] Many dispute the wisdom of making the failure to render help illegal but the moral injunction is clear: It is morally wrong to fail to prevent harm whenever we can *without serious risk of injury to ourselves.* Surgeons, therefore, cannot be expected to operate on patients with a lethal, transmissible disease if they are virtually certain to contract that disease. But surgeons cannot (morally) refuse to operate on patients who pose minimal danger. A surgeon can be expected to provide care as long as it does not entail an 'unreasonable risk'. Whether the risk is reasonable rests on two factors: its likelihood and its severity or (dis)value.

THE LIKELIHOOD OF INJURY

A priori, surgeons have a greater risk of acquiring AIDS than other physicians because they have the greatest exposure to blood and bodily fluids. Indeed surgeons have a risk of acquiring hepatitis B which is about 1.5 times that of other physicians.[6] So far, however, studies of AIDS amongst health care workers have not shown surgeons to be inordinately affected. Of 33 health care workers with AIDS and no additional risk factor, only three were surgeons. Nine were nursing assistants, seven housekeeping or maintenance workers, three nurses, three laboratory technicians, two physicians, one dentist, one therapist and four without patient contact.[7] This data suggests that surgeons are not at a substantially greater risk than other health care workers, perhaps because they have more opportunity for self-protection by wearing gloves, gowns and protective eye-covering.

Prospective surveillance studies of needle injuries or mucous membrane exposure to fluids from AIDS patients have shown that only 3 out of 770 health care workers became infected; none were surgeons.[8] Combining data from several studies gives a risk of HIV infection of 0.76 percent at a 95 percent confidence level. This risk might have been lower had existing guidelines been followed. When compared with other viruses, HIV is a 'weakling'[9] and the concentration of HIV particles in infected blood is low.[10] In comparison with hepatitis B, the chance of HIV infection is much lower: 25 percent compared with 0.76 percent.[11] Hepatitis is far less lethal; 90 percent of hepatitis B infections clear in less than a year and less than half of the remaining patients develop chronic disease.[12] One percent of hepatitis patients die from fulminant disease. However at least 25 to 50 percent of HIV infected patients develop AIDS and at least 85 percent of AIDS patients are dead in five years.[13]

Hagen, Meyer and Paukel[14] compared the risk for a surgeon operating on a known HIV patient with that of operating on a patient whose HIV status is unknown. They estimated that a surgeon performs 360 operations per year, with a skin puncture rate of one per every 43 cases, and the risk of infection after skin puncture with infective material between 9/10,000 and 3/10,000. This yields a risk between 1/4,500 and 1/130,000 (per year) when surgeons operate on patients who are known infective. They used a (high) prevalence rate of 1/100, reported in a Seattle hospital, and then calculated a maximal risk of 1/450,000 (per year) when HIV status is unknown. For a young surgeon with a 30 to 40 year career the risk becomes 1/88,000 providing the prevalence remains unchanged. But, for a surgeon operating on 10 HIV infected patients per year, a likely average for some surgeons in high incidence hospitals, especially with the projected rising incidence, the risk for an entire career could be as high as 9/100. The chance of infection therefore varies tremendously, between 1/88,000 and 9/100.

Two aspects of these figures are striking. First, the risk varies enormously between high and low prevalence areas. For surgeons to be aware of their risk they need to know something about the prevalence in their hospital. This can be accomplished with routine, periodic, random and blind screening. Secondly, surgeons who refuse to care for HIV infected patients increase the risk to their colleagues by 'forcing' them to provide the needed services. A small number of refusals over a long time produces a substantial risk. This enhances the safety of a few by increasing the risks for others. If this produces psychological or physical incapacity on the part of the surgeons shouldering the burden of care for HIV patients, this could put added stress (finding there were no longer any surgeons available to care for the HIV patients) back onto the refusing surgeons. This creates a kind of Prisoner's Dilemma wherein what seems best for one person (the refusing surgeon) individually becomes worse for him overall because he has failed to take into consideration the impact on his fellow surgeons. Getting out of a Prisoner's Dilemma requires cooperation and selecting an alternative which will be best for everyone.[15]

THE (DIS)VALUE OF INJURY

Determining whether the risk is 'reasonable' however depends on more than the probabilities. It also requires a value judgment which has both personal and cultural dimensions. The need for personal assessment becomes obvious when one considers the difference between danger and fear. Danger, an objective property, and fear, a psychological response, are inconsistently related. For one person, a given situation produces paralyzing anxiety while for another the same situation evokes confidence and enhanced effectiveness. Fear of AIDS might incapacitate one surgeon while another operates with alacrity. Despite the existence or reality of personal differences, the need for a reliable system of medical care requires a stable, non-idiosyncratic estimate of danger. A 'reasonable' degree of danger therefore has to be based on the response of most surgeons to a situation. An excessive response becomes unacceptable when assuming the role of a 'surgeon'.

Surgeons as a group, like policemen, firemen and soldiers, voluntarily accept greater risks. One might explain this in terms of reward: surgeons are rewarded because they are at greater risk. Another explanation invokes ability: because surgeons are better able to perform operations without self-injury they can sustain a higher risk. But the fundamental explanation relies on the moral notion of a profession: it is the duty of a physician to help patients. The professional performs his duty because of his commitment rather than 'in trade' for pay.

Does the fact that surgeons accept higher risks mean they are obligated to take the risk of caring for HIV patients? The answer to this question must consider the medical-social costs of AIDS and the benefits which surgeons can provide. Personal commitment[16] heroism,[17] self-effacement[18] and fear of legal reprisal[19] are important but insufficient. Surgeons must take the risk when the consequences of refusing are too great. . . .

SURGICAL SETTING

The following undramatic example of a routine surgical encounter emphasizes how the HIV problem connects to the entire system of medical care delivery. It is an actual situation selected because it illustrates the network of concerns that need to be addressed in order to ensure effective medical care for a future with many more HIV patients.

A single 35 year old man with an extensive history of drug abuse was undergoing emergency cholecystectomy for acute cholecystitis. Near the end of the operation, a pronged retractor, used earlier, was passed from the nurse to the surgeon. One of the prongs tore the nurse's glove and produced a small abrasion. The nurse immediately screamed: "My god, what I am doing here? What does this man have? Nursing is dangerous to your health!" The abrasion was cleaned with an antiseptic, the glove changed and the nurse was advised to report to the hospital infection control committee.

In this instance another medical disorder, acute cholecystitis, completely unrelated to HIV infection, was the reason for surgical treatment. The patient refused to have an HIV blood test postoperatively, but his history of parenteral drug use meant there was a considerable chance of infection. Prior testing would have been useless since the result would not have been available in time to be helpful. The injury occurred during a routine maneuver, one that would not *a priori* seem risky, and was inflicted by a commonly used instrument which could be modified to reduce the risk. Also, the injury occurred near the end of the operation when there is less likelihood of exposure to large quantities of blood and less intensity of concentration. Finally, it was the assistant, not the surgeon, who was injured.

These findings suggest that all operations deserve careful scrutiny to avoid injuries, not just those, like venous access and node and lung biopsies, commonly done in HIV infected patients. Prior testing will have limited utility. Physicians, nurses and technicians should continuously review procedures and instruments to enhance safety in light of the HIV risk. All participants should remain alert to the small maneuvers which put each other, not just the patient, at risk. Previous operating room customs have focused almost entirely on the patient; this need not be relaxed but rather extended to explicitly include the surgical team. Finally, non-surgeons may be at as much risk as surgeons for such injuries and this means that the question the surgeon needs to ask is not just: "Should I operate on this patient?" but "Should we operate on this patient?" Indeed the 'we' in this interrogatory should refer to the entire health care system; the micropractices in the operating room should be based on a larger social policy regarding the care of HIV infection. . . .

PERMISSIBLE DISTINCTIONS

Permissible distinctions share two features: an appropriate basis and consistent application. In medical practice, diagnoses are distinctions made for the purpose of providing benefit. The diagnosis of AIDS appropriately influences some medical choices: e.g. using pentamidine for pneumonia. But choosing less effective or suboptimal measures just to avoid the risk of transmission is unwarranted. In addition, diagnoses are overlapping approximations rather than neat, rigid categories. AIDS patients can have heart disease, gastrointestinal problems and neurological difficulties in addition to being infected with HIV. Treating patients with the latter problems plus AIDS suboptimally means denying them a benefit. Not doing a cholecystectomy for acute cholecystitis because the patient has HIV infection, as in the case presented, could not be condoned unless there were obvious benefit to the patient or overwhelming danger to the staff. HIV infection should not lead to inferior care.

Using the HIV test preoperatively is hindered by the inconsistency of false negatives and positives.[20] If an infected patient tests negative, this creates a false sense of security, perhaps reducing attention to inconvenient and tedious details that might reduce transmission. During the 'window' between infection and seropositivity, patients can transmit HIV. False positives create problems when alternative, non-standard therapies are chosen in order to reduce risk and especially in cases in which test results become available to employers, insurance carriers, housing authorities or other agencies who use it unjustly to limit rights or benefits. While the number of false negatives and positives is small, routine pre-operative testing would have to show that the benefit to care-givers outweighed these detriments.

Furthermore, the universal precautions recommended by the CDC provide protection and at the same time do not threaten to limit care.[21] These measures include gloves, gowns and protective eye-covering whenever coming in contact with bodily fluids. Should additional measures (e.g. double gloving, not using a power saw) be used when operating on someone known to be infected? In many instances these measures would be acceptable but one must be careful to avoid the hazards of a new, unfamiliar, non-standard technique since deviations from routine protocol can increase the chance of an accident. In addition, such deviations could reduce the impetus to develop more suitable universal precautions. Thus, from both a practical and ethical point of view, surgery should be done in the same way whenever possible, whether an HIV test is negative or positive.

THE SURGEON'S SOCIAL RESPONSIBILITY

Surgeons, like other physicians, must bear in mind that their actions are likely to influence public opinion. Public anxiety about AIDS, due, in part, to unwarranted skepticism concerning scientific information,[22] has led to the mistreatment of children and adults. Measures like widespread education directed at modifying high-risk behavior, the use of HIV testing for epidemiologic purposes, and funding for research are reasonable based on present data while a general quarantine, isolation of infected individuals in the school or workplace, and mandatory blood screening offer no hope of benefit. Yet legislators and other policy-makers are not sure whether to rely on recommendations based on scientific data or seek what seems like immediate and definite security. Since surgeons represent 'the scientific community,' their refusal to care for HIV infected patients encourages further public distrust of science. On the other hand, providing universal care regardless of HIV status and avoiding impermissible distinctions encourages confidence in science and helps allay public anxiety and the possibility of mistreatment.

Finally, taking the refusals of surgeons seriously means that, even though the likelihood of infection is low, we need to search for ways to reduce it even further. HIV is exquisitely sensitive to many common antiseptic agents. Perhaps operating personnel should scrub routinely after, as well as before, every operation for their own protection. Research directed at materials and methods to protect care-givers should be promoted as well as research to find agents to treat HIV infection. Other materials for gloves and gowns might offer better protection than those currently available. Surgeons should play an active role in establishing and reviewing policies for safety and efficiency in the operating room.

In conclusion, refusals by individual surgeons to operate on HIV infected patients threaten a fundamental right to treatment with equal concern and respect, as well as a dependable system of health care delivery essential for an epidemic. Surgeons cannot be expected to take unreasonable risks, but 'reasonableness' is not a matter of personal preference. Reasonableness must be defined in terms of the likelihood of injury, its adversity, the group (or role) involved and the public benefit to be gained. Responsible surgeons act on the basis of a policy with universal rules and appropriate distinctions. Surgeons also have a respon-

sibility to support the available scientific data on AIDS and fulfill their obligation to the surgical team.

REFERENCES

The author would like to thank Dr. Leon Eisenberg for numerous reviews and helpful suggestions in the preparation of this article.

1. L. Gruson, "AIDS fear spawns ethics debate as some doctors withhold care," *New York Times* 1987; July 11: 1; S. Starer, "Fear of AIDS," *American Medical News* 1987; October 2: 1; P. J. Guy, "AIDS: A Doctor's Duty," *British Medical Journal* 1987; 294: 445.

2. "AIDS in the Operating Room," *Surgical Practice News* 1987; August: 5–11.

3. R. Gillon, "Refusal to Treat AIDS and HIV Positive Patients," *British Medical Journal* 1987; 294: 1332–3.

4. "Prevention and Control of Acquired Immunodeficiency Syndrome," *JAMA* 1987; 258: 2097–103.

5. J. Feinberg, *Harm to Others*. Oxford: Oxford University Press 1984, 127–129.

6. A. E. Dennes, J. L. South, J. E. Maynard et al., "Hepatitis B Infection in Physicians: Results of a Nationwide Seroepidemiologic Survey," *JAMA* 1978; 239: 210–12.

7. "Recommendations for Prevention of HIV Transmission in Health-Care Settings," *JAMA* 1987; 258: 1293–305.

8. G. H. Friedland, R. S. Klein, "Transmission of the Human Immunodeficiency Virus," *New England Journal of Medicine* 1987; 317: 1125–35.

9. J. E. Osborn, "The AIDS Epidemic: Multidisciplinary Trouble," *New England Journal of Medicine* 1986; 324: 779–82.

10. A. M. Geddes, "The Risk of AIDS to Health Care Workers," *British Medical Journal* 1986; 292: 711–2.

11. *Confronting AIDS: Directions for Public Health, Health Care and Research*, Washington DC: National Academy Press, 1986.

12. R. K. Ockner, "Chronic Hepatitis," In Cecil-Loeb, *Textbook of Medicine*, Philadelphia: WB Saunders, 1985; 824–7.

13. R. Rothenberg, M. Woelfel, R. Stoneburner, et al, "Survival with the Acquired Immunodeficiency Syndrome," *New England Journal of Medicine*, 1987; 212: 1297–302.

14. M. D. Hagan, K. B. Meyer, S. G. Pauker, "Routine Preoperative Screening for HIV: Does the Risk to the Surgeon Outweigh the Risk to the Patient?" *JAMA* 1988; 259: 1357–59.

15. J. Elster, *Ulysses and the Sirens: Studies in Rationality and Irrationality*, Cambridge: Cambridge University Press, 1984.

16. A. Jonsen, "Ethics and AIDS," *Bulletin of American Cell Surgeons* 1985; 70: 16–18.

17. A. Zuger and S. H. Miles, "Physicians, AIDS and Occupational Risk: Historic Traditions and Ethical Obligations." *JAMA* 1987; 258: 1924–28.

18. E. D. Pellegrino, "Altruism, Self-Interest and Medical Ethics," *JAMA* 1987; 258: 1939–40.

19. G. W. Matthews, V. S. Neshund, "The Initial Impact of AIDS on Public Health Law in the United States—1986," *JAMA* 1987; 257: 344–52.

20. *JAMA*, supra note 7.

21. P. D. Cleary, M. J. Barry, K. H. Mayer, A. M. Brandt, L. Gostin, H. V. Fineberg, "Compulsory Premarital Screenings for the Human Immunodeficiency Virus," *JAMA* 1987; 258: 1757–62.

22. L. Eisenberg, "The Genesis of Fear: AIDS and the Public's Response to Science," *Law, Medicine & Health Care* 1987; 14: 243–9.

POSTSCRIPT

Should Surgical Patients Be Screened for HIV?

The debate about screening surgical patients has a counterpart in the debate about screening surgeons and other health care workers who perform invasive procedures as well. If HIV-infected patients pose a threat to doctors, do HIV-infected doctors pose an equal or even more serious threat to patients? So far the risk of HIV transmission to surgical patients seems to be extremely low, much lower than the risk of hepatitis B transmission to patients. Dr. Frank Rhame of the University of Minnesota estimates the risk at between one in 100,000 and one in a million operations. A review of 2,160 patients of a Tennessee surgeon who died of AIDS showed that only one (an intravenous drug user) was HIV-positive and may have already had AIDS at the time of his surgery (*Journal of the American Medical Association*, July 25, 1990). Other retrospective reviews of surgical patients of HIV-infected doctors have not uncovered any cases of transmission.

One case of health-care-worker-to-patient transmission has been reported by the CDC. Although there is no conclusive evidence, it was reported that a woman with no other risk factors was infected during a dental procedure and developed symptoms of HIV disease two years later.

Most medical professional organizations reject routine screening of physicians and call for individualized decisions about whether an HIV-infected doctor should continue to perform particular invasive procedures. There is, however, little guidance on which to base these case-by-case decisions. Dr. Rhame, for example, suggests that such doctors avoid performing surgery that requires blind, by-feel manipulation of sharp instruments but not other types of surgery.

For a moving account of a young physician's experiences of discrimination and illness after becoming infected on the job, see Hacib Aoun, "When a House Officer Gets AIDS," *The New England Journal of Medicine* (September 7, 1989). In "HIV-Infected Physicians and the Practice of Seriously Invasive Procedures," *Hastings Center Report* (January/February 1989), Lawrence Gostin calls for professional guidance to protect patient safety and the privacy of infected physicians.

For more information on screening surgical patients, see Michael D. Hagen, Klemens B. Meyer, and Stephen G. Pauker, "Routine Preoperative Screening for HIV: Does the Risk to the Surgeon Outweigh the Risk to the Patient?" *Journal of the American Medical Association* (March 1988), and Paul M. Arnow et al., "Orthopedic Surgeons' Attitudes and Practices Concerning Treatment of Patients with HIV Infection," *Public Health Reports* (March/April 1989).

ISSUE 11

Do Physicians Have an Ethical Duty to Treat AIDS Patients?

YES: Albert R. Jonsen, from "The Duty to Treat Patients with AIDS and HIV Infection," in Lawrence C. Gostin, ed., *AIDS and the Health Care System* (Yale University Press, 1990)

NO: James W. Tegtmeier, from "Ethics and AIDS: A Summary of the Law and a Critical Analysis of the Individual Physician's Ethical Duty to Treat," *American Journal of Law & Medicine,* vol. 16, nos. 1 and 2 (1990)

ISSUE SUMMARY

YES: Philosopher Albert R. Jonsen asserts that refusing to provide treatment in specific cases, because it is inconvenient, risky, or burdensome, casts a shadow on the most precious value of medicine, its commitment to service.
NO: Attorney James W. Tegtmeier asserts that it is improper to assert that physicians have an ethical duty to treat individuals with AIDS because the grounds for imposing such a duty are too weak to support that conclusion.

In March 1987 Dr. W. Dudley Johnson, a prominent cardiac surgeon, announced that he would not operate on acquired immunodeficiency syndrome (AIDS) patients or those infected with the human immunodeficiency virus (HIV). A few months late the press quoted another cardiac surgeon: "I've got to be selfish. . . . It's an incurable disease that's uniformly fatal, and I'm certainly at a high risk of getting it. I've got to think about myself; I've got to think about my family. That responsibility is greater than to the patient."

These attitudes are common. In August 1990 the National Commission on AIDS described as "shocking" the number of physicians reluctant to take care of people living with HIV infection and AIDS. New York City has had over 25,000 cases of AIDS, more than any other city in the world, and yet the Gay Men's Health Crisis, the largest volunteer AIDS agency, has a referral list of just 45 qualified private physicians in Manhattan who are willing to take patients. Only one or two doctors in the other four boroughs, which have half the city's cases, are willing to take private AIDS patients. The Physicians Association for AIDS Care, a national organization, has a referral list of only 2,000 physicians, out of the country's 600,000 licensed doctors.

How have physicians behaved in past epidemics? The record is mixed. Galen, the great classical physician, fled Rome when plague struck in A.D.

166. In the fourteenth century, when the bubonic plague, known as the Black Death, killed one quarter of the population of Europe, some physicians stayed to treat patients, for both financial gain and civic loyalty. Many others, however, fled in fear or locked themselves in their houses and refused to come out. During the Great Plague of London, which occurred in 1665, physicians responded in similarly divergent ways. The public apparently had no greater respect for either category: those who left were called "deserters"; those who stayed only to provide useless treatments were called "quacks."

In America, the yellow fever epidemic in Philadelphia in 1793 was the first great test for physicians. While three of the best-known doctors retreated to the countryside, most others remained, some to become sick and die themselves. Largely in order to establish public confidence in physicians, the first code of medical ethics of the American Medical Association (AMA), newly formed in 1847, declared: " . . . and when pestilence prevails, it is [physicians'] duty to face the danger, and to continue their labors for the alleviation of the suffering, even at the jeopardy of their own lives." This formal statement of professional obligation remained in the AMA's Code of Ethics until 1957, when it was deleted, mostly because epidemics of contagious diseases seemed a remote danger in an age of antibiotics and miracle drugs.

AIDS has presented a challenge to the dual professional traditions of individual autonomy and social responsibility. In the United States, private physicians are not legally obligated to treat anyone unless they have already established a physician-patient relationship. Even in that case, physicians can terminate the relationship unilaterally by providing a suitable substitute or giving the patient sufficient notice to find an alternative source of care. Physicians employed by public hospitals do not have such discretion, nor do physicians in emergency rooms, although they can refuse care if they believe an emergency does not exist or if the patient would be better served by a transfer.

The selections that follow present two views of physicians' ethical (as opposed to legal) responsibility. Albert R. Jonsen states that the strength of the professional obligation to care for the sick comes from the nature of illness and the nature of professional care. The obligation is reinforced by the importance of the work of the health professions in the AIDS epidemic. James W. Tegtmeier states that the reasons advanced for an ethical obligation to treat patients with AIDS are not well grounded; if there is to be such a duty, it must be enacted into law.

YES
Albert R. Jonsen

THE DUTY TO TREAT PATIENTS WITH AIDS AND HIV INFECTION

The father of modern surgery, Ambroise Pare, once reflected on the danger of caring for persons infected with plague. "[Surgeons] must remember," he wrote, "that they are called by God to this vocation of surgery: therefore they should go to it with high courage and free of fear, having firm faith that God both gives and takes our lives as and when it pleases Him."[1] These reflections of a sixteenth century Frenchman, expressed in religious terms, may seem foreign to our times, but they remind us of a question that seems to haunt physicians, surgeons, and other providers of health care perennially: at what danger or cost to myself must I carry out my work? Throughout history, many have answered as did Pare: something morally compelling about being a healer, whether divinely given or not, requires one to take even great risks in caring for the sick. Others, although they rarely assert so in writing, seem to have viewed their work more prosaically and felt no greater or lesser obligation than any decent person who must balance the risks of living against the goods of livelihood.[2]

The AIDS epidemic revives that perennial question in vivid ways. The sudden appearance of a lethal infection, the rapid spread of infection to more than a million Americans, the death of thousands of those infected, and the expected death of many more have thrust American health care providers into an epidemic that caught them unprepared. Remarkably, the scientific unpreparedness ceded to a rapid mobilization of several biomedical disciplines—virology, immunology and epidemiology—leading to identification of the causative agent and the modes of transmission. Clinical care developed more slowly, but research on therapies and preventative interventions is now intense. The social, ethical, and psychological unpreparedness lingers on, however, being met by sporadic and incomplete responses.[3]

Among the lingering issues is the troubling question of the duty to treat the HIV-infected person. Because this question is a contemporary version of the perennial question stated above, it will never be definitively answered; still, professional providers of care must form their consciences honestly and

From Albert R. Jonsen, "The Duty to Treat Patients with AIDS and HIV Infection," in Lawrence C. Gostin, ed., *AIDS and the Health Care System* (Yale University Press, 1990). Copyright © 1990 by Yale University. Reprinted by permission.

firmly. Failure to do so can lead to deterioration of care, discrimination, and distrust between patients and providers.

Although most physicians, nurses, and technicians in American health care seem to have accepted the duty to provide suitable care even in the face of risk, the constant stresses arising from the perception of risk to self and from the difficulties of caring for AIDS patients can erode the general dedication to serve. The erosion may appear in a variety of ways. Subtle evasion of certain forms of interaction with patients and the discovery of excuses and exceptions, sometimes cloaked with pseudoscientific rationales, can lead to a deterioration of quality of care. Even the most dedicated providers can find their ability to care eroded by the constant exposure to perceived risks. Questions arise regularly about the desirability of screening all patients, or all surgical and obstetrical patients, or anyone seeking elective surgery. It is asked whether the physician has the right to refuse to perform certain risky procedures that might not be strictly necessary for the patient. There are continuing reports of an anecdotal nature about providers actually refusing needed care and about inappropriate referrals and transfers of patients suspected of HIV infection. Occasionally, refusals of care are reported to government agencies or advocacy groups as complaints of discrimination.

Relatively few physicians and nurses have encountered these patients up until now, because AIDS has been concentrated in large metropolitan areas. But in the next decade these patients will begin to appear throughout the American health care system. Many physicians and nurses will see them for the first time. The lessons already learned in the major centers of the epidemic must be communicated to those professionals who will be called to care for patients in the near future. The special features of health care outside major metropolitan areas must also be taken into consideration in designing policies and programs.

At the center of all educational efforts stands the fundamental moral question, is it ethically permissible for a provider of health care to refuse to care for a patient with AIDS or who has positive test results for antibody to HIV?

This is a question of conscience, a question posed by an individual to himself or herself in order to decide how his or her conduct should reflect certain values and principles. It is a deeply personal question, but it goes beyond personal choice to the acceptance or rejection of values and principles beyond the private self and deriving from social, cultural, and religious sources that surround the individual. Answering it expresses the willingness to be identified with and by a certain course of action and to bear the burdens of being so identified. Thus, in this chapter I will say little about the legal obligations to treat discussed at length in other essays, although the question of conscience might sometimes involve the legal, insofar as each person must decide whether or not to obey the law.[4] In this essay I define the duty to treat as a moral rather than a legal obligation.

This particular question of conscience is not familiar for most modern health professionals. They generally go about their work, caring for the patients that come into their hands in various ways, rarely having to ask themselves, "Do I have a duty to treat this person?" Occasionally, the question will arise in a peculiar circumstance, such as the extremely noncompliant patient or the very demanding and difficult patient. Occasionally, the question will occur as a matter of policy, such as the decision to provide uncompensated care to indigent patients. In general, however, physicians take it for granted that they have duties to care for patients that they, or their institutions, have accepted. Nurses assume that they have the duty to care for the patients to whom they are assigned.

So, the problem of conscience with regard to patients with HIV infection is particularly difficult because it is unfamiliar to those struggling to resolve it. They may be unclear about the terms of the problem, about the reasons it is a problem, and about the principles that might be used to reflect upon it. I will attempt to state the terms of the problem. Ultimately, resolution depends on the conscientious judgment of individuals.

REASONS FOR THE PROBLEM

The problem of conscience has at least four salient components: the perception of serious risk, the influence of prejudice, the burden of caring for AIDS patients, and the presumption of professional freedom of choice. Some professionals will be bothered by all of these components; others by only one or two of them. Any review of the problem must consider them all.

Health providers are at risk of infection when they are engaged in providing medical and nursing care to persons with HIV infection. The virus can be transmitted from an infected to an uninfected party even before any symptoms of AIDS are recognized. The modes of transmission of the virus are well understood: exposure to the blood and bodily fluids of an infected person, usually through sexual intercourse, the sharing of drug needles, or transfusion of infected blood. The fetus can be infected by maternal blood. Health professionals are at risk of exposure by accidental punctures or cuts incurred while caring for patients or by contact with hemorrhage through spills or splashes of blood. A small number of health professionals are known to have been infected in this way. Serious efforts have been made to quantify the risk of infection for providers of care, and in general, the risk is apparently low—in the range of 0.4 percent after exposure to infected blood by sharp needle injury. The risk after exposure to infected blood in other ways (for example, contact with mucous membranes or nonintact skin) "is probably considerably less and cannot be measured with existing data."[5] Health professionals, particularly those whose work puts them into frequent contact with patient's blood and fluids, may know the statistical facts about their risks but may remain deeply concerned. Their concern has two sound bases: even low risks are real, and the low risk has a serious outcome—lethal disease.

Formation of one's conscience must take account both of facts, in the form of statistics and other data, and of fears and apprehensions. While it is often difficult and sometimes impossible to dispel fears and apprehensions entirely (some professionals, of course, seem immune to them), still a conscientious judgment about a duty to treat in face of risk must ask whether the risks, as well as the fears, are reasonable. We shall return to this consideration.

A second component in the problem of the duty to treat is the peculiar epidemiology of the disease—namely, prevalence among homosexual men and abusers of intravenously injected illicit drugs. Both of these groups are viewed in a negative light by American society: the former because many deeply disapprove of their sexual preferences; the latter because they are involved in a criminal and destructive activity. Both are the object of what sociologists call stigmatization. This term designates a complex social and psychological process whereby certain persons are perceived as without social value and even as threatening to the dominant society. They are marked (hence, the word *stigma*, which in derivation evokes the branding of a criminal) for exclusion from certain social benefits and interactions. The stigma goes far beyond the actual features of the stigmatized and creates a negative social image that extends into all aspects of judgment about them, making it difficult to be objective about their behavior and their needs.

Health professionals have long honored an ethic of objectivity about their patients; they try not to allow their personal opinions about the values, lifestyle, and morality of their patients to influence their professional judgments about the patients' health care needs. Yet, this honored ethic sometimes comes under stress. Some professionals may find certain persons so repugnant that they will not accept them as patients or, if they must serve them, do so reluctantly and sometimes negligently. This latter course is rightly condemned as unethical, even when the former may be implicitly tolerated. Stigmatization influences the judgments of individuals in more subtle ways than overt dislike and frank prejudice. Professionals may disvalue the stigmatized in ways they hardly recognize. Even when professionals believe they are not prejudiced, they may perceive and treat stigmatized persons differently from others. For example,

providers who have never seriously balked at the risk of infection from hepatitis B (which still causes a number of deaths each year) are fearful of the risk of HIV infection (which has yet to cause the death of an exposed provider). This makes one wonder whether submerged prejudices enhance the apprehension of danger.[6]

In addition to the perception of risk and the problem of prejudice, health professionals may find the care of AIDS patients a demanding task. The disease itself is devastating, no cure is presently available, and death is the inevitable outcome. Many patients come largely from groups with whose life-style the health professional may be unfamiliar and even unsympathetic. On the other hand, the patients are predominantly young adults whose lives are cut short; some of these have great promise. Such patients as the female partners of intravenous drug users, infants born infected, and unknowing recipients of transfusions of infected blood inspire particular compassion. With these patients, the provider of care may be deeply sympathetic, even emotionally identified. In general, caring for AIDS patients imposes notable stress on professionals. The psychological phenomenon known as burnout is all too familiar to those who have dedicated themselves to the care of these patients.[7] This phenomenon itself, or the anticipation of it, may be a component in the problem of conscience.

Thus, as health professionals are exposed to increasing numbers of persons who are infected with HIV, their sense of responsibility toward these patients may be influenced by their perception of the risks involved in caring for such patients, their overt prejudices and covert complicity with stigma, and the stresses they actually experience, or expect to experience, in dealing with AIDS patients.

A final component cannot be discounted—namely, the strong value that Americans of all sorts, including health professionals, place on freedom of choice. There has long been, in the United States, a reluctance to force one person to provide services to another against his or her will. The Principles of Ethics of the American Medical Association state that a physician may choose those whom he or she wishes to serve.[8] American law does not require physicians to provide services to any particular patient, unless some special relationship already exists.[9] Nurses are in a different situation, since they are usually employees of hospitals and are rarely given the opportunity to select their patients. Still, the right to refuse to care for a particular patient, either by not accepting that person as a patient or by discharging oneself from responsibility in a recognized way, is deeply embedded in the ethos of American medicine. It is difficult to challenge this ethos by stating that physicians or other providers have an obligation that prohibits them from exercising such a presumed moral right.

THE SOURCES OF OBLIGATION

How does one go about forming one's conscience? Does one do so merely by deciding whether or to what extent one wishes to participate in so problematic a business? Formation of conscience, I believe, is more than an expression of personal preference. It is an exercise in which one tests personal preferences against the importance of what one is asked to do. For the pious Ambroise Pare (whose motto was, "I dressed his wounds but God cured him"), a divine vocation

to surgery was the measure of importance. But in an era when such faith is rare, measures of importance must be discovered, and they must be such as to persuade many, if not all, of the concerned parties that caring for the sick without discrimination and regardless of personal risk and inconvenience is intimately bound up with the profession and the work of health care.

This conclusion may not attain the stance of an absolute moral principle. Indeed, philosophers may cavil at designating it a moral principle at all, since the inference from importance to moral imperative is not strictly logical. Still, whether we call it important or imperative, the work of caring for the seriously ill even under adverse circumstance for the provider cannot be casually dismissed. Individuals should exempt themselves only for the most serious reasons, and public policies should not sanction practices that undermine such commitment.

The discovery of importance requires a careful look at the nature of the work of health care. That look should begin with an inquiry into the history and tradition of this work with a view to answering the questions: Have those who engaged in health care in the past considered it important to undertake their work in the face of personal danger and inconvenience? If so, how seriously did they take this task? Are there circumstances in which a physician may refuse to respond to a person's need? Was caring for the sick at danger to oneself considered an ethical duty and were those who refused or refrained judged unethical practitioners?

Scholars have reviewed the evidence that might indicate whether physicians in many times and cultures have acknowledged a moral duty to treat the sick even at risk to themselves and contrary to their inclinations. The historical record is mixed. First, the problem is raised only occasionally. When it is, the distinction between actual behavior and the affirmation of a duty is not often made. Still, it appears that, as long as a distinct and self-defined class of healers has existed in our culture, they have faced the perennial problem in some form or another. The problem of caring for strangers and enemies was sometimes debated; the problem of caring for those who could not pay has been an enduring issue. . . .

In the recent literature on the subject of professional responsibility, philosophers, physicians, and historians have sought to go deeper. They have attempted to articulate a basic principle that applied to the very work of providing help to the sick. Some have found it in the nature and character of the physician's role, still others in the reciprocal obligations between society and the profession.[10] The former line of argument suggests that undertaking the profession implies a commitment to certain virtues associated with medicine and healing and among these is the duty to care for the sick. The second line of argument stresses the implicit contract between a profession to which society grants a monopoly on the healing arts and the society whose needs it serves. A short article by Edmund Pellegrino states the case in favor of a strong obligation most comprehensively. He suggests that three things specific to medicine impose an obligation that subordinates the physician's self-interest to a duty of altruism. First, medical need itself constitutes a moral claim on those who are equipped to help because illness renders the patient uniquely vulnerable and dependent. Physicians invite trust

from those in a position of relative powerlessness. Second, the physician's knowledge is not proprietary, since it is gained under the aegis of the society at large for the purpose of having a supply of medical personnel. Those who acquire this knowledge hold it in trust for the sick. Third, physicians in entering the profession, enter a covenant with society to use competence in service of the sick. These three reasons, Pellegrino argues, support the conclusion that physicians, collectively and individually, have a moral obligation to attend the sick.[11] There are, then, multiple reasons—tradition, the solemn declarations of professionals, the nature of the profession itself and its virtues, the conditions of the sick and their relationship to providers, the expectations of society as a whole, and its social contract with professions—to support the affirmation that service to the sick at risk and inconvenience to oneself is a matter of great importance. All of these reasons, as John Arras points out in an excellent article,[12] are open to some critical comment, but taken together they converge to the same point, namely that there appears to be a stringent and serious moral obligation, closely bound up with the very profession of being a physician or other provider of health care.

At the same time, all commentators allow that even this stringent and serious obligation has certain limitations and exceptions. The ethical principle of attending the sick cannot be interpreted as an obligation on the physician to respond to any and every request for help; that would be physically impossible and financially ruinous for the practitioner. Providers do not present themselves to society (to use the terms in the title of a paper by George Annas)[13] as saints, whose personal lives are totally subordinated to a higher ideal, but as healers with an important but limited skill. They offer to help, but they and the society recognize their finitude.

Thus, if there is such a principle, it must be limited in some way. Some limitations are generally accepted without question. Most obvious among these are the choice of a speciality, the selection of a geographical area, the establishment of a practice, and the determination of prices for service. Under special circumstances, such as the dearth of physicians in an area or speciality, even these generally accepted limitations might be questioned. Certain other limits that a physician might set on his or her service are ethically dubious, such as serving only the rich or persons of one race or religion. These sorts of limits make a mockery of the overall principle, since being rich or white or Catholic, for example, have nothing to do with medical need.

The most problematic sort of limitation would be the exclusion of certain sorts of genuine, treatable medical needs because the physician finds something unacceptable about the need or the needy. For example, the disease renders the patient physically repugnant, the disease is associated with behavior the physician considers immoral, or—and this is the case with AIDS—the disease is dangerous to the physician. Refusing service for the first two reasons is clearly reprehensible. But is personal risk a reasonable excuse from service?

Until quite recently, physicians regularly exposed themselves to serious risk when they treated patients with infectious diseases. Even when the principle of accepting risk in order to help those in need is acknowledged, however, certain rules of thumb guide its application.

Those rules are the familiar ones defining the circumstances in which a person has a moral obligation to aid another person who is in danger: the reasonableness of the risk, the feasibility of help, the urgency of the need, and the absence of less risky alternatives.

The reasonableness of the risk in caring for patients with AIDS is the question in this case. Reasonableness refers to such things as evidence that the activity is actually dangerous, the probability that harm will occur, and the magnitude of the harm for oneself and for others. Each of these elements must be assessed in light of the best available information and the best common sense about the situation at hand.

In the ordinary course of life, activities are usually designated as high risk because the *frequency* of adverse events is high. We engage almost unthinkingly in many activities in which the adverse effects rarely occur but may be very serious, indeed lethal, when they do, such as driving to work and engaging in sports activities. In the case of AIDS, the frequency of the adverse event, seroconversion after accidental occupation exposure, is very low.[14] At the same time, the magnitude of the harm is great: there is strong probability that infection will proceed to disease and that disease will lead to death.

Thus, the moral quandary: Should I undertake an action that I have presumed duty to perform, if the action has a low probability of resulting in harm to me (and others, for example, my spouse) of great magnitude? In general, one could respond to that quandary by reflecting that a life ruled by the strategy of avoiding the low probabilities of even great harm would be a paralyzed life. Usually, however, our reflection on this question turns to the importance of the work to be done or the activity to be performed. We ask ourselves whether "it's worth it."

One way of asking whether some activity is worth the risk is to reflect on certain features of the actual case in question. These features are included in the traditional "rules of rescue," namely, the urgency and feasibility of helping and the existence of alternatives. The seriousness of the obligation to which physicians are held can be mitigated by demonstrating cases in which the medical intervention is not urgent, such as a request for cosmetic surgery only to enhance one's image, a procedure that is unlikely to benefit the patient, such as inserting a shunt to dialyse a patient whose death is imminent under any circumstances, or a medical intervention that would be as useful as a surgical one. In some situations a plausible case might be made that an intervention be omitted. The rationale is that the intervention is actually not needed at this time or under this form. It does not constitute a rescue in any significant sense. But it is obvious that in such cases, psychological, and emotional factors can distort this judgment by exaggerating the sense of danger, magnifying perceived risks, or trivializing the need or urgency of treatment. Scrupulous honesty and courage are indispensable adjuncts to such evaluation. Excusing oneself from so serious an obligation as service to those one is professionally committed to serve cannot be done lightly. These sorts of cases are debatable, and the best approach to their resolution is debate or, at least, open discussion with the patient and one's colleagues.

A question less dramatic than actual refusal to treat is the proposal to require an HIV antibody test of all patients or of all surgical patients. In addition to the problems about the behavior of the test in low-risk populations and about interpretation of the test, it is crucial to ask what decisions might be faced and what procedures initiated on the basis of information gained by that test. Are there specific maneuvers that might be modified if the patient is antibody-positive? For example, would the surgeon staple rather than suture, use a different technique for hemostasis, proceed more slowly and cautiously, pass instruments differently? If there are safer procedures that could be employed in the more dangerous (to the surgeon) situation, what increase in risk to the patient can be tolerated? Clearly, such reasoning might be part of a rational approach to care. If reasonable modification might decrease the risk to the operator without increasing risk to the patient, voluntary preoperative testing might be justified. In the absence of any practical modification of procedure, information about the patient's infective state could lead to unjustified refusal of needed care.

The point of the preceding discussion is to demonstrate the stringency of the physician's duty to treat by examining the allowable exceptions. Even when exceptions and limitations to the duty to treat are admitted, they are limited and narrow. If made more generous and wide, these exceptions would evacuate the obligation itself to all meaning. I conclude, then, that there is a strong imperative on physicians to respond to the need of the sick and that the imperative does allow certain limitations, but that a refusal to serve based on fear of disease, burden of care, or inconvenience is not easy to justify. Only the most sound and serious reasons, together with scrupulously honest reasoning, may excuse a refusal to provide to the HIV-infected patient any service that would be rendered to noninfected patients with similar needs. Even then, the justification of such a refusal holds only in the particular cases in which the facts meet the ethical tests mentioned above. Policies that allow providers easy outs or designate broad classes of refusable patients or services should be repudiated.

THE IMPORTANCE OF THE WORK

The strength of the professional obligation to care for the sick comes from the nature of illness and from the nature of professional care. The obligation is reinforced by the importance of the work of the health professions in the AIDS epidemic. The epidemic is among the most important challenges faced by physicians, nurses, and the health care system in the twentieth century. The challenges arise not merely in the number of patients who will require care (although the numbers will be great and in some localities overwhelming) but touch the very roots of modern health care as a science and as a practice. All persons who identify themselves as health professionals share in the task of meeting those challenges.

When the AIDS epidemic began, the science of medicine had progressed to the point where several branches—virology and immunology—made possible the identification and characterization of the causative agent. Unlike any previous infectious disease, this disease attacks the immune system itself. It forces scientists to rethink the very basis of medical understanding of the immunological process. Similarly, because AIDS seems to render impotent the mighty tool for prevention of infectious disease, immunization, it creates unique problems in prevention and therapy. In this way, AIDS challenges medicine at its scientific roots. Would it not be ironic if medicine claimed to have the intellectual resources to meet that challenge and, at the same time, tolerated the refusal of practitioners to care for patients? Historians tell us that, during the plague epidemics in Europe, physicians would stand outside the hospitals and shout their medical orders to the monks and nuns within who cared for the patients. A contemporary medical science that would study AIDS but not care for its patients would be replicating that cowardly and ridiculous practice.

This consideration bears on the burdensome and stressful aspect of caring for many patients with a disease so devastating and inevitably lethal. A disease so medically and scientifically significant must be pursued, even though doing so is burdensome and stressful. To do otherwise would be to discount the importance of the disease itself. Even more ethically compelling should be the recognition that those who suffer the disease, who are living instances of AIDS, deserve care even if that care imposes burdens and causes stress in their care providers. To reject the living instances of the disease would represent one of the most serious ethical errors of modern medicine: attending to the disease and ignoring the patient. Every effort should be made to reduce the burden and stress of providers (which usually falls on the most dedicated) and thereby eliminate this as a specious reason to neglect their care.

The "biopsychosocial" nature of the disease also makes it strikingly challenging to modern medicine. It was quickly recognized that the mode of transmission of HIV was deeply embedded in complex human behaviors. Public health officials realized that education leading to behavioral change was the best, indeed the only, preventive strategy. They argued repeatedly that the imposition of traditional public health measures, such as quarantine and isolation, would be counterproductive. In addition, the disease itself is embedded in complex psychosocial reactions to aspects of human life other than the disease, such as sexuality and addiction, and its prevalence among already stigmatized populations colors our understanding of it in significant ways. This epidemic, then, is manifestly a biopsychosocial phenomenon that outreaches by far the virally induced pathology itself. Ancient Hippocratic medicine described "the epidemic constitution," which meant the peculiar conjunction of climate and locale that bred disease. Similarly, AIDS has a modern "epidemic constitution"—the peculiar configuration of ideas, prejudices, and emotions that surround its existence.

The application of modern medical technology to the disease requires a better understanding of the biopsychosocial nature of AIDS than medicine now possesses. Unlike the providential mastery of virology and immunology that allowed medicine to identify the disease and agent, medical understanding of the psychological and social constituents of health and disease is sadly anemic. The AIDS epidemic forces medicine to strengthen its appreciation of these constituents and to use this stronger understanding as a diagnostic, therapeutic, and preventative instrument. This will expand medical understanding of medicine itself.

This consideration is relevant to the problem of stigmatization. Part of the biopsychosocial nature of AIDS is its presence in groups that are already disadvantaged and excluded from certain social goods. Physicians and other providers might find these patients personally repugnant and perceive them within the categories of the stigma attached to them. If providers of care cannot untangle the webs of myth, falsehood, and misinterpretation that stigma spins around persons, the nature of the disease and its transmission, as well as the education needed to contain and eliminate it, will remain obscure and confused, to the detriment, not only of the stigmatized themselves, but of the entire society.

Again, it would be ironic if the disease that thrust medicine into a deeper appreciation of this dimension of all disease were also the disease that medicine avoided. One of the principal features of understanding the psychology and sociology of health and disease is understanding the response of practitioners to forms of disease. If irrational fear, stress, misinformation, and prejudice characterize the response of health professionals to HIV-infected persons, and if remedying those responses proves futile, medicine will fail one of the most significant challenges it has faced in this century.

Finally, in the United States, a strong presumption in favor of physicians' freedom of choice to select those whom they will serve prevails. This is congruous with the American philosophy of liberty and is reflected in law and social practice. It is restricted with reluctance. Yet, this epidemic may be one time when reluctant restriction is advisable. Certainly, the broad scope of that right need not be constrained: physicians should still be able to select their specialities and their place of practice. But all providers who engage themselves to work in institutions abdicate in some sense the particular form of that right that allows them to select among individual patients. People who come as patients to those institutions deserve full service. Even providers in private practice, who retain the right to select patients, must form their consciences and decide whether to restrict their own freedom. The reasons for doing so are worth considering.

In the next decade, the numbers of patients and the magnitude of their need will grow, placing heavy burdens on the profession, on health care, and on society. If some members of the health professions exempt themselves from caring for these patients, they ignore the most serious task posed to their talents in this era. They would calmly contemplate from a distance the sight of thousands of sick and dying left unattended or attended only by those courageous professionals whose risks are now multiplied by their erstwhile colleagues who have retired to the sidelines. Boccaccio's De-cameron described with biting sarcasm such a reaction to the plague of Florence in 1348: "Those who were alive and well took a very inhuman precaution, namely to run away and avoid the sick, by which means they thought their own health would be preserved. . . . having withdrawn to a comfortable abode where there were no sick persons, they locked themselves in and settled down to a peaceable existence."[15]

The refusal or reluctance of one surgeon here and one nurse there may seem insignificant, but the occasional refusal, once tolerated, establishes a new and perverse principle in health care: individuals may ethically ignore those in need of care. Such a principle fosters the perception that medicine is in no way different from a business, setting up shop where safe profits can be made. Admitting into medicine a principle that would allow the health professionals to rescue themselves from caring for sick persons because that care might cause them harm, especially at a time of major crisis and challenge, hovers on the verge of massive hypocrisy. It says to society the equivalent of, "Believe in medicine and its powers; yet do not expect medical practitioners to use those powers when they are needed, but only when it is safe and practical for them to do so."

This perception is a serious threat to the reputation of the profession and all of its practitioners. Refusing treatment in specific cases casts a shadow on the most precious value of medicine, its commitment to service. A London apothecary who stayed to treat patients during the plague in London in 1665 wrote eloquently about those who deserted their charges. His words are worth recalling even today: "Every man that undertakes to be of a profession or takes upon him any office must take all parts of it, the good and the evil, the pleasure and the pain, the profit and the inconvenience altogether and not pick and choose, for ministers must preach, captains must fight and physicians attend the sick."[16]

NOTES

1. C. E. A. Winslow, *The Conquest of Epidemic Disease: A Chapter in the History of Ideas.* (Madison: University of Wisconsin Press, 1980), 118.

2. D. W. Amundsen, "Medical Deontology and Pestilential Disease in the Middle Ages." *Journal of the History of Medicine and Allied Sciences* 32 (1977):402–421.

3. C. F. Turner, H. G. Miller, L. E. Moses, eds., *AIDS: Sexual Behavior and Intravenous Drug Use.* (Washington, D.C.: National Academy Press, 1989), chapters 6, 7.

4. G. Annas, "Not Saints but Healers: A Health Care Professional's Legal Obligation to Treat," *American Journal of Public Health* 78 (July 1988); 844–849; T. Brennan, "Occupational Trans-

mission of HIV," chapter 10, [*The Duty to Treat Patients with AIDS and HIV Infection*].

5. D. M. Bell, "HIV Infection in Health Care Workers," chapter 8, [*The Duty to Treat Patients with AIDS and HIV Infection*]; J. R. Allen, "Health Care Workers and the Risk of Transmission," *Hastings Center Report* (April 1988), 2–4.

6. J. A. Kelly, J. S. St. Lawrence, S. Smith, et al., "Stigmatization of AIDS Patients by Physicians." *American Journal of Public Health* 77 (July 1987); 789–791.

7. R. M. Wachter, "The Impact of AIDS on Medical Residency Training." *New England Journal of Medicine* 314 (1986); 177–179.

8. AMA Council on Ethical and Judicial Affairs, *Current Opinions*, 1986, Principle VI, 9.11.

9. Annas, supra note 4.

10. A. Zuger, S. H. Miles, "Physicians, AIDS, and Occupational Risk: Historical Traditions and Ethical Obligations." *Journal of the American Medical Association* 258 (1987); 1924–1928; E. Emmanuel, "Do Physicians Have an Obligation to Treat Patients with AIDS?" *The New England Journal of Medicine* 318 (1988); 1686–1688; J. D. Arras, "The Fragile Web of Responsibility: AIDS and the Duty to Treat." *Hastings Center Report* (April 1988), 10–20; L. M. Peterson, "AIDS: The Ethical Dilemma for Surgeons." *Law, Medicine & Health Care* 17 (1989); 139–144; L. Walters, "Ethical Issues in Prevention and Treatment of HIV Infection and AIDS." *Science* 239 (1988); 597–603; E. Pellegrino, "Altruism, Self-Interest and Medical Ethics." *Journal of the American Medical Association* 258 (1988); 1939–1940.

11. Pellegrino, supra note [10].

12. Arras, supra note [10].

13. Annas, supra note 4.

14. Bell, supra note 5.

15. Boccaccio, *The Decameron*, trans. G. H. McWilliams (London: Penguin), 53.

16. W. Boghurst, *Limographia*, ed. J. F. Payne (London, 1894), 61.

NO

James W. Tegtmeier

ETHICS AND AIDS: A SUMMARY OF THE LAW AND A CRITICAL ANALYSIS OF THE INDIVIDUAL PHYSICIAN'S ETHICAL DUTY TO TREAT

Persons afflicted with acquired immune deficiency syndrome (AIDS) or its preceding medical conditions face a potential problem with assured access to basic threshold medical care. Subject to certain limitations, there is no guarantee that a physician will fulfill the health care needs of any population of patients. Individuals with AIDS, thus, have a considerable interest in the development of a duty on behalf of physicians to provide treatment. This Note first highlights the limits of the legal duty to treat. It then examines the theoretical impetus propelling an ethical duty to treat. The Note concludes that the grounds for imposing an ethical duty on physicians are too weak to support the result, but the creation of an AIDS-specific legal duty is a viable alternative.

> That is no country for old men. The young
> In one another's arms, birds in the trees
> —Those dying generations—at their song,
> The salmon-falls, the mackerel-crowded seas,
> Fish, flesh, or fowl, commend all summer long
> Whatever is begotten, born, and dies.
> Caught in that sensual music all neglect
> Monuments of unaging intellect.[1]

I. INTRODUCTION

Historically, individual physicians have experienced little constraint on their autonomy. This autonomy is particularly evident with respect to the physician's ability to accept or reject patients. Thus, commentators have recently documented several instances where physicians refused to treat certain classes of individuals during epidemics.[2] During the fourteenth and seven-

From James W. Tegtmeier, "Ethics and AIDS: A Summary of the Law and a Critical Analysis of the Individual Physician's Ethical Duty to Treat," *American Journal of Law & Medicine*, vol. 16, nos. 1-2 (1990). Copyright © 1990 by the American Society of Law & Medicine. Reprinted by permission.

teenth century outbreaks of bubonic plague throughout Europe and in London, the majority of physicians fled the cities or locked themselves in their houses.[3] When the nineteenth century cholera and yellow fever epidemics swept the United States, the combination of the increased number of sick and the decreased number of physicians willing to treat the diseases forced civic authorities to employ mercenary "plague doctors" from surrounding communities.[4] Therefore, from the individual physician's perspective, health care has been largely a product of the free market, carrying with it no obligations binding physicians to treat those needing medical attention.[5]

After a lengthy period of relatively little pestilence in Europe and the United States, physician autonomy is now under attack. The reason for this new challenge is the advent of the modern pandemic, acquired immune deficiency syndrome (AIDS).[6] This attack often is based explicitly or implicitly on the alleged existence of an ethical, as opposed to a legal, duty to treat.

Unfortunately, those commentators who espouse an ethical duty to treat persons with AIDS, AIDS-related complex (ARC) or human immunodeficiency virus (HIV) infection generally have few substantial arguments with which to support their position. In the absence of such support, those theories of ethical duty have little or no logical foundation.

This Note explores and challenges the basis and wisdom of imposing on physicians an ethical duty to treat under these circumstances. It concludes that there is presently no solid basis upon which to assert the existence of an ethical duty for physicians to treat patients who are infected with HIV. Therefore, such a duty should not arise solely under an ethical

framework. Rather, any asserted duty to treat should take shape as an extension of current legal principles, either judicially made or legislatively enacted. Developed in this way, the asserted duty will receive the degree of scrutiny which is needed prior to its application to physicians.

II. BACKGROUND: THE CURRENT LEGAL THRESHOLDS

. . . While publicly employed physicians, such as doctors employed at state hospitals or Veterans Administration facilities, may have a legal duty to treat AIDS patients as a result of federal or state anti-discrimination laws, private physician's legal duty to provide treatment to patients with AIDS, ARC or HIV infection does not yet have a strong statutory basis. Moreover, the common law duty to treat is limited to physicians' breaches of a pre-existing, express or implied physician-patient relationship. The breach of this contract-based duty requires improper termination of treatment. Where such an improper termination occurs, the patient has a cause of action based on abandonment. Generally, these conditions unite to severely limit the individual physician's legal duty to treat patients carrying the human immunodeficiency virus.

III. RESTRAINTS ON THE ARTICULATION OF ETHICAL DOCTRINE

Because the legal duty to treat creates such a small window of physician liability, health associations, doctors and other interested parties have sought alternative bases for imposing a duty to treat in order to avert a potential medical disaster resulting from physicians' widespread refusal to treat AIDS, ARC or HIV infected individuals. Many argue, therefore, that there is an ethical duty to provide treatment to AIDS patients.[7]

Although the difference between legal and ethical duties is significant in that breaches of an ethical duty go largely unpunished or draw only mild discipline from society,[8] the relationship between the two is far from trivial. Ethical duties often inform the development of parallel legal duties. Furthermore, medical licensing boards have discretion to stress ethical considerations to varying degrees.[9] With respect to a duty of physicians to treat patients with HIV, for example, the recognition of an ethical duty may have a great impact on the development of anti-discrimination statutes, or it might lead medical licensing boards to require the treatment of AIDS patients as a condition of licensing. Thus, before this alleged ethical duty begins to have a real impact, there is good reason to ascertain whether the perceived duty makes good ethical sense. The overarching question is how to distinguish what is and what is not ethically sound.

A. Introductory Theory

The source of ethics is a philosophical question which does not have a single and obvious answer.[10] One perspective is that ethics are objective, external truths which humans struggle to come to know. This line of thinking had its origin in the Platonic "forms"[11] and strongly influenced such later theorists as Aquinas and Kant.[12] The opposite view is that ethics originate in the human psyche and can thus be molded and advanced or restrained in whatever way best serves humankind. This stance was

adopted by John Stuart Mill and, to a large degree, Jeremy Bentham.[13]

Regardless of which of these theories, or any of the theories in between, one adopts, the fundamental soundness and acceptability of any ethic depend upon the reasoning which supports it. One element which historically has tended to cloud the ability to intuit ethics is intense emotional debate.[14] Thus, advancing an ethical duty for physicians to provide medical treatment poses a risk to physician autonomy if the duty is based primarily on emotional argument, for such a basis may unnecessarily and unreasonably limit or eliminate that aspect of traditional physician discretion. The remaining portion of this Note will examine the degree of risk which emotional debate regarding the treatment of patients with AIDS, ARC or HIV infection can present to physician autonomy. It will then examine the current status of the search for an ethical duty in this area.

B. The Risks Inherent in Emotional Debate

One fundamental problem with emotional debate is that it invites logical deficiency in the derivation of ethical doctrine. This flaw results because emotion does not necessarily correspond with reason.[15] In itself, logical deficiency is somewhat harmful in creating an asymmetry with other ethics; that is, logical shortcomings with regard to one ethic may call into question the credibility of those other ethics which have a genuine foundation in reason. Logical deficiency, however, is also a symptom of the potential for more drastic problems. As one commentator has noted, the possibility exists that a majority, propelled by passion and emotion, will force the premature realization of an ethical duty.

This may in turn lead the majority to seek to override the minority's individual liberties and thereby trammel the minority's rights:

> [F]ear [or another intense emotion] may override normal restraint. At its most extreme this may lead to unstoppable demands that drastic measures be taken to meet the danger. . . . [T]he majority may refuse to acknowledge the attempt by the minority to exercise their [individual rights], relying not so much on [the majority's] rights as on [its] raw power.[16]

On a number of occasions, a combination of emotion and the majority's outcries arguably influenced the decisions of the judiciary.[17] For example, in *Korematsu v. United States*,[18] the Supreme Court held that the World War II internment of Japanese-Americans living on the West Coast did not constitute a violation of the Equal Protection Clause of the fourteenth amendment.[19] In addition, in *Plessy v. Ferguson*,[20] the Supreme Court upheld Louisiana's "separate but equal" railroad accommodations for black and white passengers.[21] The Court's holding in that case came long after Congress added the Civil Rights Amendments to the Constitution.[22] More recently, in *Bowers v. Hardwick*,[23] the Supreme Court upheld a Georgia law banning homosexual sodomy in private residences.[24] This opinion suspended a trend toward a broad right to privacy in the home.[25] Therefore, as these cases suggest, popular ethics grounded in flawed reasoning may again impact on the development of the law in this country.

In the case of imposing an ethical duty on physicians to treat patients carrying the human immunodeficiency virus, one private interest at stake is the autonomy of physicians. Regardless of whether this interest rises to the level of similar privacy rights which have been violated in the past, it remains true that physician autonomy is a tradition that should remain inviolate until a legislature limits it through the creation of a legal duty or until a rationally based ethical duty takes shape.

C. Balancing Ethics and Emotion

One author has divided the competing perspectives on the interplay of emotion and reason into a trichotomy.[26] At one end of this continuum lies the rationalist perspective. This position looks only to the consistency and force of rational debate, and it attempts to eliminate all emotion as irrational and misleading.[27] The rationalist's view is attractive in its striving for precision and consistency; however, it fails to consider the role that emotion will inevitably play in human decision-making. The weakness of the rationalist perspective, then, is its attempt to remove emotion completely from the decisionmaker rather than to recognize it and hedge against its undue influence.

Near the opposite end of the continuum is the mutual interactionist perspective in which reason and emotion are coexisting forces. According to this approach, a balance should exist so that reason tutors and informs emotion, while emotion, at the same time, tutors and informs reason.[28] In this way, reason never remains unduly static, and emotion never becomes irrational. The mutual interactionist perspective, however, presupposes that the requisite balance between reason and emotion can be maintained.[29] This perspective, therefore, does not answer the initial question of how to assure an acceptable balance of reason and emotion.

Between the two extremes lies an intermediate perspective which does not have the weaknesses of the more extreme perspectives. This view recognizes that, although emotion is unavoidable, it can inordinately influence reason. Thus, while emotion divines possible inadequacies in the status quo by assisting in the intuitive perception of that which seems morally repugnant, emotion is significantly more dangerous than carefully reasoned analysis. For this reason, ethics should always have an independent basis in rationality.[30] Despite its recognition of the role of emotion, this latter perspective, like the others, requires that firm distinctions be made between the emotional and rational foundations of an ethic.

The test for distinguishing reasoned ethics from emotional ethics requires a strict review of the allegedly ethical doctrine. The arguments must be coherent, and the logic must be rational. The existing literature asserting an ethical duty to treat persons with AIDS, ARC or HIV infection lacks the kind of well-reasoned proof necessary to build a strong foundation for the ethic.

Proponents of an ethical duty to treat most often advance an argument based on a social contract theory.[31] This view suggests that the medical profession owes an obligation to society as a *quid pro quo* for society's grant of a practical monopoly over the health care industry. This duty transfers down from the entire profession to the individual physician.[32] How the transfer of this duty is accomplished, however, is usually only summarily addressed.

One commentator noted that what is needed to justify the transfer of duty is a substantial bridge, such as a recognized historical acceptance of this individualized duty.[33] It is questionable, though, whether such a strong historical trend exists.[34] Thus, for example, the argument that physicians have an ethical duty to treat conflicts with pre-existing codified standards of medical ethics. Section Five of the Code of Ethics of the American Medical Association provides that "[a] physician may choose whom he shall serve. In an emergency, however, he *should* render service to the best of his ability."[35] Courts typically interpret this language to indicate that there is no ethical imperative requiring physicians to provide any person with treatment absent a contractual relationship even in emergency circumstances.[36] Moreover, most scholarly articles dealing with the history of an ethical duty to treat conclude that such a history does not exist.[37]

Certain commentators ultimately resolve this question by declaring a "folk wisdom," or oral tradition, of an historical duty to treat.[38] A persistent folk wisdom, however, even if it does exist, only minimally supports an ethical duty to treat. It is an especially weak proposition in light of the codified American Medical Association ethics and recent historical surveys suggesting a lack of historical duty.[39]

It is further asserted that the folk wisdom and certain recent accounts of medical heroism are at least sufficient to shift the burden of proof to those alleging that no duty to treat exists.[40] This shift is inappropriate, however. There is as much or more folk wisdom and historical evidence indicating a tradition of physician autonomy as there is of medical heroism.[42] Therefore, because the effect at stake is an ethical duty binding on all physicians, the resolution of the debate must not depend upon a technical burden of proof question. Rather, it should turn on the substance of the argument, particularly when both sides find equal support in the history and literature. Mere cavilling over legal form adds little to the search for an ethical truth.

In the absence of an historical foundation, two authors declare a strict "virtue-based" medical ethic.[42] This virtue-based theory is presumably based upon Aristotle's conception of virtuous acts as being the highest good,[43] and it was distilled by Scribonius Largus, a first century physician, into a principle specifically applicable to doctors.[44] According to this theory, all professions consist of two components: commitment to an end, and commitment to the functions or duties necessary to attain that end.[45] Thus, for example, undertaking to serve the end of healing obligates physicians to treat sick persons who present themselves for medical care—the function necessary to attain that end.[46]

Commentators have recognized, however, that physicians have not heeded the virtue-based principles during some of the worst recorded plagues and epidemics.[47] Thus, to contend such an ethical duty exists is tantamount to asserting an ethical duty "by fiat."[48] Such a proposal simply does not have a history of support.

Even absent historical support, it is possible that the virtue-based theory is valid but has merely lain dormant. The success of other, analogous applications of a virtue-based ethic are therefore relevant to the soundness of such an assertion here. One analogy lies in the debate over attorneys' ethical obligation to represent without fee those indigent persons whom a court directs the attorneys to represent. The American Bar Association's (ABA) Model Code of Professional Responsibility provides that: "[e]very

lawyer . . . should find time to participate in serving the disadvantaged. The rendition of free legal services to those unable to pay reasonable fees continues to be an obligation of each lawyer. . . ."[49] This strongly suggests a professional legal ethic.

Although there is a fundamental difference between physicians' general duty to treat and a professional duty to provide free care, both varieties of duty are based on ethics. Therefore, the arguments which support one should also transfer to commend the other asserted duty. Significantly, unlike the case of a physician's duty to treat, the theory that an attorney has an historic duty to represent indigents has had some success.[50] More importantly, however, among those states which do not recognize this historic duty, the acceptance of a virtue-based ethic is implicitly rejected. While a few states' courts have recognized a professional obligation based solely on virtue,[51] this theory generally is used in conjunction with the historic duty argument or in dicta.[52] Consequently, it is unclear how much independent weight the virtue-based principle actually carries. The implication is that many in a position to judge the adequacy of the virtue-based argument find it is by itself insufficient to support the proposition for which it is advanced.

Other state courts are critical of the judiciary's role in ordering gratuitous service and refuse to appoint a lawyer to such service against the lawyer's will.[53] Still others entirely refuse to appoint attorneys to represent indigents free of charge.[54] In addition to the divergent state treatment of this matter, the virtue-based ethic has little support outside of the few state courts that have mentioned it. The ABA has never recognized a *man-*

Fiat: Authorization on sanction

datory rule regarding the provision of *pro bono*, or charitable, legal services,[55] and most scholarly commentators reject both the historical and the virtue-based ethical duty regarding indigent legal representation.[56] Moreover, federal courts can only "request" that an attorney represent a person acting in an *in forma pauperis* proceeding.[57]

In summary, a virtue-based theory of professional ethics, like the historical and social contract approaches, does not have the rational qualities indicative of sound ethical doctrine. As a consequence, it is currently improper to assert that physicians have an ethical duty to treat individuals with AIDS, ARC or HIV infection.

IV. CONCLUSION

All of the theories which commentators have advanced in favor of an ethical duty to treat are susceptible to criticism regarding the soundness of the logic and principles comprising their foundation. Although this Note concludes that such formulations do not therefore deserve more than minimal consideration, the cause of those advocating a duty to treat is far from lost. There are clearly other avenues, both more compelling and more appropriate, for establishing such a duty. State and local statutory relief, for example, such as that recently enacted in Los Angeles and San Francisco, has only begun to tap the potential for a legal duty to treat.

Perhaps a simple warning against the currently proclaimed arguments in favor of an ethical duty to treat will be sufficient to ensure more productive scholarly discussion. If, however, the lessons of the past are forgotten, or if rationality is set aside for the sake of expediency, the fervor that may result could inhibit physician autonomy far beyond what is necessary to take care of the perceived crisis regarding the treatment of persons with AIDS. It is only through such reasoned analysis that the medical and legal professions can reach correct ethical conclusions, and it is only through correct ethical conclusions that the traditional freedom and autonomy of the medical profession can be safeguarded.

NOTES

1. Yeats, *Sailing to Byzantium*, in THE NORTON ANTHOLOGY OF POETRY 886–87 (3d ed. 1983).
2. *See, e.g.* Fox, *The Politics of Physicians' Responsibility in Epidemics: A Note on History*, HASTINGS CENTER REP., Apr.-May 1988, at 5 (special supp.); Zuger & Miles, *Physicians, AIDS, and Occupational Risk: Historic Traditions and Ethical Obligations*, 258 J. A.M.A. 1924 (1987).
3. Zuger & Miles, *supra* note 2, at 1924–25.
4. Fox, *supra* note 2, at 7–8.
5. The "free market" of health care is an appropriate analogy. In exchange for enduring increased risk of contracting disease, doctors historically received inflated salaries, license to subsequently practice medicine in the city and the esteem of the citizens and civic authorities. *Id.* at 9.
6. Acquired immune deficiency syndrome (AIDS) is currently a fatal medical condition for which there is no cure. Affliction with the AIDS virus is classified in three stages. The first stage is infection with the human immunodeficiency virus (HIV). HIV infection is detected through medical tests to determine the presence of HIV antibodies. This stage of the disease is often asymptomatic. The second stage involves the onset of initial symptoms and is known as AIDS-related complex (ARC). The final stage is full-blown AIDS from which death eventually results. On January 30, 1989, the Centers for Disease Control (CDC) reported 83,592 cases of AIDS in the United States. The definition of AIDS for CDC's purposes includes laboratory evidence of HIV infection. For a general discussion of AIDS' origin, development, symtomatology, testing and treatment, see 2 M. GUNDERSON, D MAYO & F. RHAME, AIDS: TESTING AND PRIVACY 9–36 (1989).
7. *See, e.g.*, [Emanuel, *Do Physicians Have an Obligation to Treat Patients with AIDS?*, 318 NEW ENG. J. MED. 1686 (1988), from the American Medical Association, *see A.M.A. Rules That Doctors Are Obligated to Treat AIDS*, N.Y. Times, Nov.

13, 1987, at A14, col. 1, and from the Surgeon General, *see Doctors Who Shun AIDS Patients Are Assailed by Surgeon General*, N.Y. Times, Sept. 10, 1987, at A1, col. 4.]

8. Banks, [*AIDS and the Right to Health Care*, 4 ISSUES L. & MED. at] 167.

9. *Id.* at 167 n.115.

10. *See generally* MacIntyre, *Why is the Search for the Foundations of Ethics So Frustrating?*, HASTINGS CENTER REP., Aug. 1979, at 16.

11. PLATO, THE REPUBLIC 168-72, 240-42 (G.M.A. Grube trans. 1974).

12. MacIntyre, *supra* note [10], at 21.

13. *Id.* at 20-21.

14. *See infra* notes [17-26 and accompanying text.

15. *Cf.* Joseph, *Civil Liberties in the Crucible: An Essay on AIDS and the Future of Freedom in America*, 12 NOVA L. REV. 1083 (1988) (discussing the irrationality of emotion and how it has on past occasions led to poor results).

16. *Id.* at 1094 (footnote omitted).

17. *Id.* at 1096-99.

18. 323 U.S. 214 (1944).

19. *Id.* at 219.

20. 163 U.S. 537 (1896).

21. *Id.* at 548.

22. U.S. CONST. amend. XII, XIV, IV.

23. 478 U.S. 186 (1986).

24. *Id.* at 196.

25. *See, e.g.*, Roe v. Wade, 410 U.S. 113 (1973); Eisenstadt v. Baird, 405 U.S. 438 (1972); Griswold v. Connecticut, 381 U.S. 479 (1965).

26. Callahan, *The Role of Emotion in Ethical Decisionmaking*, HASTINGS CENTER REP., June-July 1988 at 9.

27. *Id.*

28. *Id.* The mutual interactionist posture is adopted by Callahan. His [sic] paper is devoted to developing and clarifying this position.

29. Callahan notes the need for "personal equilibrium" but does not suggest how this balance is attained or maintained.

30. *Id.*

31. *See, e.g.*, Emanuel, *supra* note [7], at 1686.

32. *Id.*

33. Arras, *The Fragile Web of Responsibility: AIDS and the Duty to Treat*, HASTINGS CENTER REP., Apr.-May 1988, at 10, 12 (special Supp.).

34. *See supra* notes 2-5 and accompanying text.

35. AMERICAN MED. ASS'N., CODE OF ETHICS § 5 (1980) (emphasis added); *see* Hiser v. Randolph, 126 Ariz. 608, 610 n.1, 617 P.2d 774, 776 n.1 (1980) and accompanying text (citing and applying Section Five of the AMA Code of Ethics).

36. *Hiser*, 126 Ariz. at 610 n.1, 617 P.2d at 776 n.1.

37. *See* Arras, *supra* note [33], at 13-14; *see also* Fox, *supra* note 2, at 9; Zuger & Miles, *supra* note 2, at 1924; *but cf.* Amundson, *Medical Deontology*

and Pestilential Disease in the Late Middle Ages, 32 J. HIST. MED. ALLIED SCI. 403 (1977).

38. Arras, *supra* note [33], at 14.

39. These recent historical surveys are set forth in *supra* notes 2-4 and accompanying text.

40. Arras, *supra* note [33], at 14.

41. *See, e.g.*, Zuger & Miles, *supra* note 2, at 1926; *see generally* Fox, *supra* note 2, at 5.

42. Zuger & Miles, *supra* note 2, at 1927.

43. ARISTOTLE, NICHOMACHEAN ETHICS 17 (M. Ostwald trans. 1962).

44. *See* Arras, *supra* note [33], at 13; Zuger & Miles, *supra* note 2, at 1927.

45. Zuger & Miles, *supra* note 2, at 1927.

46. *Id.*

47. Arras, *supra* note [33], at 13.

48. *Id.*

49. MODEL CODE OF PROFESSIONAL RESPONSIBILITY EC 2-25 (1988).

50. For a general discussion, including historical considerations, of the debate over an ethical duty of attorneys to represent indigents without charging a fee, see Scott v. Roper, 688 S.W.2d 757 (Mo. 1985) (en banc).

51. *Id.* at 763 (citing State v. Ruiz, 269 Ark. 331, 602 S.W.2d 625 (1980); State v. Keener, 224 Kan. 10, 577 P.2d 1182 (1978); Penrod v. Cupp, 284 Or. 417, 587 P.2d 96 (1978)).

52. *Id.*

53. *Id.* at 769.

54. *Id.* at 764 (citing Weiner v. Fulton County, 113 Ga. App. 343, 148 S.E. 2d 143 (1966); McNabb v. Osmundson, 315 N.W. 2d 9 (Iowa 1982); Honore v. Washington State Bd. of Prison Terms & Paroles, 77 Wash. 2d 660, 466 P.2d 485 (1970)).

55. *Id.* at 763-64.

56. *Id.* at 764-65.

57. 28 U.S.C. § 1915(d) (1982).

POSTSCRIPT

Do Physicians Have an Ethical Duty to Treat AIDS Patients?

Most major medical organizations have developed policy statements that reject a refusal to treat patients that is based solely on a diagnosis of AIDS or HIV infection. In 1987 the AMA's Council on Ethical and Judicial Affairs reaffirmed its earlier stand: "A physician may not ethically refuse to treat a patient whose condition is within the physician's current realm of competence solely because the patient is seropositive (i.e., tested positive for HIV infection)." Other organizations that have issued strong statements in support of an ethical obligation to treat patients with AIDS are the American College of Physicians, the Association of American Medical Colleges, the Infectious Disease Society of America, the American Dental Association, and the Academy of General Dentistry.

A few groups, however, have taken a different position. The Texas Medical Association and the Arizona Board of Medical Examiners have not found a refusal to treat AIDS patients a breach of any ethical duty. While the American College of Surgeons has not issued a policy statement, Dr. John G. Bartlett, writing in the *American College of Surgeons' Bulletin* in March 1988, observed: "It is clear that the profession is obliged to care for patients, but it is also clear that both the law and the American Medical Association's Code of Ethics (section 6) permit the physician to 'choose whom to serve,' except in emergencies."

In a review of AIDS litigation, Lawrence O. Gostin describes an increasing number of cases of discrimination by health care workers and predicts that this trend will continue ("The AIDS Litigation Project: A National Review of Court and Human Rights Commission Decisions, Part II: Discrimination," *Journal of the American Medical Association*, April 18, 1990). For a historical overview that concludes that treating patients with AIDS or HIV infection is a virtuous act, rather than a professional obligation or a social contract, see Abigail Zuger and Steven H. Miles, "Physicians, AIDS, and Occupational Risk: Historic Traditions and Ethical Obligations," *Journal of the American Medical Association* (October 9, 1987). Articles that generally support an ethical obligation to treat, though with different rationales, are: Ezekiel J. Emanuel, "Do Physicians Have an Obligation to Treat Patients with AIDS?" *The New England Journal of Medicine* (June 23, 1988); Gregory P. Gramelspacher and Mark Siegler, "Do Physicians Have a Professional Responsibility to Care for Patients With HIV Disease?" *Issues in Law and Medicine* (Winter 1988); Diane Geraghty, "AIDS and the Physician's Duty to Treat," *Journal of Legal Medicine* (March 1989); and Bernard Lo, "Obligations to Care for Persons with Human Immunodeficiency Virus," *Issues in Law and Medicine* (Winter 1988). Also see "AIDS: The Responsibilities of Health Professionals," a Special Supplement of the *Hastings Center Report* edited by Kathleen Nolan and Ronald Bayer (April/May 1988), especially the article "The Fragile Web of Responsibility: AIDS and the Duty to Treat," by John D. Arras.

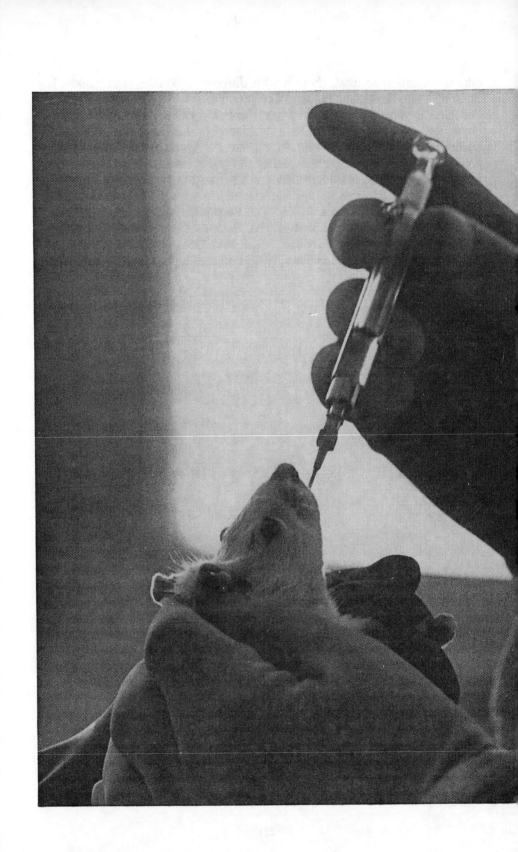

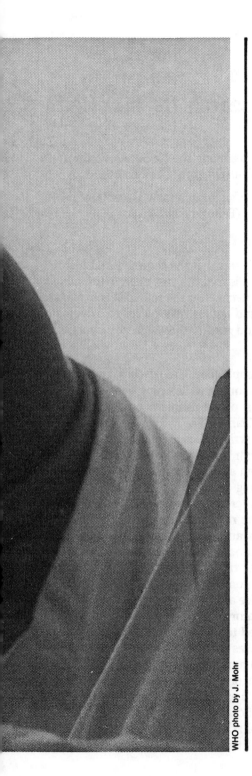

PART 4

Human and Animal Experimentation

The goal of scientific research is knowledge that will benefit society. But achieving that goal may subject humans and animals to some risks. Is it ethical, for example, to cause embarrassment and anguish to an experimental subject by deceiving him in the hope of adding considerably to our store of knowledge concerning human behavior? Questions arise not only about how research should be conducted, but whether it should be conducted at all, such as in the use of animals or the performance of animal organ implants. These questions transcend national boundaries and raise questions of whether research can be "ethical" in one country and not in another. This section contends with issues that will shape the future of experimental science.

Can Deception in Research Be Justified?

Should Ethical Standards of International Research Be "Culturally Relevant"?

Is It Ethical to Implant Animal Hearts in Humans?

Should Animal Experimentation Be Permitted?

ISSUE 12

Can Deception in Research Be Justified?

YES: Stanley Milgram, from "Subject Reaction: The Neglected Factor in the Ethics of Experimentation," *Hastings Center Report* (October 1977)

NO: Diana Baumrind, from "Research Using Intentional Deception: Ethical Issues Revisited," *American Psychologist* (February 1985)

ISSUE SUMMARY

YES: Psychologist Stanley Milgram believes that the central moral justification for allowing deceptive experiments is that the vast majority of subjects who take part in them find them acceptable after the rationale is explained.
NO: Social psychologist Diana Baumrind argues that the costs of deception research to subjects, the profession, and society outweigh any benefits.

Imagine the following situation: Two people come to a psychology laboratory to participate in a study about memory and learning—specifically, the researcher explains, about the effects of punishment on learning. One subject is a teacher, and the other is a learner. The learner is strapped into a chair with an electrode attached to his wrist. He is told to memorize a list of word pairs; whenever he makes an error he will be given electric shocks of increasing intensity. The teacher is then seated before an impressive shock generator, which has switches ranging from 15 volts to 450 volts. The researcher explains that when the learner gives a correct answer to a word pair, the teacher should move on to the next item. But when the answer is incorrect, the teacher must give him an electric shock—and at a higher voltage each time. As the experiment proceeds, the learner makes more and more mistakes and responds to the electric shocks with increasing protests, cries of pain, and finally screams of agony.

This experiment was real. It took place at Yale University in the early 1970s in Stanley Milgram's psychology laboratory. But the learner was an actor. He received no shocks and only pretended to be in pain. The teacher was the true subject of the experiment, which was not about learning at all but about obedience and authority. How far, Milgram wanted to know, would people go in following orders to inflict pain on someone who protests? A few people, he found, defied the researcher's orders. Most, despite obvious stress and discomfort, cooperated to a significant degree.

Much psychological and other social science research, particularly in the field of social psychology, is based on the use of deception to achieve its goals. Milgram's obedience experiments are particularly dramatic, but by no means rare. The moral dilemma posed by such research is: Is it justifiable to deceive subjects, thereby violating a basic ethical principle of truth-telling, in order to conduct a scientific experiment? Those who defend deception, such as Philip Zimbardo of Stanford University and Charles Smith of City University of New York, claim that deception produces beneficial knowledge that could not be obtained any other way. They point out that deception may be the only way to ensure that the subjects' responses are valid; that the only harms involved are temporary feelings of embarrassment or anger; and that after subjects are debriefed or told the true purpose of the experiment, they do not object to it.

On the other side are those, such as Donald Warwick and Herbert Kelman of Harvard University and Thomas Murray of Case Western Reserve University, who believe that in principle it is unethical to deceive others, even for a scientific goal. Deception, they say, *wrongs* subjects (that is, it deprives them of the right to decide freely whether to participate in an experiment or not) even when it does not harm them physically or even psychologically. Research can be designed without deception to achieve the same answers, they argue. Furthermore, they believe that many subjects are reluctant to describe their true feelings about the research and in any case ought to be protected from "inflicted insights" (knowledge about oneself that one would rather not know—such as one's capacity to inflict pain on others). These opponents contend that deception research destroys trust in the researcher and in science itself, and makes it difficult to find truly naive or unsuspecting subjects.

The two selections that follow present the views of two social scientists with personal experience in deception research. Stanley Milgram describes the aftermath of his experiments and concludes that the main justification for his method was the subjects' own ultimate acceptance of it. Diana Baumrind, on the other hand, emphasizes that the violation of trust between subject and researcher, especially when the subject is a student, harms the larger enterprise of science itself.

YES
Stanley Milgram

SUBJECT REACTION:
THE NEGLECTED FACTOR
IN THE ETHICS OF EXPERIMENTATION

Social psychology is concerned with the way in which individual behavior, thoughts, and action are affected by the presence of other people. Although experimentation is not the only way of garnering knowledge in the discipline, it is a major tool of inquiry. As experiments in social psychology typically involve human subjects, they necessarily raise ethical issues, some of which I will discuss here.

INFORMED CONSENT

Many regard informed consent as the cornerstone of ethical practice in experimentation with human subjects. Yet social psychology has until now been unable to assimilate this principle into its routine experimental procedures. Typically, subjects are brought into an experiment without being informed of its true purpose. Indeed, sometimes subjects are misinformed. Is such a procedure ever justifiable?

Herbert Kelman[1] has distinguished two quite different explanations for not informing the potential subject of the nature of the experiment in which he is to take part. One might term the first the motivational explanation; that is, if one told the subject what the experiment was to be like, he might refuse to participate in it. Misinforming people to gain their participation appears a serious violation of the individual's rights, and cannot routinely constitute an ethical basis for subject recruitment.

The second, more typical, reason for not informing a subject is that many experiments in social psychology cannot be carried out if the subject knows about the experiment beforehand.

Consider in this connection Solomon Asch's class study[2] of group pressure and conformity. The subject is told that he is to take part in a study on the perception of lines. He is asked to make a judgment as to which of three lines

From Stanley Milgram, "Subject Reaction: The Neglected Factor in the Ethics of Experimentation," *Hastings Center Report*, vol. 7, no. 5 (October 1977). Copyright © 1977 by The Hastings Center. Reprinted by permission.

is equivalent in length to a standard line, but he does so in the presence of other individuals who, unknown to him, are working for the experimenter and give wrong answers. The experimenter's purpose is to see whether the subject will go along with the erroneous group information or resist the group and give the correct answer.

Clearly the subject is misinformed in several respects. He is told that he is to take part in an experiment on perception rather than group pressure. He is not informed that the others present are working for the experimenter, but is led to believe that they have the same relationship to the experimenter as he. It is apparent that if a subject were informed of the true purpose before participating in the study, he could not experience the psychological conflict that is at the crux of Asch's study. The subject is not denied the information because the experimenter fears he would not participate in the study, but for strictly epistemological reasons, that is, for somewhat the same reason the author of a murder mystery does not reveal to the reader who the culprit is: to do so would undermine the psychological effects of the reading experience.

A majority of the experiments carried out in social psychology use some degree of misinformation. Such practices have been denounced as "deception" by critics, and the term "deception experiment" has come to be used routinely, particularly in the context of discussions concerning the ethics of such procedures. But in such a context, the term "deception" somewhat biases the issue. It is preferable to use morally neutral terms such as "masking," "staging," or "technical illusions" in describing such techniques, because it is not possible to make an objective ethical judgment on a practice unless it is described in terms that are not themselves condemnatory.

Is the use of technical illusions ever justified in experiments? The simplest response, and the one that is most socially and ethically comfortable, is to assert unequivocally that they are not. We all know that honesty and a fully informed relationship with the subject is highly desirable and should be implemented whenever possible. The problem is that many people also believe strongly in the value of inquiry into social psychology, of its potential to enlighten us about human social behavior, and ultimately to benefit us in important ways. Admittedly, this is a faith, but one which impels us to carefully examine whether the illusions and misinformation required by experiments have any claim to legitimacy. We know that illusions are accepted in other domains without affronting our moral sensibilities. To use a simple-minded example, on radio programs, sound-effects of prancing horses are typically created by a sound-effects man who uses split coconut shells; rainfall is created by sand falling on metal sheets, and so forth. A certain number of listeners know about this, some do not; but we do not accuse such programs of deceiving their listeners. Rather we accept the fact that these are technical illusions used in support of a dramatic effort.

Most experiments in social psychology, at least the good ones, also have a dramatic component. Indeed, in the best experiments the subjects are brought into a dramaturgical situation in which the script is only partially written: it is the subject's actions that complete the script, providing the information sought by the investigator. Is the use of technical illusions to be permitted in radio programs, but not scientific inquiry?

There are many instances in everyday life in which misinformation is tolerated or regarded as legitimate. We do not cringe at the idea of giving children misinformation about Santa Claus, because we feel it is a benign illusion, and common sense tells us it is not harmful. Furthermore, the practice is legitimized by tradition. We may give someone misinformation that takes him to a surprise party. The absolutists may say that this is an immoral act, that in doing so one has lied to another person. But it is more important to focus on the person who is the recipient of this information. Does he find it a demeaning experience, or a delightful treat?

One thing is clear: masking and technical illusions ought never to be used unless they are indispensible to the conduct of an inquiry. Honesty and openness are the only desirable basis of transaction with people generally. This still leaves open the question of whether such devices are permissible when they cannot be avoided in a scientific inquiry.

There is another side to this issue. In the exercise of virtually every profession there may be some exemption from general moral practice which permits the profession to function. For example, although a citizen who has witnessed a murder has a moral obligation to come forth with this information, lawyers have a right—indeed an obligation—of "privileged communication." A lawyer may know that his client has committed a murder, and is obligated not to tell the authorities. In other words, a generally accepted moral obligation is suspended and transformed in the case of legal practice, because in the long run we consider this exemption beneficial to society.

Similarly, it is generally impermissible to examine the genitals of strange women. But it is a technical requirement for the practice of obstetrics and gynecology. Once again, for technical reasons, we suspend a general moral rule in the exercise of a profession, because we believe the profession is beneficial to society.

The question arises: is there any comparable exemption due the social scientist because of technical requirements in the kind of work he does, which in the long run, we believe will benefit society? It is true that most often the individual participant in an experiment is not the beneficiary. Rather it is society as a whole that benefits, or at least, that is the supposition of scientific inquiry.

Still another side to the staging by social psychologists is frequently overlooked. The illusions employed by most experiments are usually short-term. They are sustained only insofar as they are required for the purpose of the experiment. Typically, the subject is informed of the experiment's true character immediately after he has participated in it. If for thirty minutes the experimenter holds back on the truth, at the conclusion he reaffirms his confidence in the subject by extending his trust to him by a full revelation of the purpose and procedures of the experiment. It is odd how rarely critics of social psychology experiments mention this characteristic feature of the experimental hour.

From a formal ethical standpoint, the question of misinformation in social psychology experiments is important, because dissimulation subverts the possibility of informed consent. Indeed, the emphasis on "deception" has virtually preempted discussion of ethics among social psychologists. Some feel it is a misplaced emphasis. Support is given to this view by a recent study by Elinor Mannucci.[3] She questioned 192 laymen concerning their reaction to ethical aspects of psychology experiments, and found that they regarded deception as a relatively minor issue. They were far more concerned with the quality of the experience they would undergo as subjects. For example, despite the "deceptive" elements in the Asch experiment the great majority of respondents in Mannucci's study were enthusiastic about it, and expressed admiration for its elegance and significance. Of course, the layman's view need not be the final word, but it cannot be disregarded, and my general argument is that far more attention needs to be given to the experiences and views of those who actually serve as subjects in experiments.

NEGATIVE EFFECTS

Is an experiment that produces some sort of negative, aversive, or stressful effect in the subject justified? In this matter, two parameters seem critical: first, the intensity of the negative experience, and second, its duration. Clearly, the discussion that follows refers to effects that do not permanently damage a subject, and which most typically do not exceed in intensity experiences which the subject might encounter in ordinary life.

One thing is clear. If we assert categorically that negative emotions can never ethically be created in the laboratory, then it follows that highly significant domains of human experience are excluded from experimental study. For example, we would never be able to study stress by experimental means; nor could we implicate human subjects in experiments involving conflict. In other words, only experiments that aroused neutral or pos-

itive emotions would be considered ethical topics for experimental investigation. Clearly, such a stricture would lead to a very lopsided psychology, one that caricatured rather than accurately reflected human experience.

Moreover, historically, among the most deeply informative experiments in social psychology are those that examine how subjects resolve conflicts, for example: Asch's study of group pressure studies the conflict between truth and conformity; Bibb Latané and John Darley's bystander studies[4] create a conflict as to whether the subject should implicate himself in other peoples' troubles or not get involved; my studies of obedience[5] create a conflict between conscience and authority. If the experience of conflict is categorically to be excluded from social psychology, then we are automatically denying the possibility of studying such core human issues by experimental means. I believe that this would be an irreparable loss to any science of human behavior.

My own studies of obedience were criticized because they created conflict and stress in some of the subjects. Let me make a few comments about this. First, in this experiment I was interested in seeing to what degree a person would comply with an experimental authority who gave orders to act with increasing harshness against a third person. I wanted to see when the subject would refuse to go on with the experiment. The results of the experiment showed first that it is more difficult for many people to defy the experimenter's authority than was generally supposed. The second finding is that the experiment often places a person in considerable conflict. In the course of the experiment subjects sometimes fidget, sweat, and break out in nervous fits of laughter. I have dealt with some of the ethical issues of this experiment at length elsewhere,[6] but let me make a few additional remarks here.

SUBJECT REACTION: A NEGLECTED FACTOR

To my mind, the central moral justification for allowing my experiment is that it was judged acceptable by those who took part in it. Criticism of the experiment that does not take account of the tolerant reaction of the participants has always seemed to me hollow. I collected a considerable amount of data on this issue, which shows that the great majority of subjects accept this experiment, and call for further experiments of this sort. The table below shows the overall reaction of participants to this study, as indicated in responses to a questionnaire. On the whole, these data have been ignored by critics or even turned against the experimenter, as when critics claim that "this is simply cognitive dissonance. The more subjects hated the experiment, the more likely they are to say they enjoyed it." It becomes a "damned-if-they-like-it and damned-if-they-don't" situation. Critics of the experiment fail to come to grips with what the subject himself says. Yet, I believe that the subject's viewpoint is of extreme importance, perhaps even paramount. Below I shall present some approaches to ethical problems that derive from this view.

Some critics assert that an experiment such as mine may inflict a negative insight on the subject. He or she may have diminished self-esteem because he has learned he is more submissive to authority than he might have believed. First, I readily agree that the investigator's responsibility is to make the laboratory session as constructive an experience as possible, and to explain the experiment to the subject in a way that allows his performance to be integrated in an insightful way. But I am not at all certain that we should hide truths from subjects, even negative truths. Moreover, this would set experimentation completely apart from other life experiences. Life itself often teaches us things that are less than pleasant, as when we fail an examination or do not succeed in a job interview. And in my judgment, participation in the obedience experiment had less effect on a participant's self-esteem than the negative emotions engendered by a routine school examination. This does not mean that the stress of taking an examination is good, any more than the negative effects of the obedience experiments are good. It does mean that these issues have to be placed in perspective.

I believe that it is extremely important to make a distinction between biomedical interventions and those that are of a purely psychological character, particularly the type of experiment I have been discussing. Intervention at the biological level *prima facie* places a subject "at risk." The ingestion of a minute dose of a chemical or the infliction of a tiny surgical incision has the potential to traumatize a subject. In contrast, in all of the social psychology experiments that have been carried out, there is no demonstrated case of resulting trauma. And there is no evidence whatsoever that when an individual makes a choice in a laboratory situation—even the difficult choices posed by the conformity or obedience experiments—any trauma, injury, or diminution of well-being results. I once asked a government official, who favored highly restrictive measures on psychology experiments, how many cases of actual trauma or injury he had in his files that would call for such measures. He indicated that not a single such case was known to him. If this is true, then much of the discussion about the need to impose government restrictions on the conduct of psychology experiments is unrealistic.

Of course, one difficulty in dealing with negative effects is the impossibility of proving their nonexistence. This is particularly true of behavioral or psychological effects. It seems that no matter what procedures one follows—interviewing, questionnaires, or the like—there is always the possibility of unforeseen negative effects, even if these procedures do not uncover them. Therefore, in an absolute sense, one can never establish the absence of negative effects. While this is logically correct, we cannot use this as a basis for asserting that such effects necessarily follow from psychological experimentation. All we can do is rely on our best judgment and assessment procedures in trying to establish the facts, and formulate our policies accordingly.

IS ROLE PLAYING A SOLUTION?

Given these problems and the particular requirements of experiments in social psychology, is there any way to resolve these issues so that the subject will be protected, while allowing experimentation to continue? A number of psychologists have suggested that role playing may be substituted for any experiment that requires misinformation. Instead of bringing the subject into a situation whose true purpose and nature were kept from him, the subject would be fully informed that he was about to enter a staged situation, but he would be told to act *as if it* were real. For example, in the obedience

experiment subjects would be told: "Pretend you are the subject performing an experiment and you are giving shocks to another person." The subject would enter the situation knowing the "victim" was not receiving shocks, and he would go through his paces.

I do not doubt that role playing has a certain utility. Indeed, every good experimenter employs such role playing when he is first setting up his laboratory situation. He and his assistants often go through a dry run to see how the procedure flows. Thus, such simulation is not new, but now it is being asked to serve as the end point, rather than the starting point of an experimental investigation. However, there is a major scientific problem. Even after one has had a subject role play his way through an experimental procedure, we still must wonder whether the observed behavior is the same as that which a genuine subject would produce. So we must still perform the crucial experiment to determine whether role-played behavior corresponds to nonrole-played behavior.

Nor is role playing free of ethical problems. A most striking simulation in social psychology was carried out by Philip Zimbardo at Stanford University.[7] Volunteers were asked to take part in a mock prison situation. They were to simulate either the role of the prisoner or guard with the roles chosen by lot. They were picked up at their homes by local police cars, and delivered to Zimbardo's mock prison. Even in the role-playing version of prison, the situation became rather ugly and unpleasant, and mock guards acted cruelly toward the mock prisoners. The investigator called off the simulation after six days, instead of the two weeks for which it had been planned. Moreover, the simulation came under very heavy ethical criticism. The ethical problems that simulation was designed to solve did not all disappear. The more closely role-playing behavior corresponds to real behavior, the more it generates real emotions, including aversive states, hostile behavior, and so on. The less real emotions are present, the less adequate the simulations. From the standpoint of the aversive emotions aroused in a successful simulation, ethical problems still exist.

Kelman aptly summarized the state of simulation research when he stated that simulation is not so useless a tool of investigation as its critics first asserted, nor as free of ethical problems as its proponents believed.[8]

PRESUMPTIVE CONSENT

Recall that the major technical problem for social psychology research is that if subjects have prior knowledge of the purposes and details of an experiment they are often, by this fact, disqualified from participating in it. Informed consent thus remains an ideal that cannot always be attained. As an alternative, some psychologists have attempted to develop the doctrine of *presumptive consent*. The procedure is to solicit the view of a large number of people on the acceptability of an experimental procedure. These respondents would not themselves serve in the experiment, having been "spoiled" in the very process of being told the details and purposes of the experiment. But we could use their expressed views about participation as evidence of how people in general would react to participation. Assuming the experiment is deemed acceptable, new subjects would be recruited for actual participation. Of course, this is, ethically, a far weaker doctrine than that which relies on informed consent of the participant. Even if a hundred people indicate that they would be willing to take part in an experiment, the person actually chosen for participation might find it objectionable. Still, the doctrine of the "presumed consent of a reasonable person" seems to me better than no consent at all. That is, when for epistemological purposes the nature of a study cannot be revealed beforehand, one would try to determine in advance whether a reasonable person would consent to being a subject in the study and use that as a warrant either for carrying out the investigation or as a basis for modifying it.

Perhaps a more promising solution is to obtain *prior general consent* from subjects in advance of their actual participation. This is a form of consent that would be based on subjects knowing the general types of procedures used in psychological investigations, but without their knowing what specific manipulations would be employed in the particular experiment in which they would take part. The first step would be to create a pool of volunteers to serve in psychology experiments. Before volunteering to join the pool people would be told explicitly that sometimes subjects are misinformed about the purposes of an experiment, and that sometimes emotional stresses arise in the course of an experiment. They would be given a chance to exclude themselves from any study using deception or involving stress *if they so wished*. Only persons who had indicated a willingness to participate in experiments involving deception or stress would, in the course of the year, be recruited for experiments that involved these elements. Such a procedure might reconcile the technical need for misinformation with the ethical problem of informing subjects.

Finally, since I emphasize the experience of the person subjected to procedures as the ultimate basis for judging whether an experiment should continue or not, I wonder whether participants in such experiments might not routinely be given monitoring cards which they would fill out and submit to an independent monitoring source while an experiment is in progress. An appropriate monitoring source might be a special committee of the professional organization, or the human subjects' committee of the institution where the experiment is carried out. Such a procedure would have the advantage of allowing the subject to express reactions about an experiment in which he has just participated, and by his comments the subject himself would help determine whether the experiment is allowable or not. In the longrun, I believe it is the subject's reaction and his experience that needs to be given its due weight in any discussion of ethics, and this mechanism will help achieve this aim.

REFERENCES

1. Herbert Kelman, "Remarks made at the American Psychological Association," New Orleans, 1974.

2. Solomon E. Asch, *Social Psychology* (New York: Prentice Hall, 1952).

3. Elinor Mannucci, *Potential Subjects View Psychology Experiments: An Ethical Inquiry,* Unpublished Doctoral Dissertation. The City University of New York, 1977.

4. Bibb Latané and John Darley, *The Unresponsive Bystander: Why Doesn't He Help?* (New York: Appleton, 1970).

5. Stanley Milgram, *Obedience to Authority: An Experimental View* (New York: Harper and Row, 1974).

6. Stanley Milgram, "Issues in the Study of Obedience: A Reply to Baumrind," *American Psychologist* 19 (1964), 848-52.

7. Philip Zimbardo, "The Mind is a Formidable Jailer: A Pirandellian Prison," *The New York Times Magazine* (April 8, 1973), p. 38.

8. Kelman, "Remarks."

NO

Diana Baumrind

RESEARCH USING INTENTIONAL DECEPTION

If deceit is used to obtain consent, by definition it cannot be informed. Deceptive instructions logically contradict the informed consent provision contained in all federal and professional ethical guidelines. Yet these guidelines do permit each of the provisions guaranteeing informed consent to be waived provided that some or all considerations such as the following pertain:

(a) The research objective is of great importance and cannot be achieved without the use of deception; (b) on being fully informed later (Principle E), participants are expected to find the procedures reasonable and to suffer no loss of confidence in the integrity of the investigator or of others involved; (c) research participants are allowed to withdraw from the study at any time (Principle F), and are free to withdraw their data when the concealment or misrepresentation is revealed (Principle H); and (d) investigators take full responsibility for detecting and removing stressful aftereffects of the experience (Principle I). (American Psychological Association, 1982, p. 41)

No strategic guidelines are included to assure that these considerations pertain. Institutional review boards (IRBs), as well as investigators, are at liberty to set their own.

Neither the incidence nor the magnitude of deception reported in social psychological research appears to have decreased since 1973. . . .

RULE-UTILITARIAN OBJECTIONS TO DECEPTION RESEARCH

The cost-benefit analysis arising from the metaethical justification called *act-utilitarianism* (Frankena, 1963) is used to justify these exceptions. By contrast, *deontological* or *rule-utilitarian* metaethical positions do not lend themselves to justification of the use of deceptive research practices. From both these more stringent metaethical positions, if informed consent is a right of participants

From Diana Baumrind, "Research Using Intentional Deception: Ethical Issues Revisited," *American Psychologist*, vol. 40, no. 2 (February 1985), pp. 165-174. Copyright © 1985 by the American Psychological Association. Reprinted by permission.

and intentional deception a necessary violation of that right, then intentional deception is to be avoided in the research setting.

The thesis of act-utilitarianism is that a particular act is right if, and only if, no other act the agent could perform at the time would have, on the agent's evidence, better consequences. From an act-utilitarian stance, if in the opinion of the investigator, the requirements of the research demand that the participants be kept unaware that they are being studied or deception must be used to create a psychological reality in order to permit valid inference, then failure to obtain informed consent, concealment, and deception could be justified. The decision would be made by the investigator applying a cost-benefit calculus to the specific situation. Act-utilitarianism, by comparison with rule-utilitarianism, falls short as a metaethical system of justification because (a) it fails to consider the substantive rights of the minority, (b) it fails to take long-range costs into account, and (c) it is subjective and not generalizable. It takes little to convince a researcher or a review board of his or her peers that the long-range benefits of a clever bit of deceptive manipulation outweigh the short-range costs to participants of being deceived. The long-range costs to subjects and society are unknown and therefore are easy for investigators and review boards to dismiss. It is difficult to imagine more extreme instances of deception than those provided by Zimbardo's experiments, and yet both were approved by the Stanford IRB, subsequent to 1973, just as Milgram's experiments had been reviewed favorably at Yale prior to 1973.

Deontological moralists (e.g., Wallwork, 1975) claim that the basic judgments of obligation are perceived as being given intuitively without recourse to consideration of what serves as the common good. For deontologists such as Kant, the principle of justice or truth or the value of life stands by itself without regard to any balance of good over evil for self, society, or the universe. By contrast, I hold, with Waddington (1960), that the function of ethical beliefs is to mediate human evolution so that there can be no principles, including preservation of life, distributive justice, and trustworthiness that are absolutely inviolable.

I ground my judgment that intentional deception in the research setting is morally wrong not in act-utilitarianism (which is too relativistic) or in a deontological categorical imperative (which is too dogmatic), but rather in rule-utilitarianism, the view that an act is right if, and only if, it would be as beneficial to the common good in a particular social context to have a moral code permitting that act as to operate under a rule that would prohibit that act. In Western society, as a result of innate or learned behaviors associated with optimum survival for our community, most of us elevate rules of social living that maximize the opportunity for self-determination so that we may hold each other accountable for our actions. Also, we share strong aversions to certain types of actions. We are averse to hurting others, killing others, and telling lies, and so we feel that we must *justify* these acts if we intentionally commit them. Those of us who are rule-utilitarians grant that even actions to which we have strong moral aversions are justifiable in certain contexts. Thus, retaliative aggression may be justifiable provided that it is proportionate to the grievance; killing may be justifiable if our victim is an enemy or a murderer or a fetus under three months; telling lies may be justifiable if intended to benefit the recipient and not the liar; hurting others may be justifiable if we are dentists or surgeons. However, by justifying morally aversive acts we legitimate them, and this, too, has social consequences, because harm inflicted self-righteously may appear to demand no reparation and is not self-correcting.

Why is intentional deception in the context of the research endeavor so wrong from a rule-utilitarian perspective? At least three ethical rules generally accepted in Western society proscribe deceitful research practices: (a) the right of self-determination within the law, which translates in the research setting to the right of informed consent; (b) the obligation of a fiduciary (in this case, the researcher) to project the welfare of the beneficiary (in this case, the subject); and (c) the obligation, particularly of a fiduciary, to be trustworthy in order to provide sufficient social stability to facilitate self-determined agentic behavior. Consistent with a rule-utilitarian position, I propose to ground these rules teleologically by arguing that their adoption benefits modern Anglo-American society more than contradictory rules, thus explaining their general acceptance.

The principle of *informed consent* is a manifestation of the basic right granted each individual in Anglo-American political philosophy and tradition to be self-determining and let alone so long as the individual is not interfering with the right of other individuals or the public. According to Sir William Blackstone (1765–1769/1941), individuals surrender to society many rights and privileges that they would be free to exercise in a state of nature, in exchange for benefits that each receives as a member of society. Each citizen retains, however, certain rights and privileges that the public may not abrogate without the citizen's consent. Thus, subjects have the right to judge for themselves whether being lied to or learning something painful about themselves constitutes psychological harm for them. A violation of an individual's right of informed consent is a breach of the social contract and thus legitimates retaliative lawlessness because only in a rule-following environment may we be held fully accountable for the consequences of our actions. Therefore, social scientists must exercise their right to seek knowledge within the constraints imposed by the right to informed consent of those persons from whom they would obtain that knowledge.

Further, the basic rules of fiduciary law apply to the researcher-subject and the teacher-student relationships (Holder, 1982). A fiduciary obligation pertains when a person, called the *fiduciary*, is dealing with another under circumstances involving the placing of a special confidence. The overriding duty of the fiduciary is loyalty and trustworthiness by contrast to the principle of "caveat emptor," which may apply to some sales relations. If challenged, the burden of proof is on the fiduciary to show loyalty and trustworthiness. It is illogical for an investigator to justify the use of deceit by appealing to the special quality of the investigator-subject relationship when it is just that special quality that enables the investigator to recruit participants and establishes the fiduciary obligations of the investigator to be trustworthy in relations with them. If the rule that justifies scientific experimentation is "You shall know the truth, and the truth shall set you free," then that rule applies also in the conduct of science.

Finally, violation of trust is generally held to be immoral, and even more so in a fiduciary relationship, especially when the subject is also a student for whom the experimenter serves as a model. If the student is beguiled, his or her trust has been misplaced. If the student is not beguiled, then deceptive instructions do not undermine trust. Psychology undergraduates in heavily experimental departments expect rigged lotteries, deceptive instructions, and the use of confederates. Those who adopt a game-set are not likely to be disillusioned because they do not assume that the experimenter is trustworthy. Under those conditions, subjects may be beguiled, but they are not betrayed. The wrong done as well as the harm done is trivial. But to the extent that students routinely suspend belief, then experimental control has not been achieved by deceptive instructions, and there are no benefits to weigh against the costs. The costs include encouraging students to lie in the interests of science and career advancement.

Even from the permissive stance of an act-utilitarian cost-benefit analysis, it is the responsibility of investigators who wish to use deceptive practices that fail to conform to the informed consent provision of the ethical guidelines to demonstrate first, that the social and scientific benefits of their proposed research objectives are indeed sufficiently significant to offset the costs to participants, the profession, and society; second, that the research paradigm will effectively accomplish those objectives; and third, that those objectives cannot be accomplished equally well by using nondeceptive research paradigms. We proceed now to reexamine the costs and benefits of deception research.

COSTS OF DECEPTION RESEARCH

The costs of deceptive research practices accrue to the participants, to the scientific enterprise, and to society.

Harm Done to the Subject

A brief excerpt from an autobiographical account of a former secretary who typed my earlier articles illustrates the subtle but serious harm that can be done to subjects by undermining their trust in their own judgment and in fiduciaries as well as the reluctance many have to admit, even to themselves, that they have been duped.

This experiment [involving deceptive feedback about quality of performance relative to peers] confirmed my conviction that standards were completely arbitrary . . . because the devastating blow was struck by a psychologist, whose competence to judge behavior I had never doubted before. . . . It is not a matter of "belief" but of fact that I found the experience devastating.

I was harmed in an area of my thinking which was central to my personal development at that time. Many of us who volunteered for the experiment were hoping to learn something about ourselves that would help us to gauge our own strengths and weaknesses, and formulate rules for living that took them into account. When, instead, I learned that I did not have any trustworthy way of knowing myself—or anything else—and hence could have no confidence in any lifestyle I formed on the basis of my knowledge, I was not only disappointed, but felt that I had somehow been cheated into learning, not what I needed to learn, but something which stymied my very efforts to learn. I told literally no one about it for eight years because of a vague feeling of shame over having let myself be tricked and duped. It was only when I realized that I was not peculiar but had, on the contrary, had a *typical* experience that I first recounted it publicly. (Baumrind, 1978, pp. 22–23)

Anecdotal evidence such as this had been challenged as hearsay. A number of studies are harmed by deception experiments. The results are equivocal. However, most of these studies rely on self-report rather than behavioral evidence. About 80% of subjects, when asked, say that they were glad to have participated in the experiment. This is used illogically to establish that subjects suffered no harm. Thus, Milgram (1974, p. 195) justified his shocking procedure by citing results of a follow-up questionnaire in which 84% of subjects said they were glad to have participated in the experiment. However, as Patten (1977) pointed out, it is logically inconsistent for Milgram to use the self-reported judgments of overly acquiescent ("destructively obedient") subjects to establish the ethical propriety of his experiments. Similarly, Marshall and Zimbardo's (1979) subjects were chosen for their hypnotic suggestibility and would be expected to defer compliantly to the experimenter's expertise. After all, if self-reports could be regarded as accurate measures of the impact of experimental conditions, we could dispense entirely with experimental manipulation and behavioral measures, substituting instead vivid descriptions of environmental stimuli to which subjects would be instructed to report how they would act.

Self-report questionnaries used to assess participants' reactions are tacked on as an afterthought and generally lack psychometric sophistication. Subjects' self-reported gladness to be stressed and deceived may be explained by a variety of psychological mechanisms in addition to deferential compliance discussed above. These mechanisms include reduction of cognitive dissonance, identification with the aggressor, and masochistic obedience. It takes well-trained clinical interviewers to uncover true feelings of anger, shame, or altered self-image in participants who believe that what they say should conform with their image of a "good subject." Ring, Wallston, and Corey (1970), in their follow-up interview exploring subjective reactions to a Milgram-type obedience experiment, reported that many subjects stated that they were experiencing difficulty in trusting adult authorities. In a recently reported study of the effects of debriefing (Smith & Richardson, 1983), about 20% of 464 introductory psychology undergraduates reported experiencing harm. In the harm group, 61% had participated in a deception experiment as compared to 38% in the no-harm group. Students who had participated in deception experiments tended to perceive psychologists as less trustworthy than did nondeceived participants. Even subjects who deny other harmful effects do report decreased trust in social scientists following deception research. For example, citing instances of experimental deception:

Fillenbaum (1966) found that deception led to increased suspiciousness (even though subjects tended not to act on their suspicions), and Keisner (1971) found that deceived and debriefed subjects were "less inclined to trust experimenters to tell the truth" (p. 7). Other authors (Silverman, Shulman, & Wiesenthal, 1970; Fine & Lindskold, 1971) have noted that deception decreases compliance with demand characteristics and increases negativistic behavior. (In Wahl, 1972, p. 12)

Decreased trust in fiduciaries then is a generally acknowledged cost of deception itself. Even if we choose to accept self-report data as veridical, 20% of subjects report such harm and the proportion is highest for deception research. From an ethical and legal perspective, harm is done to *each* individual. The harm the minority of subjects report they have suffered is not nullified by the majority of subjects who claim to have escaped unscathed, any more than the harm done victims of drunk drivers can be excused by the disproportionate number of pedestrians with sufficient alacrity to avoid being run over by them.

From a rule-utilitarian perspective, the procedural issue concerns where the locus of control should rightly reside. The generally accepted principle of respect for self-determination dictates that the locus of control should reside with each participant. The subject, like the investigator, retains the right to decide whether the likely benefits to self and society outweigh the likely costs to self and society. The investigator is not privileged to weigh the costs to the subjects against the benefits to society. The principle of informed consent allows the subject to decide how to dispose of his or her person. The subject acting as sovereign agent may freely agree to incur risk, inconvenience, or pain. But a subject whose consent has been obtained by deceitful and fraudulent means has become an object for the investigator to manipulate. A subject can only regain sovereignty by claiming to have been a subject all along and not an object. Not surprisingly, subjects tend to affirm their agency by denying that they have allowed themselves to be treated as objects, and when queried by an experimenter, most will say that they were glad to have been subjects.

Harm Done to the Profession

The harm done by deception researchers accrues to the profession and to the larger society as well as to the individual. The scientific costs of deception in research are considerable. These costs include (a) exhausting the pool of naive subjects, (b) jeopardizing community support for the research enterprise, and (c) undermining the commitment to truth of the researchers themselves.

The power of the scientific community is conferred by the larger community. Social support for behavioral science research is jeopardized when investigators promote parochial values that conflict with more universal principles of moral judgment and moral conduct. The use of the pursuit of truth to justify deceit risks the probable effect of undermining confidence in the scientific enterprise and in the credibility of those who engage in it. As a result of widespread use of deception, psychologists are suspected of being tricksters. Suspicious subjects may respond by role-playing the part they think the investigator wants them to do (Orne, 1962), or pretending to be naive. The *practice* of deceiving participants and of justifying such deception undermines the investigators' own integrity and commitment to truth. Short-term gains are traded for the cumulative costs of long-term deterioration of investigators' ethical sensibilities and integrity and damage to their credibility.

Harm Done to Society

The moral norm of reciprocity proscribing deceitful social relations both acknowledges and places a positive value on the fact that the elements of social reality are reciprocally determined. The inherent cost of behaving deceitfully in the research setting is to undermine trust in expert authorities. If conduct in the laboratory or natural setting cannot be isolated from conduct in daily life, the implications are far-reaching. In a popular article entitled "Snoopology," John Jung (1975) discussed some probable effects of experimentation in real-life situations with persons who did not know they were serving as experimental subjects. These included increased self-consciousness in public places, broadening of the aura of mistrust and suspicion that pervades daily life, inconveniencing and irritating persons by contrived situations, and desensitizing individuals to the needs of others by "boy-who-cried-wolf" effects so that unusual public events are suspected of being part of a research project.

Truth telling and promise keeping serve the function in social relations that physical laws do in the natural world; these practices promote order and regularity in social relations, without which intentional actions would be very nearly impossible. By acting in accord with agreed-upon rules, keeping promises, acting honorably, and following the rules of the game, human beings construct for themselves a consistent environment in which purposive behavior becomes possible.

REFERENCES

American Psychological Association, Committee for the Protection of Human Participants in Research. (1973). *Ethical principles in the conduct of research with human participants*. Washington, DC: Author.

American Psychological Association, Committee for the Protection of Human Participants in Research. (1982). *Ethical principles in the conduct of research with human participants* (2nd ed.). Washington, DC: Author.

Baron, R. A. (1981). The "Costs of deception" revisited: An openly optimist rejoinder. *IRB: A Review of Human Subjects Research*, 3(1), 8–10.

Baumrind, D. (1964). Some thoughts on ethics of research: After reading Milgram's "Behavioral study of obedience." *American Psychologist, 19*, 421–423.

Baumrind, D. (1971). Principles of ethical conduct in the treatment of subjects: Reaction to the draft report of the Committee on Ethical Standards in Psychological Research. *American Psychologist, 26*, 887–896.

Baumrind, D. (1972). Reactions to the May 1972 draft report of the Ad Hoc Committee on Ethical Standards in Psychological Research. *American Psychologist, 27*, 1082–1086.

Baumrind, D. (1975a). It neither is nor ought to be: A reply to Wallwork. In E. C. Kennedy (Ed.), *Human rights and psychological research: A debate on psychology and ethics* (pp. 37–68). New York: Thomas Y. Crowell.

Baumrind, D. (1978). Nature and definition of informed consent in research involving deception. In *The Belmont Report: Ethical principles and guidelines for the protection of human subjects of research* (DHEW Publication No. (OS) 78-0014, 23-1-23-71). Washington, DC: The National Commission for the Protection of Human Subjects of Biomedical and Behavioral Research.

Baumrind, D. (1979). IRBs and social science research: The costs of deception. *IRB: A Review of Human Subjects Research*, 1(6), 1–4.

Berkowitz, L., & Donnerstein, E. (1982). External validity is more than skin deep: Some answers to criticisms of laboratory experiments. *American Psychologist, 37*, 245–257.

Berkowitz, L., & Geen, R. G. (1966). Film violence and cue properties of available targets. *Journal of Personality and Social Psychology, 3*, 525–530.

Blackstone, W. (1941). *Commentaries on the laws of England*. Washington, DC: The Washington Law Book Co. (Original work published 1765–1769)

Bronfenbrenner, U. (1977). Toward an experimental ecology of human development. *American Psychologist, 32*, 513–531.

Dresser, R. S. (1981). Deception research and the HHS final regulations. *IRB: A Review of Human Subjects Research*, 3(4), 3–4.

Fillenbaum, S. (1966). Prior deception and subsequent experimental performance: The "faithful" subject. *Journal of Personality and Social Psychology, 4*, 532–537.

Fine, R. H., & Lindskold, S. (1971). Subject's experimental history and subject-based artifact. *Proceedings of the Annual Convention of the American Psychological Association, 6*, 289–290.

Frankena, W. (1963). *Ethics*. Englewood Cliffs, NJ: Prentice-Hall.

Gardner, G. T. (1978). Effects of federal human subjects regulations on data obtained in environmental stressor research. *Journal of Personality and Social Psychology, 36*, 628–634.

Geller, D. M. (1982). Alternatives to deception: Why, what, and how? In J. E. Sieber (Ed.), *The* ethics of social research: Surveys and experiments (pp. 40–55). New York: Springer-Verlag.

Glass, D. C., & Singer, J. E. (1972). Urban stress: Experiments on noise and social stressors. New York: Academic Press.

Goldstein, R. (1981). On deceptive rejoinders about deceptive research: A reply to Baron. IRB: A Review of Human Subjects Research, 3(8), 5–6.

Heisenberg, W. K. (1958). Physics and philosophy. New York: Harper & Row.

Holder, A. R. (1982). Do researchers and subjects have a fiduciary relationship? IRB: A Review of Human Subjects Research, 4(1), 6–7.

Jung, J. (1975). Snoopology. Human Behavior, 4(10), 56–59.

Kane, T. R., Joseph, J. M., & Tedeschi, J. T. (1976). Person perception and the Berkowitz paradigm for the study of aggression. Journal of Personality and Social Psychology, 33, 663–673.

Keisner, R. (1971). Debriefing and responsiveness to overt experimenter expectancy cues. Unpublished manuscript, Long Island University, Long Island, NY.

Marshall, G. D., & Zimbardo, P. G. (1979). Affective consequences of inadequately explained physiological arousal. Journal of Personality and Social Psychology, 37, 970–988.

McNamara, J. R., & Woods, K. M. (1977). Ethical considerations in psychological research: A comparative review. Behavior Therapy, 8, 703–708.

Milgram, S. (1964). Issues in the study of obedience: A reply to Baumrind. American Psychologist, 19, 848–852.

Milgram, S. (1974). Obedience to authority. New York: Harper & Row.

Mills, J. (1976). A procedure for explaining experiments involving deception. Personality and Social Psychology Bulletin, 2, 3–13.

Milgram, S. (1964). Issues in the study of obedience: A reply to Baumrind. American Psychologist, 19, 848–852.

Milgram, S. (1974). Obedience to authority. New York: Harper & Row.

Orne, M. T. (1962). On the social psychology of the psychological experiment: With particular reference to demand characteristics and their implications. American Psychologist, 17, 776–783.

Page, M. M. (1973). On detecting demand awareness by post-experimental questionnaire. Journal of Social Psychology, 91, 305–323.

Patten, S. C. (1977). Milgram's shocking experiments. Philosophy, 52, 425–440.

Ring, K., Wallston, K., & Corey, M. (1970). Mode of debriefing as a factor affecting subjective reaction to a Milgram-type obedience experiment: An ethical inquiry. Representative Research in Social Psychology, 1, 67–88.

Schachter, S., & Singer, J. (1979). Comments on the Maslach and Marshall-Zimbardo experiments. American Psychologist, 37, 989–995.

Seeman, J. (1969). Deception in psychological research. American Psychologist, 24, 1025–1028.

Shanab, M. E., & Yahya, K. A. (1977). A behavioral study of obedience in children. Journal of Personality and Social Psychology, 35, 530–536.

Sieber, J. E. (1983). Deception in social research III: The nature and limits of debriefing. IRB: A Review of Human Subjects Research, 5(3), 1–4.

Silverman, I., Shulman, A. D., & Wiesenthal, D. L. (1970). Effects of deceiving and debriefing psychological subjects on performance in later experiments. Journal of Personality and Social Psychology, 14, 203–212.

Smith, S. S., & Richardson, D. (1983). Amelioration of deception and harm in psychological research: The important role of debriefing. Journal of Personality and Social Psychology, 44, 1075–1082.

Waddington, C. H. (1960). The ethical animal. Chicago: University of Chicago Press.

Wahl, J. M. (1972, April). The utility of deception: An empirical analysis. In Symposium on Ethical Issues in the Experimental Manipulation of Human Beings, Western Psychological Association, Portland, Oregon.

Wallwork, E. (1975). In defense of substantive rights: A reply to Baumrind. In E. C. Kennedy (Ed.), Human rights and psychological research (pp. 103–125). New York: Thomas Y. Crowell.

White, L. A. (1979). Erotica and aggression: The influence of sexual arousal, positive affect, and negative affect on aggressive behavior. Journal of Personality and Social Psychology, 37, 591–601.

Zimbardo, P. G., Andersen, S. M., & Kabat, L. G. (1981, June). Induced hearing deficit generates experimental paranoia. Science, 212, 1529–1531.

POSTSCRIPT

Can Deception in Research Be Justified?

The American Psychological Association's Ethical Principles, as revised in 1981, permit deception in research but only under certain conditions: The research problem must be important; deception must be necessary in order to carry out the study; subjects must consider it reasonable after they have been debriefed; subjects must have the right to withdraw freely; and the aftereffects must be minimized by the researcher. The latest (1981) federal regulations governing research with human subjects do not specifically mention deception. However, they do state that the requirements for informed consent can be waived or altered "if the research could not practicably be carried out without the waiver or alteration." This provision has been widely interpreted as a way of permitting deception research to be approved by an institutional review board, a committee that considers the ethical aspects of research conducted at the institution.

In 1989 a new controversy about deception in research surfaced when the National Association of Social Workers (NASW) brought charges of unethical conduct against William M. Epstein. In a study designed to examine bias in the peer review practices of professional social work journals, Epstein submitted a pseudomanuscript purporting to test the value of a social work intervention. In one version the manuscript concluded that the intervention was effective, while in another version the intervention was deemed a failure. Epstein's thesis was that research that fails to support the effectiveness of social work intervention would be less likely to be accepted for publication.

The NASW claimed that informed consent should have been obtained from the journal editors because they "incurred nontrivial costs" such as time and inconvenience. The charge was rejected by the NASW Board of Directors, which said that there were no explicit violations of its Code of Ethics. For Epstein's view of the case, see his article "Studying Journal Editors: The Worst Heresy," *IRB: A Review of Human Subjects Research* (September/October 1989), and the more general article by Joan E. Sieber in the same issue of *IRB*, "On Studying the Powerful (or Fearing to Do So): A Vital Role for IRBs."

The results of Stanley Milgram's experiments and a fuller description of his method can be found in his book *Obedience to Authority: An Experimental View* (Harper & Row, 1974). For another controversial case of deception research

232

involving clandestine observations of homosexual activity in a public rest-room, see Laud Humphrey's *Tearoom Trade* (Aldine, 1970). A generally sympathetic account is "Research through Deception," by Morton Hunt, *New York Times Magazine* (September 12, 1982). For critiques of deception by social scientists, see Donald Warwick, "Social Scientists Ought to Stop Lying," *Psychology Today* (February 1975), and Thomas J. Murray, "Learning to Deceive," *Hastings Center Report* (April 1980). Also see Joan E. Sieber, ed., *The Ethics of Social Research: Surveys and Experiments* (Springer-Verlag, 1982), and Tom L. Beauchamp et al., eds., *Ethical Issues in Social Science Research* (Johns Hopkins, 1982).

Robert J. Levine has analyzed all the arguments for and against deception in his book *Ethics and Regulation of Clinical Research*, 2nd ed. (Yale University Press, 1988). He disapproves of deception, yet the Institutional Review Board that he chairs occasionally approves studies involving deception.

ISSUE 13

Should Ethical Standards of International Research Be "Culturally Relevant"?

YES: Michele Barry, from "Ethical Considerations of Human Investigation in Developing Countries," *The New England Journal of Medicine* (October 20, 1988)

NO: Marcia Angell, from "Ethical Imperialism? Ethics in International Collaborative Clinical Research, *The New England Journal of Medicine* (October 20, 1988)

ISSUE SUMMARY

YES: Physician and researcher Michele Barry believes that basic ethical principles of human investigation must be appropriately reinterpreted when applied to different cultures, many of which were unfamiliar to the international bodies that originally formulated these principles.

NO: Physician and journal editor Marcia Angell argues that just as scientific standards cannot be compromised because of local traditions, so too with ethical standards.

In 1945, in the aftermath of World War II, several Nazi doctors were put on trial before an international court in Nuremberg, Germany, for "crimes against humanity." These physicians, who had been among the most respected members of the German medical community, were eventually convicted of conducting brutal experiments on unconsenting prisoners. In the name of "science" and the military needs of the Third Reich, many inmates died or were horribly maimed. They were mostly Jews, gypsies, homosexuals, and others deemed "unfit for life" by the Nazi regime.

The revelations at Nuremberg created an international furor and led to a series of codes and regulations designed to prevent such abuses. The Nuremberg Code, for example, states as its first principle: "The voluntary consent of the human subject is absolutely essential." Most nations adopted several international codes. In the 1960s and 1970s the American public learned that serious abuses of research subjects were prevalent in the United States, although they were not as systematic or brutal as the Nazi experiments. American researchers were also accused, with some justification, of using people in Third World countries as the subjects of research that was risky or that would lead to the development of drugs that would benefit only wealthy nations.

Against this background of scandal and abuse, the U.S. federal government has set standards for research that emphasize the autonomy of individual subjects, protection from risk, written informed consent, and equity in the selection of subjects so that particular groups or individuals do not unfairly bear the burdens or reap the benefits of research. These standards are implemented through local Institutional Review Boards made up of scientists and nonscientists who review every proposed study to ensure that subjects' rights and welfare are protected.

These protections of human subjects (now often called "trial participants" to eliminate the negative connotations of "subjection") have worked reasonably well in the United States. Their applicability to research conducted abroad, however, is controversial. Some research must be conducted abroad for scientific reasons; for example, it is not feasible to study drugs to treat malaria or other tropical diseases in the United States. Other reasons may be even more influential. Scientists are moving studies to countries where it is cheaper to do studies, where the health care system is not so fragmented, and where the regulatory constraints are considered to be less onerous.

As drug trials move overseas, for whatever reason, the question of what ethical standards should be applied inevitably arises. Many of the populations from which subjects are drawn come from cultural, religious, and educational backgrounds that differ significantly from those in the West. Using the example of HIV/AIDS research, the following two selections present sharply differing views. Based on her experiences in sub-Saharan Africa, Michele Barry argues that research ethics should take into account cultural factors such as concepts of individualism and community. Marcia Angell counters with the view that human subjects in any part of the world should be protected by an "irreducible set of ethical standards."

YES

Michele Barry

ETHICAL CONSIDERATIONS OF HUMAN INVESTIGATION IN DEVELOPING COUNTRIES: THE AIDS DILEMMA

As pressure mounts within the scientific community to find a vaccine and develop strategies for the treatment of human immunodeficiency virus (HIV) infection, researchers are turning to developing countries, especially in sub-Saharan Africa, where large patient populations at risk for HIV infection can be identified and studied. Research funding is being offered by the National Institutes of Health and other agencies to establish collaborative study units, and American and European investigators, often unfamiliar with the culture, customs, and economic pressures within these developing countries, are designing large-scale studies. Although there is an urgent need to control the acquired immunodeficiency syndrome (AIDS), consideration must be given to the ethical implications and cultural obstacles involved in conducting research in developing nations.

The basic ethical principles that guide human investigation, as defined by the Helsinki Declaration and the Nuremberg Code,[1] need to be interpreted and applied within different cultural settings, many of which were unfamiliar to the international bodies that originally formulated these principles. The basic bioethical principles may have very different meanings in such settings; foreign investigators need to be sensitive to these different perspectives before conducting studies. Given the urgency of research on AIDS and the difficulties that are being encountered and will undoubtedly persist, I believe that a careful examination of cross-cultural bioethics is critical at this time. In this paper, the immediate problems associated with AIDS research in developing countries are reviewed in the context of four principles—autonomy, beneficence, nonmaleficence, and justice.

AUTONOMY AND INFORMED CONSENT

"Autonomy" is a term derived from the Greek *autos* ("self") and *nomos* ("rule"). In present-day American society, personhood is conceived in terms

From Michele Barry, "Ethical Considerations of Human Investigation in Developing Countries," *The New England Journal of Medicine*, vol. 319, no. 16 (October 20, 1988), pp. 1083-1086. Copyright © 1988 by the Massachusetts Medical Society. Reprinted by permission.

emphasizing autonomy—i.e., individual rights, self-determination, and privacy.[2] The Nuremberg Code requires that participation in biomedical research be based on freedom of individual choice, with no element of coercion or constraint. It dictates further that a person should understand the subject matter of the research sufficiently to make an enlightened decision.[1] Thus, the nature, duration, and purpose of an experiment, the methods of experimentation, the possible effects on health, and all the inconveniences entailed by the experiment need to be made known to a participant.

Applying the concept of autonomy and the requirement of informed consent may present difficulties in cultures where personal choice is extremely limited. For example, in some central African cultures the concept of personhood differs so fundamentally from that in Western cultures that many Bantu languages lack terms corresponding to the English word "person."[2] Personhood is defined by one's tribe, village, or social group. Whereas in Western terms selfhood emphasizes the individual, in certain African societies it cannot be extricated from a dynamic system of social relationships, both of kinship and of community as defined by the village.[2] Thus, an investigator seeking informed consent from persons in such a setting may need to approach community elders for their consent before attempting to obtain informed consent from individual persons. Clearly, the question of who gives informed consent—heads of households, elders, individual persons, the tribe, the ministry of health, or the government—needs to be asked with cultural sensitivity.

Ideally, each potential research subject should comprehend the nature of the investigation before providing valid informed consent.[1] This information should be communicated and interpreted culturally so that it does not become overwhelming and senseless. Unfortunately, when language barriers exist and such concepts as germ theory or viral agents are alien, a description of an AIDS-related investigation, even a simple seroprevalence study, becomes difficult to relay to participants. Illiteracy may be a problem as well, but it must never be confused with lack of intelligence.[3] Often investigators write detailed descriptions of studies to demonstrate to American human-investigation committees that informed consent is being pursued, yet they bypass the important step of making the information culturally comprehensible. I favor local community involvement, and when appropriate the oral and pictorial depiction of concepts. When possible, cultural and societal precepts should be incorporated into the information supplied to participants and into public education about high-risk behavior and AIDS.

NONMALEFICENCE AND BENEFICENCE

The principle of nonmaleficence is associated with the maxim of *primum non nocere*—"first, do no harm." The principle of beneficence requires not only that we refrain from harming patients but also that we contribute to their general welfare and health. Risk–benefit assessment for collaborative research in AIDS may be different when it is interpreted in the context of different cultures and political settings. As the Helsinki Declaration emphasizes, during human investigations the interests of science and society should never take precedence over considerations of a subject's well-being.[1] Yet in nonautonomous populations, health policy decisions and risk-benefit analyses often place state interests above concern for the individual. For example, during a recent study in Tanzania with which I was associated, on HIV seroprevalence in pregnant women and infant cord blood, health officials insisted that the women not be told what they were being tested for, or given the results. The host country's decision was based on the judgment that the results could provoke hysteria within the population about a disease with no cure and for which limited resources were available, even for palliative treatment. The American collaborator was placed in an ethical quandary about whether to continue the field study, because the American protocol, approved by a human-investigation committee, called for informed consent and the dissemination of test results. At the host country's request, serum samples were collected anonymously, but because of ethical concerns analysis of the samples in the United States has not been completed. Certainly, large studies of seroprevalence have been conducted in the United States without disclosure, but typically they have had the informed consent of the participating study group. Although no one is overtly harmed by closed studies, the beneficent treatment of research subjects should include, at a minimum, educational programs and access to the results of anonymous testing.

Limited resources may compound the risk-benefit dilemma for a developing nation. Since many countries cannot afford costly confirmation by Western blotting during large studies of seroprevalence, should asymptomatic subjects be informed of a single positive enzyme-linked immunosorbent assay? On the other hand, large seroprevalence studies with no disclosure withhold information that might lead to a change in high-risk behavior and thus save lives. Funding agencies should try to make confirmation by Western blotting possible during collaborative studies in Africa. Full disclosure—ideally with Western blot confirmation—permits self-protection, the protection of others, and the possibility of treatment should future therapeutic breakthroughs occur.[4]

The risk-benefit assessment of AIDS-related research in the developing world may involve political as well as cultural and ethical concerns. American investigators must be aware of the political and economic ramifications of their research. For countries in which the chief industry is tourism, adverse or false publicity about AIDS can disrupt fragile economies.[5] For example, the 1987 *Fodor's Kenya*[6] speculates that in some African countries the HIV infection rate may be 30 percent of the total population. This statement has no scientific support, least of all in Kenya, where well-conducted studies of seroprevalence have shown much lower rates in the general population.[7] Similarly, the efforts of American researchers to locate the origins of the AIDS virus in western or central Africa have created political controversy and discrimination against African students traveling abroad.[7] The legacy of exploitation by colonialists in many developing countries engenders suspicion even when well-intentioned research on AIDS-vaccine trials is proposed. As a result, certain ministries of health in sub-Saharan Africa have banned the exportation of any body fluid or tissue culture, even if it is ostensibly unrelated to HIV study. Many developing nations rightly take pride in new scientific and laboratory achievements and find it offensive when, for expedience, American investigators take African serum samples to the United States to be examined and processed. In the past, results have often been published even before data were shared with the host country. For all the urgency of AIDS research, human research performed in a developing country without joint collaboration, training, or education can become exploitative or at least be so perceived. Too often, external interests are served with little immediate benefit to the host country or individual subject. As a result, social and racial divisions between nations can become aggravated.

JUSTICE

The principle of justice is concerned with fairness. Neither the benefits nor the burdens of research should be unjustly distributed.[8] Under the principle of justice, research subjects should be chosen for reasons directly related to the scientific question under study and not because of their easy availability, their compromised position, or their ability to be manipulated.[9,10] For example, the mere presence of a highly accessible high-risk population in Africa, for which a low-cost vaccine trial would be feasible, does not constitute sufficient justification for using Africans as subjects.[10] Although there may be scientific interest in studying groups of Africans with different transmission risks in order to evaluate the efficacy of a vaccine, it would be unethical to subject Africans to a disproportionate share of the research risks without an equal share of the benefits.[10] A financial commitment by the developed world will therefore be required to provide an affordable or subsidized vaccine to the developing world.

The principle of justice also implies that resources be allocated in the way that best benefits the society being studied. For many developing countries, AIDS morbidity and even AIDS mortality are seen to be problems less urgent than malnutrition, malaria, tuberculosis, or even the diseases preventable by available immunizations. The World Health Organization report of December 1987 describes 73,747 cases of AIDS from 129 countries. Of these, 48,138 were from the United States and 8652 were from 37 African countries.[11] Although the latter figure clearly represents underreporting, the number of deaths from nutritional diseases alone in Africa almost certainly far exceeds AIDS mortality. Preventing the deaths of skilled, productive adults from heterosexually transmitted HIV infection must become a health priority in the developing world, but should money and manpower be diverted from reducing infant mortality due to diarrhea, malaria, or diseases preventable by immunization? For the proper allocation of resources, AIDS research and educational programs must be put into perspective alongside primary health care programs. Outside investigators need to consider the health care priorities of the collaborating nation and must try to satisfy both internal and external interests. Long-term support in the form of the commitment of laboratories, the training of local staff, or the development of educational exchange programs can mitigate feelings of exploitation and benefit both nations mutually.

HUMAN-INVESTIGATION COMMITTEES AND DEVELOPING NATIONS

The provisions for the review of research involving human subjects may be influenced by politics, the existing organization of medical practice and research, and the degree of autonomy accorded to medical researchers in the field.[12] Whatever the circumstances, there is a responsibility to defend the principles of autonomy, nonmaleficence, beneficence, and justice while conducting human investigation, as emphasized in the Helsinki Declaration and the Nuremberg Code. Research protocols should be subjected to independent ethical review by the initiating country or agency, using ethical standards as stringent as those applied to research carried out within the developed country.[12] Difficulty may arise in collaborative ventures when a host country is forced to maintain foreign standards; these demands may rekindle past resentments of colonialist policy. Sensitivity to the charge of "ethical imperialism" and to health policy decisions made by the host country is important. Mutually acceptable ethical standards can be agreed on easily if a prospective review is approached jointly.

Such deliberations should include attending to the issue of patient confidentiality. Can investigators ensure confidentiality in a foreign society? Is it possible to ensure anonymity in small village settings? Will government have access to the names of persons who are HIV positive? To ensure patient rights, outside investigators should be asking such questions. Local religious, university, or community leaders can often help with the answers.

I suggest working with a local review board composed of both medical professionals and laymen qualified to represent local community, cultural, and moral values. This board should consist of people uninfluenced by the prospect of money, prestige, or personal gain from the project. If no such board exists in the developing nation, the public health ministry or host institution can help in composing one that will maintain ongoing independent review of a project. Such ongoing evaluation is important, because protocols are often revised for expedience in the field.

CONCLUSION

Clearly, AIDS is a devastating health problem for the entire world. The most recent estimate by the World Health Organization is that between 5 and 10 million people are currently infected.[11] The reality is that for all countries, AIDS research is crucial. Despite the potential problems we have described, collaborative work should be encouraged and funded. Yet investigations need to be culturally sensitive, and research ethics need to be made culturally relevant. The formulation of codified principles to guide human investigation permits just and beneficial collaborative research across cultural barriers.

REFERENCES

1. Beauchamp TL, Childress JF, eds. Principles of biomedical ethics. 2nd ed. Oxford: Oxford University Press, 1983:339–43.

2. De Craemer W. A cross-cultural perspective on personhood. Milbank Mem Fund Q 1983; 61:19–34.

3. Setiloane GM. African traditional views. In: Benatar SR, ed. Ethical and moral issues in contemporary medical practice. Capetown, South Africa: UCT Printing Department, 1986:32–5.

4. Curran WJ. AIDS research and "the window of opportunity." N Engl J Med 1985; 312:903–4.

5. Norman C. Politics and science clash on African AIDS. Science 1985; 230:1140–2.

6. Fodor's Kenya. Rev. ed. New York: David McKay, 1987.

7. Sabatier RC. Social, cultural and demographic aspects of AIDS. West J Med 1988; 147:713–5.

8. Beauchamp TL, Childress JF, eds. Principles of biomedical ethics. 2nd ed. Oxford: Oxford University Press, 1983:183–220.

9. National Commission for the Protection of Human Subjects of Biomedical and Behavioral Research. The Belmont report: ethical principles and guidelines for the protection of human subjects of research. Washington, D.C.: Department of Health, Education, and Welfare, 1979:5. (DHEW publication no. (05) 9-12065.)

10. Christakis NA. The ethical design of an AIDS vaccine trial in Africa. Hastings Cent Rep 1988; 18(3):31–7.

11. AIDS worldwide, Lancet 1988; 1:252–3.

12. Proposed international guidelines for biomedical research involving human subjects. Geneva: World Health Organization 1981:1–49.

NO

Marcia Angell

ETHICAL IMPERIALISM? ETHICS IN INTERNATIONAL COLLABORATIVE CLINICAL RESEARCH

Is it proper for Americans to insist that their ethical standards be applied to clinical research performed in other countries? Should ethical standards be substantially the same everywhere, or is it inevitable that they differ from region to region, reflecting local beliefs and custom? And do the answers to these questions depend in any way on the importance of the research to society? Underlying these concerns is the fundamental issue of whether ethical standards are relative, to be weighed against competing claims and modified accordingly, or whether, like scientific standards, they are absolute.

The dominant view in this country is that subjects of clinical research have certain rights that can be abridged only under the most unusual of circumstances. Among these are the right to have their welfare held paramount by the researchers and the right to refuse to participate. Both are protected by institutional and governmental regulations. According to these regulations, the value of research to society does not justify violating the rights of individual subjects. For example, the 1981 "Guiding Principles for Human Studies" of the Massachusetts General Hospital[1] . . . states that "concern for the individual takes precedence over the interests of science and society" and that "A study is ethical or not at its inception; it does not become ethical because it succeeds in producing valuable data." Federal regulations[2] establish the priority of individual subjects implicitly, by defining in detail their right to be informed about a study in which they are asked to participate, to refuse participation, to be informed of findings that may modify their decision as the trial proceeds, and to withdraw without penalty. Thus, in this country ethical standards are not to be relaxed because the study is important.

The federal regulations, as well as institutional guidelines, are explicit in requiring informed consent from all research subjects. Exceptions to this general requirement are extremely limited. Federal regulations, for example, permit exceptions only in unusual situations when the research involves no more than minimal risk. Institutional review boards (IRBs) are to review

From Marcia Angell, "Ethical Imperialism? Ethics in International Collaborative Clinical Research," *The New England Journal of Medicine*, vol. 319, no. 16 (October 20, 1988), pp. 1081-1083. Copyright © 1988 by the Massachusetts Medical Society. Reprinted by permission.

clinical research studies to see that they conform to ethical standards; their approval is necessary for obtaining federal funding, but it does not generally substitute for informed consent. Obviously, even informed consent cannot justify inherently unethical research—that is, research in which the risks to subjects are known to outweigh by far the benefits to them—and this is made clear in the federal regulations. It is an important constraint, since some patients might consent to nearly anything if asked by a trusted authority.

Contrary to widespread assumption, these restrictions on the use of human subjects in clinical research are not peculiar to this country. They are spelled out explicitly in several international agreements, most notably in the Nuremberg Code of 1947[3] and the World Medical Association Declaration of Helsinki, revised in 1975.[3] Indeed, these international codes are, if anything, more stringent than the U.S. federal regulations. The Nuremberg Code, for example, states that in medical experiments on human beings, "The voluntary consent of the human subject is absolutely essential." No exceptions are mentioned. The Declaration of Helsinki also requires informed consent; if researchers believe an exception is necessary, they must give specific reasons to an independent committee. The requirement in the Declaration of Helsinki that "concern for the interest of the subject must always prevail over the interests of science and society" is a more strongly worded version of the very similar statement of the Massachusetts General Hospital, quoted above.

It is often argued that, international agreements notwithstanding, insisting on certain ethical standards when doing research in another country is a form of imperialism and therefore inappropriate. Why should we believe that ethical principles that make sense in one culture are necessarily right in another? More specifically, why should researchers be expected to obtain informed consent in a society that places little value on individual autonomy? This argument has appeal to those who are concerned with tolerance and cooperation among different societies. Any notion of equality among societies, after all, demands that we recognize one another's traditions and not try to impose foreign ones. Many see this position as a step toward countering the long history of exploitation of the Third World by the developed countries. According to this view, if informed consent is not an accepted concept in a society or if a community leader customarily speaks for the members of the community, we should not insist that subjects give informed consent. To do so, it is said, would constitute ethical imperialism.

The problem with this argument is the implication that ethical standards are matters of custom, like table manners, and that their content is irrelevant as long as they are indigenous. It further presupposes that all members of a community share its dominant values. This ethical relativism gives the same weight to practices that would sharply curtail individual freedom (whether by tradition or by a community leader) as to those that would protect it. Does this make sense? Consider an analogy. Does apartheid offend universal standards of justice, or does it instead simply represent a South African custom that should be seen as morally neutral? If the latter view is accepted, then ethical principles are not much more than a description of the mores of a society. I believe they must have more meaning than that. There must be a core of human rights that we would wish to see honored universally, despite local variations in their superficial aspects. Ethical standards in medicine similarly cannot be relative; they must be judged by their substance. The force of local custom or law cannot justify abuses of certain fundamental rights, and the right of self-determination, on which the doctrine of informed consent is based, is one of them.

Furthermore, if we accept the view that ethical standards in clinical research *are* relative, we may create a situation in which Western researchers use Third World populations to do studies they could not do at home because they would be considered unethical. Researchers would be tempted to short-circuit the sometimes onerous requirements for protecting human subjects by appealing to this ethical relativism. What would follow, then, would be true imperialism in the sense of exploitation—the very opposite of what the proponents of honoring local traditions would wish.

This is not to say that Western researchers should not make appropriate accommodations to local custom. Local sensitivities should be respected. It may be necessary, for example, to obtain permission from community leaders to enroll members of the community in a clinical study or from a husband to enroll his wife. Such permission should not, however, be a substitute for informed consent from the subjects themselves or be allowed to override a refusal. Similarly, conveying the information necessary to give informed consent may be very difficult and require a good deal of ingenuity, but it must be done. In such ways, the ethical requirements of performing clinical research in Third World societies may be more, rather than less, exacting.

Fundamental principles of humane research, however, should not be compromised. Human subjects in any part of the world should be protected by an irreducible set of ethical standards, including the requirements that they not be subjected to unreasonable risks and that they be asked for informed consent to participate. When Western researchers collaborate on studies performed in the Third World, it is particularly important that they adhere to these standards. . . . Just as there can be no compromise in scientific standards based on local traditions, there can be none in ethical standards.

REFERENCES

1. Guiding principles for human studies. Boston: Massachusetts General Hospital, 1981.

2. OPRR Reports. Protection of human subjects, 45 CFR 46. Washington, D.C. Department of Health and Human Services, 1983. (GPO publication no. 0-406-756.)

3. Beauchamp TL, Childress JF, eds. Principles of biomedical ethics. 2nd ed. Oxford: Oxford University Press, 1983:338–43.

POSTSCRIPT

Should Ethical Standards of International Research Be "Culturally Relevant"?

The sharp exchange of views in *The New England Journal of Medicine* by Michele Barry and Marcia Angell was followed by further commentaries. In "Ethical Imperialism and Informed Consent," *IRB: A Review of Human Subjects Research* (May/June 1990), Lisa Newton, a professor of philosophy at Fairfield University in Connecticut, supports Barry's conclusions. Newton points out that Western individualism is coming under severe scrutiny and that it is "very questionable that it is up to standard for export." Furthermore, she questions whether "informed consent" is indeed a universal moral standard. If it is not, as she suggests, "the investigator might better stick to the research, and accept the local assessment as to adequate protection of individual rights." Also see Judith Miller, "Towards an International Ethic for Research with Human Beings," *IRB* (Nov/Dec 1988).

For a comprehensive review of the genesis and interpretation of U.S. research regulations, see Robert J. Levine, *Ethics and Regulation of Clinical Research* (2nd edition, Yale University Press, 1986). The major international agreements are: the Nuremberg Code (1947); the Helsinki Declaration (1964, modified at Tokyo, 1975, and at Venice, 1983); and the Proposed International Guidelines for Biomedical Research Involving Human Subjects endorsed by the World Health Organization and the Council for International Organizations of Medical Science (1981). The Medical Research Council of Canada sponsored an International Summit Conference on Bioethics in 1987; the proceedings were published under the title *Towards an International Ethics for Research with Human Beings.*

Specific examples of international research are explored in the case study "Informed Consent in the Developing World," with commentaries by Ebun O. Ekunwe and Ross Kessel, *Hastings Center Report* (June 1984) and Nicholas Christakis, "The Ethical Design of an AIDS Vaccine Trial in Africa," *Hastings Center Report* (June/July 1988).

There has been considerable controversy over whether the results of the Nazi experiments, obtained unethically, should be used in contemporary scientific research. Robert L. Berger has examined the records of the Dachau hypothermia experiments in which subjects were immersed in ice water and monitored for responses to various attempts at rewarming. At least 80 to 90 people died. Berger found that these experiments were scientifically worthless as well as inhumane (*The New England Journal of Medicine*, May 17, 1990).

ISSUE 14

Is It Ethical to Implant Animal Hearts in Humans?

YES: Arthur L. Caplan, from "Ethical Issues Raised by Research Involving Xenografts," *Journal of the American Medical Association* (December 20, 1985)

NO: George J. Annas, from "Baby Fae: The 'Anything Goes' School of Human Experimentation," *Hastings Center Report* (February 1985)

ISSUE SUMMARY

YES: Philosopher Arthur L. Caplan declares that because there is a serious shortage of human organs for transplantation, it is ethically defensible to allow research involving the transplantation of animal hearts to proceed in those areas where no reasonable alternative therapy exists.

NO: Attorney George J. Annas maintains that the experiment on Baby Fae did not receive adequate ethical review and appropriate consent and that it was unjustified and premature.

On October 26, 1984, Dr. Leonard Bailey and his team at Loma Linda University Medical Center, Loma Linda, California, implanted a baboon heart in a 14-day-old infant who became known as Baby Fae. She had been born with hypoplastic left heart syndrome, a fatal condition in which the left side of the heart is much smaller than the right and is unable to pump sufficient blood to sustain life for more than a few weeks. This rare defect occurs about once in every 12,000 live births; it accounts for about a quarter of all cardiac deaths in newborns.

Baby Fae was not the first person to receive a vital organ from a nonhuman primate, but she was the first newborn. Previous attempts at xenografts (cross-species transplants) had been unsuccessful in the 1960s. But Dr. Bailey believed that there might be a better chance at success with a newborn, whose underdeveloped immune system might not reject the transplant. In addition, the use of a new drug, cyclosporine, in human transplants offered some hope of preventing organ rejection, the most serious side effect of transplantation.

As soon as the transplant was announced, however, it provoked widespread controversy. Critics asked: Was there sufficient evidence from animal experimentation to justify using this procedure on a human? Who consented for the infant and what were they told? Was it ethical to sacrifice a baboon for an experiment on a human?

The debate about Baby Fae raged for the 21 days she lived after the transplant, and beyond. It raises many general questions about human experimentation, such as the criteria necessary to try something for the first time, and the balance of risks and benefits to the subject. All federally funded research protocols are now reviewed by Institutional Review Boards (IRBs) in local institutions; Loma Linda's IRB reviewed this protocol, even though the research was privately funded. But was the review adequate?

The questions are made even more difficult because Baby Fae was a newborn, unable to consent for herself. When is it ethical to experiment on a child, particularly a dying one?

All these larger debates are echoed in the following selections. Arthur L. Caplan, a philosopher, favors research involving xenografts in areas where no reasonable alternative therapy exists because of the shortage of human organs for transplantation and because no form of artificial organ replacement is likely to become available in the near future that might serve as a permanent therapeutic option. George J. Annas disagrees. He believes that the experiment on Baby Fae—"an impoverished, terminally ill newborn"—was unjustified on scientific and ethical grounds.

YES
Arthur L. Caplan

ETHICAL ISSUES RAISED BY RESEARCH INVOLVING XENOGRAFTS

THE ETHICS OF INITIATING FURTHER RESEARCH INVOLVING HUMAN SUBJECTS AT THE PRESENT TIME

A number of factors must be weighed in evaluating the case for continuing further research involving xenografts [*a tissue graft carried out between members of different species—Ed.*] in human subjects. Does the demonstrable need for an increase in the supply of organs justify ongoing research involving human beings? Have the medical profession and public officials done all that is reasonably possible to do to maximize the supply of organs that is available to those currently or soon to be in need? What alternatives to xenografts currently exist and what alternatives are likely to exist in the near and long-term future? Are the data available from animal and clinical trials suggestive enough to support further efforts involving human subjects at the present time?

There can be little doubt that a real need exists for developing a viable form of therapy for those persons afflicted with life-threatening forms of organ failure. Many critics of human experimentation involving organ replacement, via both mechanical substitutes and transplants from animal and human sources, note that a greater focus should be placed upon research that might eventuate in strategies for modifying behaviors known to produce irreversible organ failure, such as smoking and alcohol abuse (*Time*, Dec. 10, 1984, pp. 70–73; *Washington Post*, Nov. 14, 1984, p. D7). Such strategies could lead to greater decreases in morbidity and mortality at lower cost than might be possible through the development of techniques permitting organ replacements.

From Arthur L. Caplan, "Ethical Issues Raised by Research Involving Xenografts," *Journal of the American Medical Association*, vol. 254, no. 23 (December 20, 1985), pp. 3339-3343. Copyright © 1985 by the American Medical Association. Reprinted by permission.

But the development of such strategies will do nothing to help those now afflicted or soon to be afflicted with end-stage organ failure. Moreover, preventive measures will do little to benefit those born with congenital defects and dysfunctions of life-sustaining organs. While research on preventive health measures intended to produce modifications in unhealthy life-styles is critical to the reduction of morbidity and mortality in the American population, it offers little hope to those currently or soon to be afflicted with life-threatening organ failure. Nor can those who advocate greater research into public health measures aimed at modifying risk-creating life-styles or unhealthy behaviors guarantee the successful outcome of such inquires.

It is also true that national public policy has not fully addressed existing deficits in the current system for procuring solid organs from cadaver sources. While it is indisputably true that those in need of transplants are far more likely to receive therapeutic benefit from the receipt of human as opposed to animal organs, it is uncertain whether the general public and its elected representatives are willing to examine carefully the flaws and faults of a system that obtains donations from less than 20% of suitable adult donors and almost none from newborn and infant donors.

The reality facing those now or soon to be afflicted with irreversible end-stage organ failure, their physicians, and the general public is that modifications in existing public policies that might alleviate the existing shortage in human cadaver organs for transplantation are not in the immediate offing. Nor are changes in the setting of basic research priorities, which might lead to reductions in the prevalence of organ failure in the general population as a result of modifications in behavior and life-styles, known to produce life-threatening organ failure. Most importantly, even if organ procurement from human cadaver sources were to become significantly more efficient, there would still remain a gap between the available supply of human organs and the need for them.

End-stage organ failure of the heart, kidney, and liver will continue to take a toll of lives among infants, children, and adults for the foreseeable future. With the exception of end-stage kidney failure, no form of artificial organ replacement is likely to become available in the near future that might serve as a permanent therapeutic option.

At the same time scientific and technical understanding of the biology and immunology of xenografting is, at best, primitive. A great deal of research must be done on cellular and animal models in order to advance present scientific understanding of this procedure.

There would appear to exist a pool of terminally ill persons, both children and adults, for whom no therapeutic alternatives exist or are likely to exist in the near future. Many of these individuals are faced with the prospect of inevitable death or for some renal patients, a quality of life maintained by artificial means that is lower than they desire and are willing to tolerate.

Given these realities, it would appear ethically defensible to allow research involving xenografting in human subjects to proceed in those areas where no reasonable alternative therapy exists. The plight of those in need, the lack of viable therapeutic options, the low probability that public policy will be modified to enhance access to cadaver organs, and the fact that end-stage organ failure is likely to continue to be a pressing health care problem for the foreseeable future are factors that would appear to weigh heavily against prohibitions, bans, or moratoriums on clinical trials of xenografts at this time. While there are no scientific data that justify the recruitment of potential subjects for the purposes of therapy, the plight of those dying of end-stage organ failure would appear to justify allowing their participation in further clinical trials to advance scientific understanding of the feasibility of xenografting when appropriate ethical and scientific requirements have been met.

KILLING ANIMALS FOR RESEARCH INVOLVING XENOGRAFTS

One factor that might weight against the continuation of research involving the use of animals as a source of solid organs for humans afflicted with end-stage organ failure is the need to kill animals for this purpose. While it is true that prevailing public policy in the United States allows animals to be killed for a variety of reasons, including general medical research, education, safety and efficacy testing for drugs and commercial products, recreation, and eating, it is also the case that killing animals for the explicit purpose of research intended to develop therapeutic options—which would require the further killing of animals in order to benefit the terminally ill—may raise ethical problems that are unique or specific to xenografting.

In recent years a great deal of effort has been devoted by some members of the general public, the philosophic community, and even the medical and scientific communities to draw attention to questionable practices involving the use and handling of animals for scientific purposes. Some critics of animal experimentation have argued that such practices violate the rights of animal subjects, particularly when they involve significant amounts of pain and suffering for the animals involved.

This is not the place to attempt a review of the pros and cons of the ethics of animal experimentation. However, it is important to note that many of the arguments favoring the continuation of research to develop xenografts are pertinent to the assessment of arguments about the use of animals for this purpose.

If other viable alternative methods existed for generating a sufficient increase in the supply of organs available from cadaver donors, or for making available other therapeutic options for those faced with life-threatening illness or disabilities, then certainly it would be wrong to capture, breed, and kill animals systemically for purposes that might be served in some other manner. Unfortunately, for both scientific and practical reasons, the development of alternative options to benefit those in need are not likely at the present time.

This is not to say that our society is under no obligation to develop such alternatives. Rather, the immediate non-availability of such options, when combined with a moral point of view that accords greater value to an individual human life than an individual animal life, other things being equal, would appear to justify, at least for the time being, killing animals for the purposes of further research involving xenografts. However, in the long run, serious attention must be given to the morality of killing animals for this purpose if other therapeutic alternatives are possible.

THE REGULATION OF XENOGRAFT RESEARCH INVOLVING HUMAN SUBJECTS

Despite the uncertainty and ignorance that cloud current understanding of the feasibility of using animal organs as a source of transplants for human beings, continued research on cellular, animal, and human subjects would appear to be morally justified. However, the lack of empirical knowledge concerning both biological and psychosocial aspects of this surgery would appear to require that all such research, whether publicly funded or not, be conducted in accordance with strict conformity to existing federal, state, and professional society regulations concerning human experimentation.

Indeed, the vulnerability of the human subjects who might be asked to serve in further clinical trials, particularly those who are infants or children, is so compelling as to demand unusual efforts on the part of researchers and institutional review boards to respect the autonomy, rights, and dignity of potential subjects.

The vulnerability of both healthy and terminally ill human subjects involved in the earliest stages of drug testing has led the federal government to enact strict standards for monitoring research in this area. A similar system of review and monitoring would appear to be appropriate for the regulation of any further attempts involving xenografts. While the Food and Drug Administration has no mandate to extend its regulatory oversight to medical procedures that do not involve drugs or medical devices, it would seem appropriate that such a mandate be granted before further clinical trials are undertaken.

Researchers and the members of institutional review boards are under a strong obligation to make clear to potential subjects, or their surrogates in the case of children or mentally incompetent subjects, the highly experimental nature of all forms of xenografting. Potential subjects or their surrogates must have complete and comprehensible information about the limits of scientific understanding concerning the efficacy of the surgery, their right to terminate participation in the experiment at any time, any other experimental procedures that will be undertaken as part of xenograft surgery, and any and all alternatives to xenografting that are available. Researchers interested in pursuing human trials would also appear to be under a strict obligation to inform potential subjects or their surrogates that *nothing* is known as to the long-term viability of xenografts in human beings.

Only those researchers and institutions willing to subject their research protocols and human subject protections to public scrutiny ought to undertake clinical trials of xenografts. Peer review of the competency of researchers and the scientific basis for their research is a sine qua non where terminally ill subjects are concerned. While subject confidentiality and privacy must be fully honored and protected, researchers, institutional review boards, and institutional officials must understand that their primary duty is to protect the autonomy and interests of subjects who are extremely vulnerable to coercion, misunderstandings, and a failure to comprehend the rationale for undertaking a clinical trial. Subjects or their surrogates must understand that the primary goal of research involving xenografts at the present time is to demonstrate the feasibility of such surgery.

Only when it is clear to the medical community, regulatory bodies at the local and federal levels, and the general public that both researchers and their subjects or surrogates fully understand that clinical trials involving xenografts have as their primary goal the acquisition of generalizable knowledge should further research be undertaken.

The author wishes to acknowledge the support of the Health Services Improvement Fund of Blue Cross/Blue Shield of Greater New York in the preparation of this article.

NO

BABY FAE: THE "ANYTHING GOES" SCHOOL OF HUMAN EXPERIMENTATION

Was Baby Fae a brave medical pioneer whose parents chose the only possible way to save her life, or was she a pathetic sacrificial victim whose dying was exploited and prolonged on the altar of scientific progress? To answer this question we need to examine the historical context of this experiment, together with the actions and expressed motives of the parents and physicians.

In an exclusive interview in *American Medical News* ten days after he had transplanted the heart of a baboon into Baby Fae, Dr. Leonard Bailey described Dr. James D. Hardy as "my silent champion." Speaking of Dr. Hardy's transplant of a chimpanzee heart into a human being in 1964, he said, "He's an idol of mine because he followed through and did what he should have done . . . he took a gamble to try to save a human life."[1]

Dr. Hardy, of the University of Mississippi, did the world's first lung transplant on a poor, uneducated, dying patient who was serving a life sentence for murder. John Richard Russell survived the transplant for seventeen days, and died as a result of kidney problems that were expected to kill him in any event. Less than seven months later, in January 1964, Dr. Hardy performed the world's first heart transplant on a human being, using the heart of a chimpanzee. The recipient of the chimpanzee heart, Boyd Rush, did not consent to the procedure. Like Mr. Russell, he was dying and poor. Although not a prisoner, he was particularly vulnerable because he was a deaf-mute. He was brought to the hospital unconscious and never regained consciousness. A search for relatives turned up only a stepsister who was persuaded to sign a consent form authorizing "the insertion of a suitable heart transplant" if this should prove necessary. The form made no mention of a primate heart; in later written reports Dr. Hardy contended that he had discussed the procedure in detail with *relatives*, although there was only one. Mr. Rush survived two hours with the chimpanzee heart.

Dr. Hardy's justifications for using the chimpanzee heart were the difficulty of obtaining a human heart and the apparent success of Dr. Keith

From George J. Annas, "Baby Fae: The 'Anything Goes' School of Human Experimentation," *Hastings Center Report*, vol. 15 (February 1985). Copyright © 1985 by The Hastings Center. Reprinted by permission.

Reemtsma in transplanting chimpanzee kidneys into Jefferson Davis at New Orleans Charity Hospital. Mr. Davis was a forty-three-year-old poor black man who was dying of glomerulonephritis. Davis describes his consent in this transcript of a conversation with his doctors after the operation:

> You told me that's one chance out of a thousand. I said I didn't have no choice. . . . You told me it gonna be animal kidneys. Well, I ain't had no choice.[2]

The operation took place on November 5, 1963; the patient was doing well on November 18 when he was visited by Dr. Hardy. On December 18 he was released to spend Christmas at home. Two days later he was back in the hospital, and on January 6, 1964, he died.

Whatever else one wants to say about these transplants, it is doubtful that anyone would seriously attempt to justify either the consent procedures or the patient selection procedures. Both experiments took advantage of poor, illiterate, and dying patients for their own research ends. Both seem to have violated the major precepts of the Nuremberg Code regarding voluntary, competent, informed, and understanding consent; sufficient prior animal experimentation; and an *a priori* reason to expect death as a result of the experiment.

The parallels are striking. Like Russell, Rush, and Davis, Baby Fae was terminally ill; her dying status was used against her as the primary justification for the experiment. We recognize that children, prisoners, and mental patients are at special risk for exploitation, but the terminally ill are even more so, with their dying status itself used as an excuse to justify otherwise unjustifiable research.

Like these previous subjects, Baby Fae was also impoverished; subjects in xenograft experiments have "traditionally" been drawn from this population. Finally, as a newborn, she was even more vulnerable to exploitation. Three issues merit specific discussion: (1) the reasonableness of this experiment on children; (2) the adequacy of IRB review; and (3) the quality of the consent.

THE REASONABLENESS OF THE EXPERIMENT

While different accounts have been given, it seems fair to accept the formulation by immunologist Dr. Sandra Nehlsen-Cannarella: "Our hypothesis is that a newborn can, with a combination of its underdeveloped immune system and the aid of the anti-suppressive drug, cyclosporine, accept the heart of a baboon if we can find one with tissue of high enough comparability."[1] Questions that need answers are: Is there sufficient animal evidence to support this "underdeveloped immune system" hypothesis as reasonable in the human? Does the evidence give any reason to anticipate benefit to the infant? And is there any justification for experimenting on infants before we experiment on adults who can consent for themselves? The answer to all three questions seems to be no.

Only two new relevant scientific developments have occurred since the 1963–64 experiments of Reemtsma and Hardy: better tissue-matching procedures and cyclosporine. Both of these, however, are equally applicable to adults. Only the "underdeveloped immune system" theory, which posits that transplants are more likely to succeed if done in infants with underdeveloped immune systems, is applicable to newborns, and this could be tested equally well with a human heart. Without this type of prior work we are engaged, as one of my physician colleagues puts it, in "dog lab" experiments, using children as means to test a hypothesis rather than as ends in themselves. Without adult testing, there could be no reasonable anticipation of benefit for this child; the best that could be hoped for is that the parents would bury a very young child instead of an infant. There should be no more xenografts on children until they have proven successful on adults.

THE ADEQUACY OF IRB REVIEW

Since the Loma Linda IRB seems to have dealt with these concerns inadequately, we must question whether the IRB mechanism is able to protect human subjects involved in first-of-their-kind organ transplants. The record is not very good. The Utah IRB failed to protect Dr. Barney Clark from being used as a means to promote the artificial heart.[3] Likewise, the Humana Heart Institute IRB seems to have been more interested in promoting its own institutional concerns than in protecting William Schroeder. For example, its consent form requires the subject to sign over all rights he or his heirs or other parties might have in "photographs, slides, films, video tapes, recordings or other materials that may be used in newspaper, magazine articles, television, radio broadcasts, movies or any other media or means of dissemination." Very little is known about the Loma Linda IRB and its process. According to its chairman, Dr. Richard Sheldon, the twenty-three-member IRB first received the protocol in August 1983 and approved it later that year. Dr. Bailey was told to present any changes in it to the IRB when a suitable candidate was available. These were presented and approved by a nine to seven vote, two days before Baby Fae's transplant.

Some general observations about IRBs may explain their failure in these cases. First, IRBs are composed primarily (sometimes almost exclusively) of employees and staff of the research institute itself. When that institute, in addition to its basic research mission, has another common set of beliefs, based on a shared religion like Mormonism or Seventh Day Adventism, or a secular belief in the profit motive, there is a disturbing homogeneity in the IRB. This is likely to lead to approval of a project by a researcher who also shares the same belief system.

Second, IRBs are way over their heads in this type of surgical innovation. There is no history of successful IRB review of first-of-their-kind kidney, liver, or heart transplants. Ross Woolley has described the Utah IRB that approved the Barney Clark experiment as a "bunch of folks who get together and stumble around and do our thing." More courteously, Albert Jonsen, professor of ethics at The University of California School of Medicine in San Francisco, described the plight of the same IRB as akin to being "asked to build a Boeing 747 with Wright Brothers parts." Homogeneous IRBs without experience in transplant innovation are no match for surgical "pioneers."

THE CONSENT PROCESS

On day ten after Baby Fae's transplant Dr. Bailey said:

> In the best scenario, Baby Fae will celebrate her 21st birthday without the need for further surgery. That possibility exists.

This was, in fact, never a realistic or reasonable expectation, and raises serious questions both about Dr. Bailey's ability to separate science from emotion, and what exactly he led the parents of Baby Fae to expect. He seemed more honest when he described the experiment as a "tremendous victory" after Baby Fae's death. But this could only mean that the experiment itself was the primary end, and that therapy was never a realistic goal.

As of this writing the Baby Fae consent form remains a Loma Linda Top Secret Document. But the process is much more important than the form, and it has been described by the principals. Minimally, there should have been an independent patient selection committee to screen candidates to ensure that the parents could not easily be taken advantage of, could supply the child with sufficient stable support to make long-term survival possible, were aware of all reasonable alternatives in a timely manner, and were not financially constrained in their decision making.

Baby Fae's parents had a two-and-a-half-year-old son, had been living together for about four years, had never married, and had been separated for the few months prior to Baby Fae's birth. Her mother is a high school dropout who was forced to depend on Aid to Families with Dependent Children at the time of the birth of Baby Fae. Baby Fae's father had three children by a previous marriage and describes himself as a middle-aged adolescent. He was not present at the birth of Baby Fae and did not learn about it until three days later. Both felt guilty about Baby Fae's condition, and wanted to do "anything" that might "save her life."

Dr. Bailey describes the crux of the consent process as a conversation with the parents from about midnight until 7 A.M. on October 20. In Dr. Bailey's words:

Apparently, the parents had spent three or four hours in debate at home [before admitting the baby] and now, from midnight until well into the next morning, I spent hours talking to them very candidly and very frankly. While Baby Fae was resting in bed, I showed them a film and I gave them a slide show, explaining our research and our belief why a baboon heart might work.

This account, given slightly more than two weeks after the transplant, is in error. Apparently Dr. Bailey is following Dr. Hardy's precedent of exaggerating the number of "relatives" involved in the consent process. What really happened is recounted by the couple in their exclusive interview in *People* magazine. Present at the midnight explanation were not "the parents," but the mother, the grandmother, and a male friend of the mother who was staying at her home at the time of Baby Fae's birth. Baby Fae's father was *not* in attendance, although he says, "I would have been there at the meeting with Dr. Bailey if I'd known it was going to turn into a seven-hour discussion." Nonetheless, even though he missed the explanations about what was going to happen to his daughter, "when it came time to sign the agreements, I was up there."[4]

It is unclear that either of the parents ever read or understood the consent forms, but it is evident that the father was not involved in any meaningful way in the consent process.

LESSONS OF THE CASE

This inadequately reviewed, inappropriately consented to, premature experiment on an impoverished, terminally ill newborn was unjustified. It differs from the xenograft experiments of the early 1960s only in the fact that there was prior review of the proposal by an IRB. But this distinction did not make a difference for Baby Fae. She remained unprotected from ruthless experimentation in which her only role was that of a victim.

Dr. David B. Hinshaw, the Loma Linda spokesman, understood part of the problem. In responding to news reports that the hospital might have taken advantage of a couple in "difficult circumstances to wrest things from them in terms of experimental procedures," he said that if this was true, "The whole basis of medicine in Western civilization is challenged and attacked at its very roots."[5] This is an overstatement. Culpability lies at Loma Linda.

Some will find this indictment too harsh. It may be (although none of us can yet know) that the IRB followed the NIH rules on research involving children to the letter, and that the experiment *could* be fit into the federal regulations by claiming that Baby Fae's terminally ill status was justification for an attempt to save her life. But if the federal regulations cannot prevent this type of gross exploitation of the terminally ill, they must be revised. We may need a "national review board" to deal with such complex matters as artificial hearts, xenographs, genetic engineering, and new reproductive technologies. That Loma Linda might be able to legally "get away with" what they have done demonstrates the need for reform and reassertion of the principles of the Nuremberg Code.

As philosopher Alasdair MacIntyre told a recent graduating class of Boston University School of Medicine, there are two ways to be a bad doctor. One is to break the rules; the other is to follow all the rules to the letter and to assume that by so doing you are being "good." The same can be said of IRBs. We owe experimental subjects more than the cold "letter of the law."

The *Loma Linda University Observer,* the campus newspaper, ran two headline stories on November 13, 1984, two days before Baby Fae's death. The first headline read " . . . And the beat goes on for Baby Fae"; the second, which covered an unconnected social event, could have more aptly captioned the Baby Fae story: " 'Almost Anything Goes' comes to Loma Linda."

NOTES

1. This and later quotes by Dr. Bailey appear in Dennis L. Breo, "Interview with 'Baby Fae's' Surgeon: Therapeutic Intent was Topmost," *American Medical News,* Nov. 16, 1984, p. 1.
2. Material about Dr. Hardy is drawn from Jurgen Thorwald, *The Patients* (New York: Harcourt Brace Jovanovich, 1972).
3. George J. Annas, "Consent to the Artificial Heart: The Lion and the Crocodiles," *Hastings Center Report,* April 1983, pp. 20-22.
4. Information and quotes concerning Baby Fae's parents are taken from Eleanor Hoover, "Baby Fae: A Child Loved and Lost," *People,* Dec. 3, 1984, pp. 49-63. The second part of the interview appeared in the Dec. 10 issue.
5. *New York Times,* Nov. 15, 1984, p. A27.

POSTSCRIPT

Is It Ethical to Implant Animal Hearts in Humans?

Following the controversy surrounding the Baby Fae case, the National Institutes of Health (NIH) sent a team to Loma Linda University Medical Center to review the research review procedures that were followed. The team concluded that the IRB review of the xenograft protocol followed federal regulations. However, it identified some shortcomings in the consent document: it failed to include an explanation of what compensation and medical treatment was available if injury occurred; it overstated the expected benefits of the procedure by claiming that "long-term survival" is an expected possibility; and it stated that sizematched human hearts were not available, although no search had been conducted or considered.

No further xenografts have been performed, although Dr. Bailey believes that the procedure deserves further trial. In retrospect, Dr. Jack W. Provonsha, a minister and physician associated with Loma Linda, believes that the consent given by Baby Fae's mother was as "well informed as humanly possible." However, he says that "until we have thoroughly learned all our lessons from Baby Fae we shouldn't proceed with another xenograft." Since the Baby Fae case, Dr. Bailey has performed several human heart transplants in newborns. His report of the Baby Fae case was published in the *Journal of the American Medical Association* (December 20, 1985). The same issue contains other articles on xenografts. The full account of the NIH site visit was published in *IRB: A Review of Human Subjects Research* (March/April 1985), along with other articles on the case. See also "The Subject Is Baby Fae," *Hastings Center Report* (February 1985).

Other institutions are considering transplanting hearts from chimpanzees, which are rare and endangered animals but are biologically close to humans. For a case study examining this issue, see Strachan Donnelley and Willard Gayling, "Transplanting a Chimpanzee Heart," *Hastings Center Report* (January/February 1989).

ISSUE 15

Should Animal Experimentation Be Permitted?

YES: Jerod M. Loeb, William R. Hendee, Steven J. Smith, and M. Roy Schwarz, from "Human vs. Animal Rights: In Defense of Animal Research," *Journal of the American Medical Association* (November 17, 1989)

NO: Tom Regan, from "Ill-Gotten Gains," Donald Van DeVeer and Tom Regan, eds., *Health Care Ethics: An Introduction* (Temple University Press, 1987)

ISSUE SUMMARY

YES: Jerod M. Loeb, William R. Hendee, Steven J. Smith, and M. Roy Schwarz, representing the American Medical Society's Group on Science and Technology, assert that concern for animals, admirable in itself, cannot impede the development of methods to improve the welfare of humans.
NO: Philosopher Tom Regan argues that conducting research on animals exacts the grave moral price of failing to show proper respect for animals' inherent value, whatever the benefits of the research.

In 1865 the great French physiologist Claude Bernard wrote: "Physicians already make too many dangerous experiments on man before carefully studying them in animals." In his insistence on adequate animal research before trying a new therapy on human beings, Bernard established a principle of research ethics that is still considered valid. But in the past few decades this principle has been challenged by another view—one that sees animals not as tools for human use and consumption but as moral agents in their own right. Animal experimentation, according to this theory, cannot be taken for granted but must be justified by ethical criteria at least as stringent as those that apply to research involving humans.

Philosophers traditionally have not ascribed any moral status to animals. Like St. Thomas Aquinas before him, Renéscartes, a seventeenth-century French physiologist and philosopher, saw no ethical problem in experimentation on animals. Descartes approved of cutting open a full conscious animal because it was, he said, a machine more complex than a clock but no more capable of feeling pain. Immanuel Kant argued that animals need not be treated as ends in themselves because they lacked rationality.

Beginning in England in the nineteenth century, antivivisectionists, people who advocate the abolition of animal experimentation, campaigned, with varying success, for laws to control scientific research. But the internal dissensions in the movement and its frequent lapses into sentimentality made it only partially effective. At most the antivivisectionists achieved some legislation that mandated more humane treatment of animals used for research. But they never succeeded in abolishing animal research or even in establishing the need for justification of particular research projects.

The more recent movement to ban animal research, however, is both better organized politically and more rigorously philosophical. The movement, often called animal liberation or animal rights, is similar in principle to the civil rights movement of the 1960s. Just as blacks, women, and other minorities sought recognition of their equal status, animal advocates have built a case for the equal status of animals.

Peter Singer, one of the leaders of this movement, has presented an eloquent case that we practice not only racism and sexism in our society but also "speciesism." That is, we assume that human beings are superior to other animals; we are prejudiced in favor of our own kind. Experimenting on animals and eating their flesh are the two major forms of speciesism in our society. Singer points out that some categories of human beings—infants and mentally retarded people—rate lower on a scale of intelligence, awareness, and self-consciousness than some animals. Yet we would not treat these individuals in the way we do animals. He argues that "all animals are equal" and the suffering of an animal is morally equal to the suffering of a human being.

Proponents of animal research counter that such views are fundamentally misguided, that human beings, with the capacity for rational thought and action, are indeed a superior species. They contend that, while animals deserve humane treatment, the good consequences of animal research (i.e., knowledge that will benefit human beings) outweigh the suffering of individual animals. No other research techniques can substitute for the reactions of live animals, they declare.

In the selections that follow, Jerod M. Loeb, William R. Hendee, Steven J. Smith, and M. Roy Schwarz reaffirm the American Medical Association's defense of animal research because it is essential for medical progress and it would be unethical to deprive humans and animals of advances in medicine that result from this research. Tom Regan disputes the view that benefit to humans justifies research on animals. Pointing to their inherent value, he says that "whatever our gains, they are ill-gotten," and calls for an end to such research.

YES

Jerod M. Loeb, William R. Hendee, Steven J. Smith, and M. Roy Schwarz

HUMAN vs ANIMAL RIGHTS: IN DEFENSE OF ANIMAL RESEARCH

Research with animals is a highly controversial topic in our society. Animal rights groups that intend to stop all experimentation with animals are in the vanguard of this controversy. Their methods range from educational efforts directed in large measure to the young and uninformed, to promotion of restrictive legislation, filing lawsuits, and violence that includes raids on laboratories and death threats to investigators. Their rhetoric is emotionally charged and their information is frequently distorted and pejorative. Their tactics vary but have a single objective—to stop scientific research with animals.

The resources of the animal rights groups are extensive, in part because less militant organizations of animal activists, including some humane societies, have been infiltrated or taken over by animal rights groups to gain access to their fiscal and physical holdings. Through bizarre tactics, extravagant claims, and gruesome myths, animal rights groups have captured the attention of the media and a sizable segment of the public. Nevertheless, people invariably support the use of animals in research when they understand both sides of the issue and the contributions of animal research to relief of human suffering. However, all too often they do not understand both sides because information about the need for animal research is not presented. When this need is explained, the presentation often reveals an arrogance of the scientific community and an unwillingness to be accountable to public opinion.

The use of animals in research is fundamentally an ethical question: is it more ethical to ban all research with animals or to use a limited number of animals in research under humane conditions when no alternatives exist to achieve medical advances that reduce substantial human suffering and misery? . . .

From Jerod M. Loeb, William R. Hendee, Steven J. Smith, and M. Roy Schwarz, "Human vs. Animal Rights: In Defense of Animal Research," *Journal of the American Medical Association*, vol. 262, no. 19 (November 17, 1989), pp. 2716-2720. Copyright © 1989 by the American Medical Association. Reprinted by permission.

ANIMALS IN SCIENTIFIC RESEARCH

Animals have been used in research for more than 2000 years. In the third century BC, the natural philosopher Erisistratus of Alexandria used animals to study bodily function. In all likelihood, Aristotle performed vivisection on animals. The Roman physician Galen used apes and pigs to prove his theory that veins carry blood rather than air. In succeeding centuries, animals were employed to confirm theories about physiology developed through observation. Advances in knowledge from these experiments include demonstration of the circulation of blood by Harvey in 1622, documentation of the effects of anesthesia on the body in 1846, and elucidation of the relationship between bacteria and disease in 1878.[1] In his book *An Introduction to the Study of Experimental Medicine* published in 1865, Bernard[2] described the importance of animal research to advances in knowledge about the human body and justified the continued use of animals for this purpose.

In this century, many medical advances have been achieved through research with animals.[3] Infectious diseases such as pertussis, rubella, measles, and poliomyelitis have been brought under control with vaccines developed in animals. The development of immunization techniques against today's infectious diseases, including human immunodeficiency virus disease, depends entirely on experiments in animals. Antibiotics that control infection are always tested in animals before use in humans. Physiological disorders such as diabetes and epilepsy are treatable today through knowledge and products gained by animal research. Surgical procedures such as coronary artery bypass grafts, cerebrospinal fluid shunts, and retinal reattachments have evolved from experiments with animals. Transplantation procedures for persons with failed liver, heart, lung, and kidney function are products of animal research.

Animals have been essential to the evolution of modern medicine and the conquest of many illnesses. However, many medical challenges remain to be solved. Cancer, heart disease, cerebrovascular disease, dementia, depression, arthritis, and a variety of inherited disorders are yet to be understood and controlled. Until they are, human pain and suffering will endure, and society will continue to expend its emotional and fiscal resources in efforts to alleviate or at least reduce them.

Animal research has not only benefited humans. Procedures and products developed through this process have also helped animals.[4,5] Vaccines against rabies, distemper, and parvovirus in dogs are a spin-off of animal research, as are immunization techniques against cholera in hogs, encephalitis in horses, and brucellosis in cattle. Drugs to combat heartworm, intestinal parasites, and mastitis were developed in animals used for experimental purposes. Surgical procedures developed in animals help animals as well as humans.

Research with animals has yielded immeasurable benefits to both humans and animals. However, this research raises fundamental philosophical issues concerning the rights of humans to use animals to benefit humans and other animals. If these rights are granted (and many people are loath to do so), additional questions arise concerning the way that research should be performed, the accountability of researchers to public sentiment, the nature of an ethical code for animal research, and who should compose and approve the code. Today, some animal activists are asking whether humans have the right to exercise dominion over animals for any purpose, including research. Others suggest that because humans have dominion over other forms of life, they are obligated to protect and preserve animals and ensure that they are not exploited. Still others agree that animals can be used to help people, but only under circumstances that are so structured as to be unattainable by most researchers. These attitudes may all differ, but their consequences are similar. They all threaten to diminish or stop animal research.

CHALLENGE TO ANIMAL RESEARCH

Challenges to the use of animals to benefit humans are not new—their origins can be traced back several centuries. With respect to animal research, opposition has been vocal in Europe for more than 400 years and in the United States for at least 100 years.[6]

Most of the current arguments against research with animals have historic precedents that must be grasped to understand the current debate. These precedents originated in the controversy between Cartesian and utilitarian philosophers that extended from the 16th to the 18th centuries.

The Cartesian-utilitarian debate was opened by the French philosopher Descartes, who defended the use of animals in experiments by insisting the animals respond to stimuli in only one way—"according to the arrangement of their organs."[7] He stated that animals lack the ability to reason and think and are, therefore, similar to a machine. Humans, on the other hand, can think, talk, and re-spond to stimuli in various ways. These differences, Descartes argued, make animals inferior to humans and justify their use as a machine, including as experimental subjects. He proposed that animals learn only by experience, whereas humans learn by "teaching-learning." Humans do not always have to experience something to know that it is true.

Descartes' arguments were countered by the utilitarian philosopher Bentham of England. "The question," said Bentham, "is not can they reason? nor can they talk? but can they suffer?"[8] In utilitarian terms, humans and animals are linked by their common ability to suffer and their common right not to suffer and die at the hands of others. This utilitarian thesis has rippled through various groups opposed to research with animals for more than a century.

In the 1970s, the antivivisectionist movement was influenced by three books that clarified the issues and introduced the rationale for increased militancy against animal research. In 1971, the anthology *Animals, Men and Morals*, by Godlovitch et al,[9] raised the concept of animal rights and analyzed the relationships between humans and animals. Four years later, *Victims of Science*, by Ryder,[10] introduced the concept of "speciesism" as equivalent to fascism. Also in 1975, Singer[11] published *Animal Liberation: A New Ethic for Our Treatment of Animals*. This book is generally considered the progenitor of the modern animal rights movement. Invoking Ryder's concept of speciesism, Singer deplored the historic attitude of humans toward nonhumans as a "form of prejudice no less objectionable than racism or sexism." He urged that the liberation of animals should become the next great cause after civil rights and the women's movement.

Singer's book not only was a philosophical treatise; it also was a call to action. It provided an intellectual foundation and a moral focus for the animal rights movement. These features attracted many who were indifferent to the emotional appeal based on a love of animals that had characterized antivivisectionist efforts for the past century. Singer's book swelled the ranks of the antivivisectionist movement and transformed it into a movement for animal rights. It also has been used to justify illegal activities intended to impede animal research and instill fear and intimidation in those engaged in it. . . .

DEFENSE OF ANIMAL RESEARCH

The issue of animal research is fundamentally an issue of the dominion of humans over animals. This issue is rooted in the Judeo-Christian religion of western culture, including the ancient tradition of animal sacrifice described in the Old Testament and the practice of using animals as surrogates for suffering humans described in the New Testament. The sacredness of human life is a central theme of biblical morality, and the dominion of humans over other forms of life is a natural consequence of this theme.[12] The issue of dominion is not, however, unique to animal research. It is applicable to every situation where animals are subservient to humans. It applies to the use of animals for food and clothing; the application of animals as beasts of burden and transportation; the holding of animals in captivity such as in zoos and as household pets; the use of animals as entertainment, such as in sea parks and circuses; the exploitation of animals in sports that employ animals, including hunting, racing, and animal

shows; and the eradication of pests such as rats and mice from homes and farms. Even provision of food and shelter to animals reflects an attitude of dominion of humans over animals. A person who truly does not believe in human dominance over animals would be forced to oppose all of these practices, including keeping animals as household pets or in any form of physical or psychological captivity. Such a posture would defy tradition evolved over the entire course of human existence.

Some animal advocates do not take issue with the right of humans to exercise dominion over animals. They agree that animals are inferior to humans because they do not possess attributes such as a moral sense and concepts of past and future. However, they also claim that it is precisely because of these differences that humans are obligated to protect animals and not exploit them for the selfish betterment of humans.[13] In their view, animals are like infants and the mentally incompetent, who must be nurtured and protected from exploitation. This view shifts the issues of dominion from one of rights claimed by animals to one of responsibilities exercised by humans.

Neither of these philosophical positions addresses the issue of animal research from the perspective of the immorality of not using animals in research. From this perspective, depriving humans (and animals) of advances in medicine that result from research with animals is inhumane and fundamentally unethical. Spokespersons for this perspective suggest that patients with dementia, stroke, disabling injuries, heart disease, and cancer deserve relief from suffering and that depriving them of hope and relief by eliminating animal research is an immoral and unconscionable act. Defenders of animal research claim that animals sometimes must be sacrificed in the development of methods to relieve pain and suffering of humans (and animals) and to affect treatments and cures of a variety of human maladies.

The immeasurable benefits of animal research to humans are undeniable. One example is the development of a vaccine for poliomyelitis, with the result that the number of cases of poliomyelitis in the United States alone declined from 58,000 in 1952 to 4 in 1984. Benefits of this vaccine worldwide are even more impressive.

Every year, hundreds of thousands of humans are spared the braces, wheelchairs, and iron lungs required for the victims of poliomyelitis who survive this infectious disease. The research that led to a poliomyelitis vaccine required the sacrifice of hundreds of primates. Without this sacrifice, development of the vaccine would have been impossible, and in all likelihood the poliomyelitis epidemic would have continued unabated. Depriving humanity of this medical advance is unthinkable to almost all persons. Other diseases that are curable or treatable today as a result of animal research include diphtheria, scarlet fever, tuberculosis, diabetes, and appendicitis.[3] Human suffering would be much more stark today if these diseases, and many others as well, had not been amendable to treatment and cure through advances obtained by animal research.

ISSUES IN ANIMAL RESEARCH

Animal rights groups have several stock arguments against animal research. Some of these issues are described and refuted herein.

The Clinical Value of Basic Research

Persons opposed to research with animals often claim that basic biomedical research has no clinical value and therefore does not justify the use of animals. However, basic research is the foundation for most medical advances and consequently for progress in clinical medicine. Without basic research, including that with animals, chemotherapeutic advances against cancer (including childhood leukemia and breast malignancy), beta-blockers for cardiac patients, and electrolyte infusions for patients with dysfunctional metabolism would never have been achieved.

Duplication of Experiments

Opponents of animal research frequently claim that experiments are needlessly duplicated. However, the duplication of results is an essential part of the confirmation process in science. The generalization of results from one laboratory to another prevents anomalous results in one laboratory from being interpreted as scientific truth. The cost of research animals, the need to publish the results of experiments, and the desire to conduct meaningful research all function to reduce the likelihood of unnecessary experiments. Furthermore, the intense competition of research funds and the peer review process lessen the probability of obtaining funds for unnecessary research. Most scientists are unlikely to waste valuable time and resources conducting unnecessary experiments when opportunities for performing important research are so plentiful. . . .

The Use of Primates in Research

Animal activists often make a special plea on behalf of nonhuman primates, and many of the sit-ins, demonstrations, and break-ins have been directed at primate research centers. Efforts to justify these activities invoke the premise that primates are much like humans because they exhibit suffering and other emotions.

Keeping primates in cages and isolating them from others of their kind is considered by activists as cruel and destructive of their "psychological well-being." However, the opinion that animals that resemble humans most closely and deserve the most protection and care reflects an attitude of speciesism (i.e., a hierarchical scheme of relative importance) that most activists purportedly abhor. This logical fallacy in the drive for special protection of primates apparently escapes most of its adherents.

Some scientific experiments require primates exactly because they simulate human physiology so closely. Primates are susceptible to many of the same diseases as humans and have similar immune systems. They also possess intellectual, cognitive, and social skills above those of other animals. These characteristics make primates invaluable in research related to language, perception, and visual and spatial skills.[14] Although primates constitute only 0.5% of all animals used in research, their contributions have been essential to the continued acquisition of knowledge in the biological and behavioral sciences.[15]

Do Animals Suffer Needless Pain and Abuse?

Animal activists frequently assert that research with animals causes severe pain and that many research animals are abused either deliberately or through indifference. Actually, experiments today involve pain only when relief from pain would interfere with the purpose of the experiments. In any experiment in which an animal might experience pain, federal law requires that a veterinarian must be consulted in planning the experiment, and anesthesia, tranquilizers, and analgesics must be used except when they would compromise the results of the experiment.[16]

In 1984, the Department of Agriculture reported that 61% of research animals were not subjected to painful procedures, and another 31% received anesthesia or pain-relieving drugs. The remaining 8% did experience pain, often because improved understanding and treatment of pain, including chronic pain, were the purpose of the experiment.[14] Chronic pain is a challenging health problem that costs the United States about $50 billion a year in direct medical expenses, lost productivity, and income.[15]

Alternatives to the Use of Animals

One of the most frequent objections to animal research is the claim that alternative research models obviate the need for research with animals. The concept of alternatives was first raised in 1959 by Russell and Burch[17] in their book, *The Principles of Humane Experimental Technique*. These authors exhorted scientists to reduce the pain of experimental animals, decrease the number of animals used in research, and replace animals with nonanimal models whenever possible.

However, more often than not, alternatives to research animals are not available. In certain research investigations, cell, tissue, and organ cultures and computer models can be used as adjuncts to experiments with animals, and occasionally as substitutes for animals, at least in preliminary phases of the investigations. However, in many experimental situations, culture techniques and computer models are wholly inadequate because they do not encompass the physiological complexity of the whole animal. Examples where animals are essential to research include development of a vaccine against human immunodeficiency virus, refinement of organ transplantation techniques, investigation of mechanical devices as replacements for and adjuncts to physiological organs, identification of target-specific pharmaceuticals for cancer diagnosis and treatment, restoration of infarcted myocardium in patients with cardiac disease, evolution of new diagnostic imaging technologies, improvement of methods to relieve mental stress and anxiety, and evaluation of approaches to define and treat chronic pain. These challenges can only be addressed by research with animals as an essential step in the evolution of knowledge that leads to solutions. Humans are the only alternatives to animals for this step. When faced with this alternative, most people prefer the use of animals as the research model.

COMMENT

Love of animals and concern for their welfare are admirable characteristics that distinguish humans from other species of animals. Most humans, scientists as well as laypersons, share these attributes. However, when the concern for animals impedes the development of methods to improve the welfare of humans through amelioration and elimination of pain and suffering, a fundamental choice must be made. This choice is present today in the conflict between animal rights activism and scientific research. The American Medical Association made this choice more than a century ago and continues to stand squarely in defense of the use of animals for scientific research. In this position, the Association is supported by opinion polls that reveal strong endorsement of the American public for the use of animals in research and testing.[18] . . .

The American Medical Association believes that research involving animals is absolutely essential to maintaining and improving the health of people in America and worldwide.[6] Animal research is required to develop solutions to human tragedies such as human immunodeficiency virus disease, cancer, heart disease, dementia, stroke, and congenital and developmental abnormalities. The American Medical Association recognizes the moral obligation of investigators to use alternatives to animals whenever possible, and to conduct their research with animals as humanely as possible. However, it is convinced that depriving humans of medical advances by preventing research with animals is philosophically and morally a fundamentally indefensible position. Consequently, the American Medical Association is committed to the preservation of animal research and to the conduct of this research under the most humane conditions possible.[19,20]

REFERENCES

1. Rowan AN, Rollin BE. Animal research—for and against: a philosophical, social, and historical perspective. *Perspect Biol Med.* 1983; 27:1–17.
2. Bernard C; Green HC, trans. *An Introduction to the Study of Experimental Medicine.* New York, NY: Dover Publications Inc; 1957.
3. Council on Scientific Affairs. Animals in research. *JAMA,* 1989; 261:3602–3606.
4. Leader RW, Stark D. The importance of animals in biomedical research. *Perspect Biol Med.* 1987; 30:470–485.
5. Kransney JA. Some thoughts on the value of life. *Buffalo Physician,* 1984: 18:6–13.
6. Smith SJ, Evans RM, Sullivan-Fowler M, Hendee WR. Use of animals in biomedical research: historical role of the American Medical Association and the American physician. *Arch Intern Med.* 1988; 148:1849–1853.

7. Descartes R. *'Principles of Philosophy,'* *Descartes: Philosophical Writings.* Anscombe E. Geach PT, eds. London, England: Nelson & Sons; 1969.

8. Bentham J. *Introduction to the Principles of Morals and Legislation.* London, England: Athlone Press; 1970.

9. Godlovitch S, Godlovitch, Harris J. *Animals, Men and Morals.* New York, NY: Taplinger Publishing Co Inc; 1971.

10. Ryder R. *Victims of Science.* London, England: Davis-Poynter; 1975.

11. Singer P. *Animal Liberation: A New Ethic for Our Treatment of Animals.* New York, NY: Random House Inc; 1975.

12. Morowitz HJ, Jesus, Moses, Aristotle and laboratory animals. *Hosp Pract.* 1988; 23:23–25.

13. Cohen C. The case for the use of animals in biomedical research. *N Engl J Med.* 1986; 315: 865–870.

14. *Alternatives to Animal Use in Research, Testing, and Education.* Washington, DC: Office of Technology Assessment; 1986. Publication OTA-BA-273.

15. Committee on the Use of Laboratory Animals in Biomedical and Behavioral Research. *Use of Laboratory Animals in Biomedical and Behavioral Research.* Washington, DC: National Academy Press; 1988.

16. *Biomedical Investigator's Handbook.* Washington, DC: Foundation for Biomedical Research; 1987.

17. Russell WMS, Burch RL. *The Principles of Humane Experimental Technique.* Springfield, Ill: Charles C Thomas Publisher; 1959.

18. Harvey LK, Shubat SC. *AMA Survey of Physician and Public Opinion on Health Care Issues.* Chicago, Ill: American Medical Association; 1989.

19. Smith SJ, Hendee WR. Animals in research. *JAMA* 1988; 259:2007–2008.

20. Smith SJ, Loeb JM, Evans RM, Hendee WR. Animals in research and testing; who pays the price for medical progress? *Arch Ophthalmol.* 1988; 106:1184–1187.

NO

Tom Regan

ILL-GOTTEN GAINS

THE STORY

Late in 1981 a reporter for a large metropolitan newspaper (we'll call her Karen to protect her interest in remaining anonymous) gained access to some previously classified government files. Using the Freedom of Information Act, Karen was investigating the federal government's funding of research into the short- and long-term effects of exposure to radioactive waste. It was with understandable surprise that, included in these files, she discovered the records of a series of experiments involving the induction and treatment of coronary thrombosis (heart attack). Conducted over a period of fifteen years by a renowned heart specialist (we'll call him Dr. Ventricle) and financed with federal funds, the experiments in all likelihood would have remained unknown to anyone outside Dr. Ventricle's sphere of power and influence had not Karen chanced upon them.

Karen's surprise soon gave way to shock and disbelief. In case after case she read of how Ventricle and his associates took otherwise healthy individuals, with no previous record of heart disease, and intentionally caused their heart to fail. The methods used to occasion the "attack" were a veritable shopping list of experimental techniques, from massive doses of stimulants (adrenaline was a favorite) to electrical damage of the coronary artery, which, in its weakened state, yielded the desired thrombosis. Members of Ventricle's team then set to work testing the efficacy of various drugs developed in the hope that they would help the heart withstand a second "attack." Dosages varied, and there were the usual control groups. In some cases, certain drugs administered to "patients" proved more efficacious than cases in which others received no medication or smaller amounts of the same drugs. The research came to an abrupt end in the fall of 1981, but not because the project was judged unpromising or because someone raised a hue and cry about the ethics involved. Like so much else in the world at that time, Ventricle's project was a casualty of austere economic times. There simply wasn't enough federal money available to renew the grant application.

One would have to forsake all the instincts of a reporter to let the story end there. Karen persevered and, under false pretenses, secured an interview with Ventricle. When she revealed that she had gained access to the file, knew in detail the largely fruitless research conducted over fifteen years, and was incensed about his work, Ventricle was dumbfounded. But not because Karen had unearthed the file. And not even because it was filed where it was (a "clerical error," he assured her). What surprised Ventricle was that anyone would think there was a serious ethical question to be raised about what he had done. Karen's notes of their conversation include the following:

Ventricle: But I don't understand what you're getting at. Surely you know that heart disease is the leading cause of death. How can there by any ethical question about developing drugs which *literally* promise to be life-saving?

Karen: Some people might agree that the goal—to save life—is a good, a noble end, and still question the means used to achieve it. Your "patients," after all, had no previous history of heart disease. *They* were healthy before you got your hands on them.

Ventricle: But medical progress simply isn't possible if we wait for people to get sick and then see what works. There are too many variables, too much beyond our control and comprehension, if we try to do our medical research in a clinical setting. The history of medicine shows how hopeless that approach is.

Karen: And I read, too, that upon completion of the experiment, assuming that the "patient" didn't die in the pro-

cess—it says that those who survived were "sacrificed." You mean killed?

Ventricle: Yes, that's right. But always painlessly, always painlessly. And the body went immediately to the lab, where further tests were done. Nothing was wasted.

Karen: And it didn't bother you—I mean, you didn't ever ask yourself whether what you were doing was wrong? I mean . . .

Ventricle (interrupting): My dear young lady, you make it seem as if I'm some kind of moral monster. I work for the benefit of humanity, and I have achieved some small success, I hope you will agree. Those who raise cries of wrongdoing about what I've done are well intentioned but misguided. After all, I use animals in my research—chimpanzees, to be more precise—not human beings.

THE POINT

The story about Karen and Dr. Ventricle is just that—a story, a small piece of fiction. There is no real Dr. Ventricle, no real Karen, and so on. But there *is* widespread use of animals in scientific research, including research like our imaginary Dr. Ventricle's. So the story, while its details are imaginary—while it is, let it be clear, a literary device, not a factual account—is a story with a point. Most people reading it would be morally outraged if there actually were a Dr. Ventricle who did coronary research of the sort described on otherwise healthy human beings. Considerably fewer would raise a morally quizzical eyebrow when informed of such research done on animals, chimpanzees, or whatever. The story has a point, or so I hope, because, catching us off-guard, it brings this difference home to us, gives it life in our experience, and, in doing so, reveals something about ourselves, something about our own constellation of values. If we think what Ventricle did would be wrong if done to human beings but all right if done to chimpanzees, then we must believe that there are different moral standards that apply to how we may treat the two—human beings and chimpanzees. But to acknowledge this difference, if acknowledge it we do, is only the beginning, not the end, of our moral thinking. We can meet the challenge to think well from the moral point of view only if we are able to cite a *morally relevant difference* between humans and chimpanzees, one that illuminates in a clear, coherent, and rationally defensible way why it would be wrong to use humans, but not chimpanzees, in research like Dr. Ventricle's. . . .

THE LAW

Among the difference between chimps and humans, one concerns their legal standing. It is against the law to do to human beings what Ventricle did to his chimpanzees. It is not against the law to do this to chimps. So, here we have a difference. But a morally relevant one?

The difference in the legal status of chimps and humans would be morally relevant if we had good reason to believe that what is legal and what is moral go hand in glove: where we have the former, there we have the latter (and maybe vice versa too). But a moment's reflection shows how bad the fit between legality and morality sometimes is. A century and a half ago, the legal status of black people in the United States was similar to the legal status of a house, corn, a barn: they were property, other people's prop-

erty, and could legally be bought and sold without regard to their personal interests. But the legality of the slave trade did not make it moral, any more than the law against drinking, during the era of that "great experiment" of Prohibition, made it immoral to drink. Sometimes, it is true, what the law declares illegal (for example, murder and rape) is immoral, and vice versa. But there is no necessary connection, no pre-established harmony between morality and the law. So, yes, the legal status of chimps and humans differs; but that does not show that their moral status does. Their difference in legal status, in other words, is not a morally relevant difference and will not morally justify using these animals, but not humans, in Ventricle's research.

THE VALUE OF THE INDIVIDUAL

[An] alternative vision [to utilitarian value] consists in viewing certain individuals as themselves having a distinctive kind of value, what we will call "inherent value." This kind of value is not the same as, is not reducible to, and is not commensurate either with such values as preference satisfaction or frustration (that is, mental states) or with such values as artistic or intellectual talents (that is, mental and other kinds of excellences or virtues). We cannot, that is, equate or reduce the inherent value of an individual to his or her mental states or virtues, and neither can we intelligibly compare the two. In this respect, the three kinds of value (mental states, virtues, and the inherent value of the individual) are like proverbial apples and oranges.

They are also like water and oil: they don't mix. It is not only that [a man's] inherent value is not the same as, not reducible to, and not commensurate with *his* satisfaction, pleasures, intellectual and artistic skills, etc. In addition, *his* inherent value is not the same as, is not reducible to, and is not commensurate with the valuable mental states or talents of *other* individuals, whether taken singly or collectively. Moreover, and as a corollary of the preceding, the individual's inherent value is in all ways independent both of his or her usefulness relative to the interest of others and of how others feel about the individual (for example, whether one is liked or admired, despised or merely tolerated). A prince and a pauper, a streetwalker and a nun, those who are loved and those who are forsaken, the genius and the retarded child, the artist and the philistine, the most generous philanthropist and the most unscrupulous used car salesman—all have inherent value, according to the view recommended here, and all have it equally. . . .

WHAT DIFFERENCE DOES IT MAKE?

To view the value of individuals in this way is not an empty abstraction. To the question, "What difference does it make whether we view individuals as having equal inherent value, or as utilitarians do, as lacking such value, or, as perfectionists do, as having such value but to varying degree?"—our response to this question must be, "It makes all the moral difference in the world!" Morally, we are *always* required to treat those who have inherent value in ways that display proper respect for their distinctive kind of value, and though we cannot on this occasion either articulate or defend the full range of obligations tied to this fun-

damental duty, we can note that we fail to show proper respect for those who have such value whenever we treat them as if they were mere receptacles of value or as if their value was dependent on, or reducible to, their possible utility relative to the interests of others. In particular, therefore, Ventricle would fail to act as duty requires—would, in other words, do what is morally wrong—if he conducted his coronary research on competent human beings, without their informed consent, on the grounds that this research just might lead to the development of drugs or surgical techniques that would benefit others. That would be to treat these human beings as mere receptacles or as mere medical resources for others, and though Ventricle might be able to do this and get away with it, and though others might benefit as a result, that would not alter the nature of the grievous wrong he would have done. And it would be wrong, not because (or only if) there were utilitarian considerations, or contractarian considerations, or perfectionist considerations against his doing his research on these human beings, but because it would mark a failure on his part to treat them with appropriate respect. To ascribe inherent value to competent human beings, then, provides us with the theoretical wherewithal to ground our moral case against using competent human beings, against their will, in research like Ventricle's.

WHO HAS INHERENT VALUE?

If inherent value could nonarbitrarily be limited to competent humans, then we would have to look elsewhere to resolve the ethical issues involved in using other individuals (for example, chimpanzees) in medical research. But inherent value can only be limited to competent human beings by having the recourse to one arbitrary maneuver or another. Once we recognize that we have direct duties to competent and incompetent humans as well as to animals such as chimpanzees; once we recognize the challenge to give a sound theoretical basis for these duties in the case of these humans and animals; once we recognize the failure of indirect duty, contractarian, and utilitarian theories of obligation; once we recognize that the inherent value of competent humans precludes using them as mere resources in such research; once we recognize that perfectionist vision of morality, one that assigns degrees of inherent value on the basis of possession of favored virtues, is unacceptable because of its inegalitarian implications, and once we recognize that morality simply will not tolerate double standards, then we cannot, except arbitrarily, withhold ascribing inherent value, to an equal degree, to incompetent humans and animals such as chimpanzees. All have this value, in short, and all have it equally. All considered, this is an essential part of the most adequate total vision of morality. Morally, none of those having inherent value may be used in Ventricle-like research (research that puts them at risk of significant harm in the name of securing benefits for others, whether those benefits are realized or not). And none may be used in such research because to do so is to treat them as if their value is somehow reducible to their possible utility relative to the interests of others, or as if their value is somehow reducible to their value as "receptacles." What contractarianism, utilitarianism, and the other "isms" discussed earlier will allow is not morally tolerable.

HURTING AND HARMING

The prohibition against research like Ventricle's, when conducted on animals such as chimps, cannot be avoided by the use of anesthetics or other palliatives used to eliminate or reduce suffering. Other things being equal, to cause an animal to suffer is to harm that animal—is, that is, to diminish that individual animal's welfare. But these two notions—harming on the one hand and suffering on the other—differ in important ways. An individual's welfare can be diminished independently of causing her to suffer, as when, for example, a young woman is reduced to a "vegetable" by painlessly administering a debilitating drug to her while she sleeps. We mince words if we deny that harm has been done to her, though she suffers not. More generally, harms, understood as reductions in an individual's welfare, can take the form either of *inflictions* (gross physical suffering is the clearest example of a harm of this type) or *deprivations* (prolonged loss of physical freedom is a clear example of a harm of this kind). Not all harms hurt, in other words, just as not all hurts harm.

Viewed against the background of these ideas, an untimely death is seen to be the ultimate harm for both humans and animals, such as chimpanzees, and it is the ultimate harm for both because it is their ultimate deprivation or loss—their loss of life itself. Let the means used to kill chimpanzees be as "humane" (a cruel word, this) as you like. That will not erase the harm that an untimely death is for these animals. True, the use of anesthetics and other "humane" steps lessens the wrong done to these animals, when they are "sacrificed" in Ventricle-type research. But a lesser wrong is not a right. To do research that culminates in the "sacrifice" of chimpanzees or that puts these and similar animals at risk of losing their life, in the hope that we might learn something that will benefit others, is morally to be condemned, however "humane" that research may be in other respects.

THE CRITERION
OF INHERENT VALUE

It remains to be asked, before concluding, what underlies the possession of inherent value. Some are tempted by the idea that life itself is inherently valuable. This view would authorize attributing inherent value to chimpanzees, for example, and so might find favor with some people who oppose using these animals in research. But this view would also authorize attributing inherent value to anything and everything that is alive, including, for example, crabgrass, lice, bacteria, and cancer cells. It is exceedingly unclear, to put the point as mildly as possible, either that we have a duty to treat these things with respect or that any clear sense can be given to the idea that we do.

More plausible by far is the view that those individuals have inherent value who are *the subjects of a life*—who are, that is, the experiencing subjects of a life that fares well or ill for them over time, those who have *an individual experiential welfare*, logically independent of their utility relative to the interests or welfare of others. Competent humans are subjects of a life in this sense. But so, too, are those incompetent humans who have concerned us. And so, too, and not unimportantly, are chimpanzees. Indeed, so too are the members of many species of animals: cats and dogs, monkeys and sheep, ceta-ceans and wolves, horses and cattle. Where one draws the line between those animals who are, and those who are not, subjects of a life is certain to be controversial. Still there is abundant reason to believe that the members of mammalian species of animals do have a psychophysical identity over time, do have an experiential life, do have an individual welfare. Common sense is on the side of viewing these animals in this way, and ordinary language is not strained in talking of them as individuals who have an experiential welfare. The behavior of these animals, moreover, is consistent with regarding them as subjects of a life, and the implications of evolutionary theory are that there are many species of animals whose members are, like the members of the species *Homo sapiens*, experiencing subjects of a life of their own, with an individual welfare. On these grounds, then, we have very strong reason to believe, even if we lack conclusive proof, that these animals meet the subject-of-a-life criterion.

If, then, those who meet this criterion have inherent value, and have it equally relative to all who meet it, chimpanzees and other animals who are subjects of a life, not just human beings, have this value *and* have neither more nor less of it than we do. (To hold that they have less than we do is to land oneself in the inegalitarian swamp of perfectionism). Moreover, if, as has been argued, having inherent value morally bars others from treating those who have it as mere receptacles or as mere resources for others, then any and all medical research like Ventricle's, done on these animals in the name of possibly benefitting others, stands morally condemned. And it is not only cases in which the benefits for others do not materialize that are condemnable; also to be condemned are cases, such as the research done on chimps regarding hepatitis, for example, in which the benefits for others are genuine. In these cases, as in others like them in the relevant respects, the ends do not justify the means. The *many millions* of mammalian animals used each year for scientific purposes, including medical research, bear mute, tragic testimony to the narrowness of our moral vision.

CONCLUSIONS

This condemnation of such research probably is at odds with the judgment that most people would make about this issue. If we had good reason to assume that the truth always lies with what most people think, then we could look approvingly on Ventricle-like research done on animals like chimps in the name of benefits for others. But we have no good reason to believe that the truth is to be measured plausibly by majority opinion, and what we know of the history of prejudice and bigotry speaks powerfully, if painfully, against this view. Only the cumulative force of informed, fair, rigorous argument can decide where the truth lies, or most likely lies, when we examine a controversial moral question. Although openly acknowledging and, indeed, insisting on the limitations of the arguments . . . , these arguments make the case, in broad outline, against using animals such as chimps in medical research such as Ventricle's. . . .

Those who oppose the use of animals such as chimps in research like Ventricle's and who accept the major themes advanced here, oppose it, then, not because they think that all such research is a waste of time and money, or because they think that it never leads to any benefits for others, or because they view those who do such research as, to use Ventricle's, words, "moral monsters," or even because they love animals. Those of us who condemn such research do so because this research is not possible except at the grave moral price of failing to show proper respect for the value of the animals who are used. Since, whatever our gains, they are ill-gotten, we must bring to an end research like Ventricle's, whatever our losses. A fair measure of our moral integrity will be the extent of our resolve to work against allowing our scientific, economic, health, and other interests to serve as a reason for the wrongful exploitation of members of species of animals other than our own.

POSTSCRIPT

Should Animal Experimentation Be Permitted?

In a September 1988 report, written in response to the animal rights movement, the National Academy of Sciences concluded that the use of animals in research is appropriate despite the pain they may suffer. One member of the panel, a member of the Animal Welfare Institute, refused to sign the report.

In 1985, Congress passed the Health Research Extension Act, which directed the National Institutes of Health (NIH) to establish guidelines for the proper care of animals to be used in biomedical and behavioral research. The NIH regulations implementing the law require institutions that receive federal grants to establish Animal Care and Use Committees. The Office of Science and Technology Policies' "Principles for the Utilization and Care of Vertebrate Animals Used in Testing, Research and Training" (published in the *Federal Register* on May 20, 1985) serves as the basis for the U.S. government's policy. The NIH's *Guide for the Care and Use of Laboratory Animals* (revised edition, 1985) offers explicit instructions.

In May 1984 members of the Animal Liberation Front broke into the Experimental Head Injury Laboratory of the University of Pennsylvania and stole videotape records of experiments on baboons. The resulting NIH investigation led to the withdrawal of federal funding from the head trauma unit. According to the Foundation for Biomedical Research, 76 cases of vandalism have occurred at research facilities in the past eight years. Despite better regulations on animal use, activist protests have become more frequent and more aggressive; they have even designated a "World Animal Liberation Day."

For views of the animal liberation movement, see Peter Singer, *Practical Ethics* (Cambridge, 1979); Tom Regan and Peter Singer, eds., *Animal Rights and Human Obligations*, 2nd ed. (Prentice Hall, 1989); and Bernard E. Rollin, *The Unheeded Cry: Animal Consciousness, Animal Pain, and Science* (Oxford University Press, 1989).

For opposing views, see R. G. Frey, *Interests and Rights: The Case Against Animals* (Clarendon, 1980); *The Case for Animal Experimentation* by Michael Allan Fox (University of California Press, 1986); and the Office of Technology and Assessment's *Alternatives to Animal Use in Research, Testing, and Education* (U.S. Government Printing Office, 1986). Also see *Ethics and Animals*, edited by Harlan B. Miller and William H. Williams (Humana, 1983); *Of Mice, Models, and Men: A Critical Evaluation of Animal Research* by Andrew Rowan (State University of New York Press, 1984); and the Hastings Center's "Animals, Science, and Ethics," *Hastings Center Report* (May/June 1990).

For a discussion of medical accomplishments developed through research on animals, see the Council of Scientific Affairs, "Animals in Research," *Journal of the American Medical Association* (June 23/30, 1989).

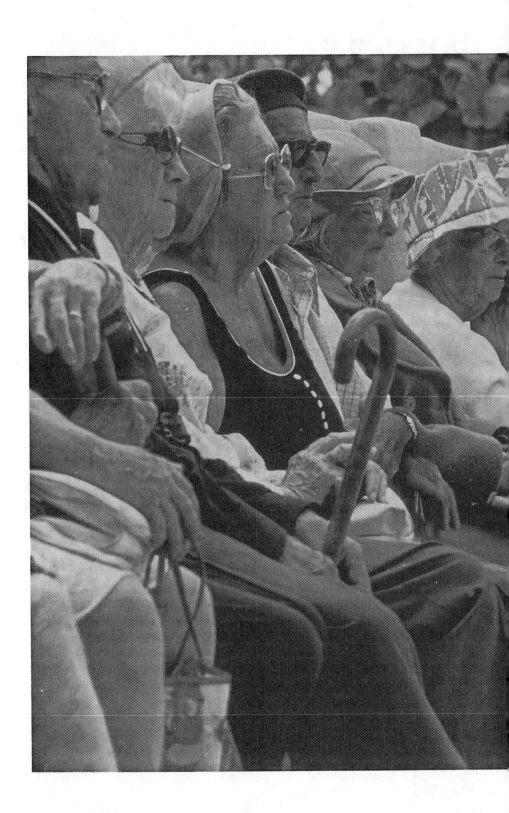

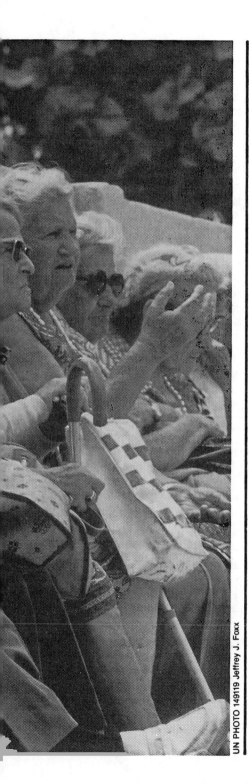

PART 5
Public Policy and Bioethics

Public policy in the field of bioethics has had to struggle to respond rapidly to scientific events and technical advances. Decisions in this field can no longer be the sole province of individual doctors or patients. The availability of advanced organ and tissue transplant technology combined with the shortage of "spare parts" has created many ethical puzzles. Financial and medical resources remain extremely limited, and society's demand is great. Can health care costs for all be contained without depriving some groups, such as the elderly, of some kinds of care? Faced with a life-threatening disease, should patients have the right to take unproven drugs? And perhaps most sweeping of all are considerations of restructuring the entire health care system to provide more equitable access. This section deals with issues that have moved to the forefront of the struggle to define social values.

Should Organ Procurement Be Based on Voluntarism?

Should Newborns Without Brains Be Used as Organ Donors?

Should There Be a Market in Body Parts?

Should Health Care for the Elderly Be Limited?

Should Dying Patients Have Greater Access to Experimental Drugs?

Should the United States Follow the Canadian Model of a National Health Program?

ISSUE 16

Should Organ Procurement Be Based on Voluntarism?

YES: Blair L. Sadler and Alfred M. Sadler, Jr., from "A Community of Givers, Not Takers," *Hastings Center Report* 14 (October 1984)

NO: Charles J. Dougherty, from "A Proposal for Ethical Organ Donation," *Health Affairs* (Fall 1986)

ISSUE SUMMARY

YES: Attorney Blair L. Sadler and physician Alfred M. Sadler, Jr., maintain that the system of encouraged voluntarism in procuring organs for transplantation increases the supply of organs without infringing on the rights of individuals and families.

NO: Philosopher Charles J. Dougherty argues that current laws should be overridden in favor of a system of routine removal, in which physicians would retrieve organs from newly dead persons unless the next of kin refuses.

Not long ago organ transplants were the stuff of science fiction. Although the first successful cornea transplant took place in 1905, the first kidney transplant (between identical twins) did not take place until 1954. The first liver transplant was performed in 1966, and the first heart transplant in 1967. Today—with the aid of better surgical techniques, better tissue-matching capabilities, and most important, new drugs that suppress the body's natural tendency to reject a transplanted organ—kidneys, hearts, pancreases, livers, lungs, spleens, and bone marrow can all be transplanted, and people are living longer with the transplanted organs than ever before. At Stanford University, for example, about 80 percent of the people who receive heart transplants now live two years or longer, while a decade or so ago only 20 percent survived as long as a year.

In the 1960s and 1970s the question was: Are these admittedly experimental operations too risky? Today the question is: Where are we going to get all the transplantable organs to fill the ever-expanding demand? A person can donate one of the body's two kidneys to a relative (assuming there is a tissue match) without endangering his or her own health, but the other organs must come from cadavers. Many people, of course, have no suitable live kidney donor in their families, and nationwide about 10,000 people are waiting for cadaver kidneys. Some cardiologists estimate that the lives of as many as 50,000 to 100,000 people could be saved each year if heart transplants were more readily available.

If medical technology has created the demand, it has also created a means to obtain the supply. For in the same period in which organ transplantation moved from experiment to therapy, medical technology also perfected techniques of maintaining heart and respiratory function in people whose brains had stopped functioning. In many states the definition of death has been changed from one that describes the cessation of heart and lung function as legal death to one that focuses on the cessation of all functions of the entire brain, often called a brain death criterion. In effect, lungs can be made to breathe, blood to circulate, and hearts to beat in dead bodies. And from dead bodies can come organs to serve the living. About 20,000 people die each year from accidents or from other causes, and they are potential organ donors—that is, they are young enough and healthy enough (except of course for the fatal injury) that their organs are suitable for transplantation.

The Uniform Anatomical Gift Act, adopted in 1968, was intended to eliminate unnecessary formalities and to make human organs available for transplantation while protecting the rights and interests of the families of the deceased. It stressed the need for informed consent before any organs or tissue were removed from a dead body. But voluntary donations, either from people who have signed organ donor cards or from families who have been approached by transplant teams when a relative has died, have not kept pace with the need. Last year only about 2,000 to 2,500 of the 20,000 potential donors actually provided organs. The main reason, it appears, is not that families are reluctant to donate (although that does occur) but that physicians and other medical personnel are reluctant to ask a grieving family.

The selections that follow examine the question of whether the voluntary system is still valid. Alfred M. Sadler, Jr., and Blair L. Sadler say that it is. They believe that public support for transplantation remains high because the principles of giving rather than taking are honored. Charles J. Dougherty argues that there would be a greater supply of organs if physicians were allowed to remove them routinely, while still offering families the right of informed refusal. He calls his proposal a "moderate alternative," fearing that a reliance on the inadequate voluntary system will lead to commercialization of organ donation or government-sanctioned taking of organs.

YES

**Blair L. Sadler and
Alfred M. Sadler, Jr.**

A COMMUNITY OF GIVERS,
NOT TAKERS

In the late 1960s, when we became involved in the questions surrounding the procurement of organs for the newly developing technology of transplantation, we and others espoused the principles of informed consent and encouraged voluntarism. The Uniform Anatomical Gift Act, drafted in 1968 by the National Conference of Commissioners on Uniform State Laws and adopted in every state and the District of Columbia by 1971, embodied those principles.[1] Despite the expansion of transplantation programs and challenges to those principles, we believe that there is no reason to discard them now. The law is doing well what it was intended to do: providing a clear mechanism for individuals and next-of-kin to consent to organ and tissue donation for humanitarian purposes. It was designed to strike a socially acceptable balance that facilitates organ donation and procurement without infringing upon other deeply held values and rights.[2]

THE TAKING OF PITUITARY GLANDS

The importance of balancing competing interests and values is not merely of theoretical interest and is underscored by the following case study. In 1963, the National Pituitary Agency, under the auspices of the National Institutes of Health (NIH), established a program to obtain cadaver pituitary glands for extraction of pituitary hormones, particularly human growth hormone. This nationwide effort enabled clinical research to be performed on human subjects who had hypopituitary dwarfism. During that period 70,000 pituitary glands were obtained annually. Because the yield of pituitary hormone from each gland was very small, the National Pituitary Agency estimated the need at up to 7,000,000 pituitary glands annually.

Two incidents in the mid-1960s highlighted the necessity to reassess the ethical and legal implications of organ removal. In Los Angeles, headlines in the *Los Angeles Times* revealed that a technician in the County Coroner's Office was accused of removing pituitary glands from cadavers during autopsy without having obtained consent. In Hennepin County, Minnesota, the coroner's authority to remove human parts for other purposes was also questioned. This information surfaced in emotionally charged newspaper articles that sharply criticized a Federal government agency's role in supporting the taking of human cadaver material without consent. This unauthorized taking, even for humanitarian purposes, was described with alarm and even horror and threatened to undermine if not destroy the enterprise. The NIH moved quickly to ensure that human cadaver material was obtained with consent only and commissioned an intensive study of the subject.

LEGAL HISTORY AND PRECEDENTS

In 1967, there was considerable variation in the law relating to dead bodies. American statutes, derived from English common law, gave next-of-kin the authority and obligation to dispose of the remains of the deceased in a timely and respectful manner. As such, kin were given possession of the body for the purposes of burial. The body was considered incapable of being owned in the commercial sense and thus could not be bought or sold. This principle was expressed in the doctrine that there were no "property rights" in the dead body. The body was not part of a deceased's estate; thus a person could not direct the disposition of his own remains.

That doctrine had been challenged in the 1950s when Grace Metalious, a well-known author, wished to donate her body to one of two medical schools and asked that no funeral services be held. Her next-of-kin objected and the matter was contested after her death. In reviewing the common law tradition, the court recognized traditional next-of-kin rights, but noted that an individual ought to have a say in his own burial and that these wishes should override next-of-kin concerns. The term "quasi-property rights" was used to identify the rights of individuals to direct the disposition of their remains.[3]

To further complicate matters, every state had adopted other laws that affected, and in some cases impinged upon, the traditional next-of-kin rights for burial. All states have autopsy laws concerning the need to determine the cause of death. Next-of-kin have authority to grant autopsy permission, and in about one-half of the states statutes allow an individual to authorize an autopsy on his or her remains.

Medical examiner or coroner's statutes define the interests of states to determine the cause of death in certain cases such as those involving crime, violence, or communicable disease. In these instances, the autopsy authority of a state overrides the objections of individuals or next-of-kin. Finally, unclaimed-body statutes specify that bodies not claimed by anyone in a defined time period can be turned over to medical schools for medical science. Does the medical examiner's authority to perform an autopsy in order to determine the causes of death include authority to remove other tissues for medical purposes? Strictly speaking, no, but the practice had apparently been going on unobserved for years in some parts of the country.[4]

CONSENT UNDER THE UNIFORM ANATOMICAL GIFT ACT

After the successful transplantation of corneas in the 1950s, states began to enact donation statutes that allowed individuals to make testamentary gifts of all or parts of their bodies for medical, scientific, or therapeutic purposes. By 1965, forty-four states had adopted some type of donation law. Four others permitted the donation of eyes only and three states had no donation statute. Each law was different: some required that a donation be made as part of a will; others said nothing about next-of-kin; some required three witnesses; still others, none. To redress this disparity, the National Conference of Commissioners on Uniform State Laws (CUSL) drafted a model law called the Uniform Anatomical Gift Act. This model was designed to foster national organ donation and tissue-matching programs. It was recognized that as transplantation became more successful, a nationwide pool for tissue typing and organ matching would be required.

A special committee of the CUSL, chaired by E. Blythe Stason, former dean of the University of Michigan Law School, worked for two years to develop a suitable law. The Uniform Anatomical Gift Act (UAGA) was completed on July 30, 1968, and was approved by the American Bar Association on August 7. A national meeting, called by the National Research Council in September, brought together representatives of the medical schools and major scientific organizations involved in this field.[5] Articles were published in law reviews and medical journals; the Commissioners, three from each state, took the model law back to the state legislatures for consideration. Forty-four state legislatures met in 1969 and forty-one adopted the law. By 1971, just three years after completion, all fifty states and the District of Columbia had adopted the model with no major modifications.[6] In the ninety-year history of the CUSL, no uniform act has ever done so well.

The Act authorizes persons eighteen years or older to donate all or part of their body for medical purposes to take effect after death. It also gives next-of-kin authority to donate if an individual before death has not given any contrary directions. A clear order of priority of next-of-kin is established. The Act specifies who can receive donations and the mechanisms by which donations can be made, including a simple card to be carried on the patient's person. Provisions are made to streamline the next-of-kin consent mechanism by authorizing a simple written statement or recorded telephone message. The act specifies that its provisions are subject to state laws governing autopsies.

Why did the law pass so quickly? First, the principles of informed consent and voluntary donation were protected. If one is opposed to organ removal, one simply does not give consent. In 1968, a Gallup Poll showed that 90 percent of Americans would be willing to donate if asked. Second, public interest in transplantation was widespread. Just as the law neared completion, Dr. Christiaan Barnard performed the first heart transplant. Many of these issues became front-page news when the model law emerged.

Comprehensive organizational efforts followed. After the act was adopted, a meeting of concerned organ donation groups was convened and a uniform donor card developed.[7] At no time was it expected that the donor card would provide all or even a large percentage of cadaver organs because many people do not bother to fill out the card. It was recognized that next-of-kin consent would remain a major part of the donation process, but the donor card could serve a very important educational function among family members. As people discuss organ donation and one family member fills out a donor card, the wishes of that person become known and shared.

ALTERNATIVES TO CONSENT

What are alternatives to consent and encouraged voluntarism? In 1968, Jesse Dukeminier and David Sanders proposed that "routine salvaging of cadaver organs" was preferable to consent.[8] Arthur Caplan has now resurrected the Dukeminier and Sanders approach. They proposed that cadaver organs be removed routinely unless an objection is entered before removal (presumed consent). The burden of action would be on the person who did not want his or her organs removed to enter an objection. Under this system, a person could object during life to the taking of his or her organs after death. The next-of-kin could also object to the use of the deceased's organs before removal if the deceased did not specifically authorize donation. These writers would shift the burden from the surgeon to obtain consent to the individual or the next-of-kin to object. In so doing, they believe that more cadaver material would become available.

We believed that the "routine salvaging" argument was dubious in 1968 and we believe it is dubious now. Next-of-kin will have an opportunity to object only if a duty is placed on the physician or hospital to notify them that a family member has died or is facing imminent death. In the absence of such notice, important constitutional problems (discussed below) might invalidate the system. Adequate notice is fundamental to the protection of constitutional rights. Without a notice requirement, the next-of-kin could forcefully argue that because they were not aware of their relative's death they could not exercise their authority to object.

To obviate the notice problem, a central registry for recording objections was proposed. Practically, a registry is fraught with major problems. The first and most important concerns the temporary nature of next-of-kin relationships. Through marriage, divorce, and death, family relationships change. Each change requires a fresh entry for the registry. Second, under this system modifying the scope of the gift is cumbersome: each time an individual wishes to change the gift, he or she must report back to the registry. Third, the creation and maintenance of such a registry will be costly. Finally, a registry forces physicians to go through an additional mechanism, which may not be up-to-date, rather than rely on a donor card or deal directly with the family.

One solution to the notice problem is to place a legal duty upon the physician or hospital to give notice to the next-of-kin so that they can object. This eliminates constitutional problems relating to freedom of religion and due process. However, the obligation of the physician or hospital to give notice to the family (that a kidney or other organ will be taken for transplant purposes unless they object) is little different from the obligation under consent statutes to request permission. We conclude that if a physician is required by law to give adequate notice that an organ will be taken, the gains for transplantation over the consent approach are illusory.

A more extreme approach authorizes compulsory removal of cadaver organs as needed for medical purposes. A compulsory removal law could be drawn narrowly and be limited to therapy such as transplantation, which is directly lifesaving. There is no doubt that a compulsory removal statute would yield more organs than either of the other systems.[10] However, it would do so at the expense of the legally protected interests previously discussed. This is important in terms of: (a) its effect on public attitudes toward medical therapeutic innovation in general and transplantation in particular; (b) its likelihood of enactment by state legislatures; and (c) its possible conflict with constitutional principles. (In the last case, the statute would be invalid.) Individuals challenging a compulsory statute could reasonably raise at least two issues of constitutional dimension: freedom of religion and due process. A detailed analysis of these issues has been presented elsewhere and will not be repeated here.[11]

THE PHILOSOPHICAL BASIS FOR CONSENT

Philosophical and humanistic principles strongly support a system based on consent. Put simply, we believe most people would prefer a community of givers rather than takers. In 1970, Paul Ramsey articulated a preference for the voluntary donation of organs over the "routine salvage" approach and concluded: "A society will be a better human community in which giving and receiving is the rule, not taking for the sake of good to come." He asserted that "the civilizing task of mankind is the fostering, the achievement, or the shoring up of consensual community" and that in "answering the need for gifts by encouraging real givers," the consent approach "meets the measure of authentic community among men. . . . The moral sequels that might flow from education and action in line with the proposed Gift Acts may be of far more importance than prolonging lives routinely. The moral history of mankind is of more importance than its medical advancement, unless the latter can be joined with the former in a community of affirmative consent."[12]

Hans Jonas, also writing at this time, stressed the need for public confidence in physicians relating to respect for life and warned: "The patient must be absolutely sure that his doctor does not become his executioner, and that no definition (of death) ever authorizes him to become one." He continues, "His right to this certainty is absolute, and so is his right to his own body with all its organs. Absolute respect for these rights violates no one else's rights, for no one has a right to another's body." Jonas further distinguishes "between the moral or emotional appeal of a cause that elicits volunteering and a right that demands compliance, for example . . . between the moral claim of a common good and society's right to that good and to the means of its realization. A moral claim cannot be met without consent; a right can do without it." Finally, Jonas reminds us that making any such choice between the "rights" of the individual and the "interests" of society requires "a careful clarification of what the needs, interests, and rights of society are, for society—as distinct from any plurality of individuals—is an abstract and as such is subject to our definition."[13]

Sir Harold Himsworth wrote in the *Daedalus* volume in which Jonas's article appeared "that the public at large must be kept involved and informed about the cost and other factors related to medical advancements." He continues that "without favorable public opinion and support, medical research and therapeutic intervention would be curtailed." He states the primary duty of the physician is to "act always to increase trust." We doubt that trust can be fostered by taking organs for transplantation.

After careful analysis, William May concluded in a similar vein: "While the procedure of routine salvaging may, in the short run, furnish more organs for transplants, in the long run, its systemic effect on the institutions of medical care would seem to be depressing and corrosive of that trust upon which acts of healing depend."[14]. . .

Any comprehensive review of the implications of alternative legal systems requires an understanding of the scientific and organizational barriers to transplantation. As was true fifteen years ago, the major barriers are: the scientific problems of donor/recipient matching and organ preservation, the educational needs of informing the public and key medical personnel, the logistical constraints of procuring and transporting organs throughout the country twenty-four hours a day and the extraordinary cost of transplantation programs.

Equally important in the long term is the recognition that transplantation represents at best a halfway technology. It will never be a substitute for curing or preventing the underlying diseases that currently lead to transplantation. The case study of pituitary gland procurement is applicable here. Scientific advances have allowed the synthesis and production of human growth hormone via genetic engineering and thus the need for cadaver pituitary procurement programs is disappearing.

In conclusion, laws based on voluntary donation and consent have accomplished their major objective. The rights of individuals and families are clear and simplified mechanisms of consent are in place under the Uniform Anatomical Gift Act. Equally important, considerable public support for transplantation continues to exist because the principles of giving rather than taking are maintained.

In the absence of convincing evidence that presumed consent legislation makes considerably more organs available for transplantation and in light of the substantial nonlegal barriers listed above, we believe it is unwise to consider dismantling the present consent system.

REFERENCES

1. A. M. Sadler, Jr., B. L. Sadler, E. B. Stason, and D. L. Stickel, "Transplantation: A Case for Consent," *New England Journal of Medicine* 280 (1969), 862–67.

2. A. M. Sadler, Jr., B. L. Sadler and E. B. Stason, "Uniform Anatomical Gift Act: A Model for Reform," *Journal of the American Medical Association,* 206 (1968), 2501–06.

3. *Holland v. Metalious*, 105 N.H. 290, 198 A. 2nd 654 (1964).

4. A. M. Sadler, Jr. and B. L. Sadler, "Transplantation and the Law: The Need for Organized Sensitivity," *Georgetown Law Journal* 57 (1968), 5–54.

5. R. E. Stevenson,, W. J. Burdette, M. Head, J. E. Murray, A. M. Sadler, Jr., and B. L. Sadler, "A Report to the Committee on Tissue Transplantation of the National Academy of Sciences—National Research Council from the Ad Hoc Committee on Medical-Legal Problems" (1968).

6. A. M. Sadler, Jr., B. L. Sadler and E. B. Stason, "Transplantation and the Law: Progress Toward Uniformity," *New England Journal of Medicine* 282 (1970), 717–23.

7. A. M. Sadler, Jr., B. L. Sadler and G. E. Schreiner, "A Uniform Card for Organ and Tissue Donation," *Modern Medicine* 37 (1969), 20-23.

8. D. Sanders and J. Dukeminier, Jr., "Medical Advance and Legal Lag: Hemodialysis and Kidney Transplantation," *UCLA Law Review* 15 (1968), 357-413; J. Dukeminier and D. Sanders, "Organ Transplantation: Proposal for Routine Salvaging of Cadaver Organs," *New England Journal of Medicine* 279 (1968), 413-19.

9. A. L. Caplan, "Organ Transplants: The Costs of Success," *Hastings Center Report* 13 (December 1983), 23-32.

10. Note, "Compulsory Removal of Cadaver Organs," *Columbia Law Review,* 69 (1969), 693-705.

11. B. L. Sadler and A. M. Sadler, Jr. "Providing Cadaver Organs: Three Legal Alternatives," *Hastings Center Studies,* 1 (1973), 13-26.

12. Paul Ramsey, *The Patient as a Person* (New Haven: Yale University Press), 1970, p. 210.

13. Hans Jonas, "Philosophical Reflections on Experimenting with Human Subjects," *Daedalus* 98 (1969), 221.

14. William May, "Attitudes Toward the Newly Dead," *Hastings Center Studies* 1 (1973), 6.

NO

Charles J. Dougherty

A PROPOSAL FOR
ETHICAL ORGAN DONATION

The current system of organ donation in the U.S. does not supply all the organs that are needed, even though transplantable organs exist . . . [T]here is little reason to expect that the "voluntary opt in" system, where donation of cadaveric organs for transplantation requires a voluntary act of donation either by the donor while he or she was alive or after death by the next of kin, will keep up with the demand.

Two factors help account for the present and predictable failure of the current system. Most of us, for deep-seated psychological and cultural reasons, are unwilling to contemplate our own deaths and the circumstances of our bodies after death. Consequently, too few people take the steps necessary while alive to plan for donation of organs at death. This means that appeals for cadaveric organs must then be made to the decedent's next of kin. But asking the next of kin for a voluntary choice to donate the body parts of a loved one in what are often tragic circumstances, accidental death of an otherwise healthy mate, for example, can be exceptionally difficult. From the relatives' perspective such a request can be devastating. By way of illustration, one woman described herself as "astounded and utterly appalled" when asked to donate her late husband's kidneys. "To make such a decision for oneself is hard enough," she reported, "but to be asked to make it on behalf of another, while one is so shocked and grief stricken is both harrowing and cruel." In sum, the problems with the current system stem from personal reluctance to consider one's own death and from the poignant circumstances in which next of kin are often placed at the time of a request to voluntarily opt into donation of a recently dead loved one's body parts.

Several proposals have been made to address these problems. Two suggestions are especially extreme. The first proposal is to give people an economic incentive to donate organs by creation of a market for buying and selling body parts. The second extreme suggestion is to give the state the authority to take needed body parts, at least in circumstances where relatives do not initiate objections to this taking. Both proposals would likely increase the

Reprinted, with changes, from Charles J. Dougherty, "A Proposal for Ethical Organ Donation," *Health Affairs* (Fall 1986), pp. 105-111. Copyright © 1986 by *Health Affairs*. Reprinted by permission.

supply of organs suitable for transplantation, but both are, I think, ethically unacceptable. . . .

REALISTIC ALTERNATIVES FOR REFORM

If these two extreme proposals for the commercialization and pricing of organs and for government sanctioned taking organs are ethically unacceptable, must we tolerate the weakness of the present system? Not necessarily, since there are two more moderate alternatives for reform. The first is a system of required request for donation. The second is one of routine removal of organs, but with the right of informed refusal by the next of kin.

A required request system would have one or both of two features. The first would require a response to the question of organ donation by all adult citizens, perhaps by a mandatory checkoff on a driver's license application, a tax return, or into some ad hoc national registry. The state of Colorado now mandates such a choice during application for a driver's license. This response would then be made available to medical personnel at the time of death. The second feature would require that in all cases of the death of a potential donor, a request for organ donation be made directly to the decedent's family by someone on the medical team. Laws mandating request for donation are now in place in twelve states.

With respect to the first element of required request, experience with the Uniform Anatomical Gift Act in the U.S. and with government sanctioned taking in France suggests that medical personnel will still likely turn for approval to the next of kin, regardless of the existence of the decedent's checkoff authority to salvage organs. And there is the practical concern that a forced choice for or against donation outside of any pertinent context may not result in an increase in organ donation. With the sense of others' needs and the inevitability of one's own death only theoretical realities at the time, it is just possible that this choice will not receive the thoughtful attention that it deserves. Further, since the choice will be forced, resentment may well develop, issuing in more refusals to donate than proponents of this scheme expect.

The other element of required request is probably the more feasible of the two, and it has met with some considerable success in the states where it is the law. But required request to the next of kin does nothing to help deal with the apparently shocking cruelty of such a request to the family that is not prepared, that has never discussed this issue in advance of tragic events. Thus, required request will probably still produce many instances of refusals born out of the pathos within which an affirmative choice to donate must be made. It is therefore unlikely that required request will allow the supply of cadaveric organs for transplantation to keep pace with increased demand.

The second option, routine removal with a right of informed refusal, has a better chance of success. This approach would reverse the burden of proof in organ donation, from the present one in which a voluntary choice must be made to opt into donation to one in which a voluntary choice would have to be made to opt out. At death, each person would be presumed to be a willing organ donor unless he or she was carrying a card indicating otherwise, was a member of a religion or group known to oppose organ donation, or the next of kin refuses permission to remove organs. This last qualification is of major significance because, unlike the system of government sanctioned taking, routine removal with a right of informed refusal would require that the next of kin be alerted to three things before any organ removal takes place: First, the next of kin must be told that it is standard procedure in these cases to remove suitable cadaveric organs for transplant to needy others. Second, unless he or she refuses to allow removal, needed organs will be removed in this case. And third, he or she can refuse permission for donation for any reason or for no reason at all, and such a refusal will be respected without penalty or prejudice.

This system would still be charitable since the transfer of organs would be neither a selling and buying nor a simple taking; it would remain an act of giving. It would still be voluntary because in every case the next of kin would be given the option to prevent donation in a free and informed manner. The advantage this system would have over the present voluntary opt in system and the required request approach is that next of kin acquiescence rather than active preference would suffice to secure needed organs for transplant. This would make the psychology of approaching bereaved next of kin easier and a decision on their part to allow donation less burdensome as well. Rather than presenting a shocking and potentially cruel request for a loved one's organs, under this system medical personnel would merely be seeking passive acceptance of doing what would then be normal. From the next of kin's point of view, this system would ask them only if they refuse or they believe that the de-

ceased would have refused to do what is usually done. The vexing question of whether or not donation is or would have been actively preferred would be put aside by a public presumption in favor of routine removal.

No doubt approaching a grieving next of kin would still be difficult, but it would surely be easier than the approach mandated under required request schemes. If it is in fact easier for all involved, it would likely lead to an enhanced supply of needed cadaveric organs for transplant. In France, where in spite of the law allowing governments sanctioned taking, something like a system of routine removal with a right of informed refusal is practiced, less than 10 percent of families approached raised objections. This would likely mean a dramatic increase in the supply of transplantable organs in the U.S. . . . [A] 90 percent rate of access to suitable cadaveric organs would more than satisfy all present need and might adequately anticipate future need for transplantable kidneys. This system would still be respectful of individual freedom as it would allow anyone to opt out for any reason. And it would enhance the common good because it would create an institutional presumption in favor of people helping people in one of the most intimate ways possible.

But some, perhaps many, will not agree. They will reject this proposal on its fundamental assumption, that the burden of proof can be reversed so as to presume everyone's willingness to donate their organs after death. Isn't this to assume, they might well ask, that the public has some claim over an individual's body? Even if an individual or next of kin can override this claim by an informed refusal, isn't it wrong to allow even a presumptive public claim over such a private entity? If anything is intimately and privately a person's and only a person's, isn't it his or her own body?

Certainly there is a truth here. We very much are our own bodies. They are the foundations of our privacy. And if it even makes sense to separate ourselves from our bodies enough to meaningfully say this, our bodies are our most intimate possessions. Yet there are equally compelling social dimensions to the human body. Our bodies represent the genetic achievements of generations of human and prehuman ancestors living together socially. We are each the immediate result of the union of two other human bodies. Each of our bodies has been a beneficiary of the many medical advances made possible by the sacrifices of countless others and of the social institutions which have sustained medical research, prevention and treatment of disease, rehabilitation, and care for the sick and dying. Because many are un-aware of these social debts does not make them any less compelling. It seems fitting in light of these very real debts to others in general, and to the institutions of health care in particular, to presume a willingness to contribute to others after death. And a system of routine removal with a right to informed refusal provides ample protection of individual freedom.

It is time to give this alternative careful consideration. The future will surely bring increased demand for transplantable organs and a public seeking policies to effect this. If required request does not allow us to meet future organ needs, the unacceptable alternatives of buying and selling human organs and of government taking will become more attractive in spite of themselves. Routine removal with a right of informed refusal is a policy alternative that can satisfy genuine human needs without turning our bodies into commodities or surrendering them to the government.

POSTSCRIPT

Should Organ Procurement Be Based on Voluntarism?

In 1985 New York became the first state to enact a "required request" law, which mandates that physicians ask families if they will consent to organ retrieval. All other states have similar laws in various stages of implementation. In New York the number of donations has doubled since the law took effect, but there is still a shortage of transplantable organs. A critique of required request laws and a response by Arthur L. Caplan, who advocate such laws, is found in "Reconsidering Required Request," *Hastings Center Report* (April/May 1988).

Bone marrow transplants have created particularly acute ethical and emotional problems. Bone marrow transplants come from living donors, and the procedure, while not life-threatening, is painful and can be risky. Since tissue-matched transplants are most likely to come from relatives, family members are often under great pressure to donate. In one recent case, a California woman became pregnant specifically to bear a child who might be a suitable bone marrow donor for her 17-year-old daughter who has leukemia.

The question of whether Americans should receive priority over foreigners in obtaining organs is debated in the case study "In Organ Transplants, Americans First?" *Hastings Center Report* (October 1986).

Two classic articles on the question of organ retrieval are Willard Gaylin, "Harvesting the Dead," *Harpers* (September 1974), and William May, "Attitudes Toward the Newly Dead," *Hastings Center Studies* (No. 1 for 1973). Also see James F. Childress, "Who Shall Live When Not All Can Live?" *Soundings* (Winter 1970). A good summary of organ shortages is John K. Iglehart, "Transplantation: The Problem of Limited Resources," *The New England Journal of Medicine* (July 14, 1983). The problem of coercing a potential donor is discussed in "Mrs. X and the Bone Marrow Transplant," *Hastings Center Report* (June 1983). Also see Dale H. Cowan et al., eds., *Human Organ Transplantation: Societal, Medical-Legal, Regulatory, and Reimbursement Issues* (Health Administration Press, 1987), and Thomas E. Starzl et al., "A Multifactorial System for Equitable Selection of Cadaver Kidney Recipients," *Journal of the American Medical Association*, vol. 257, no. 22 (June 12, 1987).

See also Kathleen S. Andersen and Daniel M. Fox, "The Impact of Routine Inquiry Laws on Organ Donation," *Health Affairs* (Winter 1988), and James F. Blumstein and Frank A. Sloan, *Organ Transplantation Policy: Issues and Prospects* (Duke University Press, 1989). A special issue of *Transplantation Proceedings* (June 1989) reviews "Patient Selection Criteria in Organ Transplantation: The Critical Questions." A series of articles on religious views of organ donation is contained in the *Delaware Medical Journal* (September 1988).

ISSUE 17

Should Newborns Without Brains Be Used as Organ Donors?

YES: Michael R. Harrison, from "Organ Procurement for Children: The Anencephalic Fetus As Donor," *The Lancet* (December 13, 1986)

NO: John D. Arras and Shlomo Shinnar, from "Anencephalic Newborns As Organ Donors: A Critique," *Journal of the American Medical Association* (April 15, 1988)

ISSUE SUMMARY

YES: Pediatric surgeon Michael R. Harrison believes that if anencephalic newborns were treated as brain-dead, rather than as brain-absent, their organs could be transplanted and their families could be offered the consolation that their loss has provided life for another child.

NO: Philosopher John D. Arras and pediatric neurologist Shlomo Shinnar argue that the current principles of the strict definition of brain death are sound public policy and good ethics.

There are too few organs for donation for all categories of persons in need, but one of the most poignant situations occurs in newborns and infants. Only small organs are suitable for these young patients, and appropriate organs become available only when other young patients die.

Today several thousand children could benefit from transplants. Those on dialysis regimens could be given the chance to lead more normal lives with kidney transplants. Those suffering from liver failure face certain death without transplants. Others are born with heart defects so severe that only new hearts can save their lives.

The technical problems in transplanting small organs are rapidly being overcome, but the ethical problems persist. Anencephalic babies are one potential source of organs for pediatric patients. These are babies who are born without brains; they may survive for a few hours or days, or even weeks, but no longer. This condition occurs about once in every 1,000 to 2,000 births and can be detected through screening of the mother's blood and confirmed through sonograms, which reveal the baby's organs in utero. About 2,000 such babies are detected each year.

The parents of these babies are faced with a difficult choice: they can choose abortion (even in the third trimester) or they can carry the pregnancy to term, knowing that their baby is doomed to die. A few parents in this situation have asked for a third option: to donate the organs of their baby so that they can feel that some good for another family has come out of their personal tragedy.

If these babies had no brain activity at all, that is, if they were brain-dead, there would be no ethical problem. Their parents could consent for the removal of their organs, just as the next of kin of a brain-dead adult can consent to organ donation. But these babies, though lacking higher brain activity, do have some rudimentary brain-stem activity. Though doomed to die, they are not yet dead. If physicians wait until the babies are brain-dead, their organs may not be suitable for transplantation.

The ethical questions thus center around the justifiability of treating anencephalic newborns as if they were brain-dead in order to achieve the goal of salvaging their organs. Is the distinction between brain-absent and brain-dead a legal technicality or does it go to the essence of human existence?

In the selections that follow, Michael R. Harrison declares that the ability to transplant fetal organs may now give us the chance to recognize the contribution of the doomed anencephalic fetus to mankind. He favors treating anencephalics legally as brain-dead. John D. Arras and Shlomo Shinnar offer a critique of this view. They believe that the attempt to reconcile the use of anencephalic newborns as organ donors with the current principles of brain death violates principles of ethics and public policy. They believe that the strict criteria for whole-brain death must be satisfied and that vital organs may not be taken from the living to benefit others.

YES
Michael R. Harrison

ORGAN PROCUREMENT FOR CHILDREN: THE ANENCEPHALIC FETUS AS DONOR

Organ transplants could give an increasing number of children with fatal childhood diseases the chance of a full life.[1, 2] However, most children die waiting for an appropriate donor organ.

THE DYING CHILD: PROMISE AT A PRICE

The need for small organs is acute and the demand is likely to grow. In the United States 300–450 children with end-stage renal disease could be taken off dialysis regimens if they received renal transplants.[3, 4] The only hope for the 400–800 children with liver failure (biliary atresia, cholestatic syndromes, and inherited metabolic defects) is liver transplantation;[5, 6] for the 400–600 children with certain forms of congenital heart disease such as hypoplastic left heart syndrome it may be cardiac transplantation;[7, 8] and for an increasing number with childhood haemopoietic and malignant diseases, it is bone-marrow transplantation.[9, 10] Finally, enzymatic, immunological, and endocrine deficiencies may be corrected by the use of cellular (rather than whole-organ) grafts.[11, 14]

For many childhood diseases, biological tissue replacement may be the only satisfactory solution because the transplant must be able to grow and adapt to increasing functional demand over the potentially long life span of the recipient. But the logistics of organ transplantation are very demanding for the young recipient, in whom rapid organ failure and lack of interim support measures make the "time window" for transplantation narrow.

The present system of obtaining vital organs from "brain-dead" accident victims cannot meet the demand for small organs. It is also logistically complex and very expensive. The cost of a new heart or liver often exceeds $100,000. Unless donor material becomes simpler and less costly to procure and transplant, these life-saving procedures will have to be rationed.

AVAILABILITY OF ANENCEPHALIC ORGANS AND TISSUES

Fetuses with defects so hopeless that they meet the requirements for pregnancy termination at any gestational age may be ideal donors. With anencephaly termination is justifiable even in the third trimester,[15] and vital organs other than the brain are usually normal. It occurs once in every 1000–2000 births,[16] is easily detected by screening for raised alphafetoprotein levels in maternal serum and amniotic fluid, and can be confirmed by sonography. When screening programmes capable of detecting 90% of all anencephalic fetuses are instituted, we can expect to detect around 2000 anencephalic fetuses in the United States each year. Even if only a small proportion proves suitable as source of donor material, it could go a long way towards satisfying estimated needs.

CAN IMMATURE ORGANS WORK?

It is unlikely that a functionally immature fetal organ can immediately replace and sustain vital organ function in a child; continued partial function of the native organ or availability of interim external support for organ function will be crucial. With support by dialysis, kidneys transplanted from newborn babies with anencephaly can show remarkable growth in size and function.[17] Technical difficulties with small-vessel anastomoses are now surmountable. Since there is no method of providing good interim support for failing liver and cardiac function, total orthotopic replacement with fetal heart or liver would be limited to neonatal recipients and near-term donors. The fetal organ would have to be large enough to fit the recipient and func-

tionally mature enough to immediately replace life-sustaining function. But traditional whole-organ orthotopic replacement may not be necessary or even desirable. Auxiliary transplantation of immature organs that can develop until they take over the life-sustaining function of the failing native organ may prove safer, simpler, and less expensive.

Fetal liver has tremendous potential for growth and functional adaptation. We have shown experimentally that auxiliary heterotopic liver transplantation is technically feasible and physiologically sound.[18, 19] A small liver allows auxiliary placement without the elaborate manoeuvres required for enlarging a child's abdomen or reducing donor liver size.[20] And the obvious disadvantage of small vessels may be offset by circulatory peculiarities of fetal liver—eg, portal inflow can be provided via the large umbilical vein, which carries all the fetal cardiac output, rather than via the small and delicate portal vein, which carries only 20% of liver blood flow in utero.[21] Also, the ductus venosus is patent for a short time after birth and this may help to adjust the haemodynamic pressure gradient across the grafted fetal liver.[18]

Orthotopic replacement of the fetal heart, like that of the liver, is limited to late-gestation donors and neonatal recipients. But use of the small immature fetal heart as a heterotopic assist device is a promising prospect. We have developed a simple way of inserting a fetal heart in neonatal animals as a right ventricular assist (vena cava to pulmonary artery) to bypass congenital right ventricular outflow obstruction, and as a left ventricular assist (left atrium to aorta) to correct hypoplastic left heart syndrome (unpublished). Thus auxiliary heterotopic placement, which has been effective in adults,[22] may be simpler and safer than orthotopic replacement for treating both right and left hypoplastic heart syndromes in children.

FETAL TISSUES AND "SELECTIVE" TRANSPLANTATION

Perhaps the most promising use of fetal tissue is for selective cellular grafts, which do not require surgical revascularisation.[2] Suspensions of fetal thymus have been used to correct immunodeficiencies,[23] and bone-marrow grafting can restore immunocompetence and haemopoietic function.[9,10] However, the rejection and graft-versus-host disease seen with grafts from mature donors are less likely with immature haemopoietic stem cells harvested from fetal marrow or liver. Since many inherited defects (eg, thalassaemia) that may be correctable by cellular grafts can be diagnosed in the first half of gestation, it may be advantageous to reconstitute a deficient cell-line by in-utero transfusion.[11] We have shown experimentally that haemopoietic stem cells given by intraperitoneal injection in the first trimester can produce lasting haemopoietic chimerism.[24]

The difficulty of separating islets from exocrine pancreatic tissue and the rejection encountered with islet-cell transplantation, which can lead to cure of experimentally induced diabetes mellitus, may be ameliorated by the use of fetal pancreas.[13, 25] Transplantation of immature pituitary tissue[21] is also promising. Furthermore, there is the possibility that a functioning organ can be "grown" in a recipient by implanting a very primitive fetal organ as a non-vascularised free graft; fetal intestine, for example, may one day be used to treat infants with the short bowel syndrome.[26] Corneal grafts may restore sight, and fetal ventricular outflow tract has been used as a homograft valved conduit.[27]

ADVANTAGES OF USING FETAL ORGANS AND TISSUES

If fetal organs prove suitable, transplantation for children may be greatly simplified biologically, technically, and logistically. But the most important potential advantage is that use of fetal organs may need less immunosuppression than will use of mature organs. Fetal organs are not less "antigeneic" and thus less subject to rejection than mature organs because histocompatibility antigens are expressed early in fetal life. However, fetal grafts in general survive longer than do more mature grafts,[28, 29] and the use of fetal donors allows the immunological manipulations that improve graft survival. The fetus can be tissue-typed by examining amniotic fluid or fetal blood,[30] so the best possible recipient can be chosen by cross-matching. In addition, recipients can be pre-treated with donor cells (amniotic fluid or blood) by the same strategy that has led to improved graft survival in clinical renal transplantation.[31]

In the future, perhaps the unique immunological relation between mother and fetus can be exploited to facilitate graft acceptance. When the need for transplantation can be predicted before birth (eg, hypoplastic left heart, thalassaemia) it may be possible to induce specific unresponsiveness in the potential recipient antenatally, for transplantation either before or after birth. Although transplantation immunity develops early in all mammals, in early gestation the fetus is uniquely susceptible to induction of tolerance by donor cell suspensions.[32] Also, graft rejection and graft-versus-host disease may be less likely if grafting is done before the recipient becomes immunocompetent and/or the donor organ becomes populated by "passenger" leucocytes.

RISKS AND BENEFITS OF ALLOWING FETAL ORGAN DONATION

The diagnosis of fetal anencephaly is always devastating. Once the family has worked through their grief and decided how the pregnancy will be managed, the possibility of organ donation may be brought up. In my experience families are surprisingly positive about donation; they clutch at any possibility that something good might be salvaged from a seemingly wasted pregnancy. Sometimes families even bring up the subject themselves, or they become upset when organs cannot be donated because of a legal ambiguity (see below).

Would allowing organ procurement from an anencephalic fetus increase maternal risk? To be successfully transplanted, the organs must be oxygenated and perfused until harvest. If labour were induced by the usual techniques (for example, by cervical dilatation and ripening, pitocin) rather than by the more violent techniques often used in late abortions (for instance, prostaglandin injection), most anencephalic fetuses can be delivered vaginally without increased risk to mother.[33] Caesarean delivery would ordinarily not be considered except for maternal indications, even when labour is difficult to induce, or when the anencephalic fetus seems to be in distress.

ETHICAL AND LEGAL ISSUES

If further research and clinical experience shows that use of fetal organs is a biologically sound and cost-effective treatment for otherwise hopeless childhood diseases, society will have to decide what attitude to adopt towards the anencephalic fetus.

One attitude is that the anencephalic baby is a product of human conception incapable of achieving "personhood" because it lacks the physical structure (forebrain) necessary for characteristic human activity; and thus can never become a human "person". The idea that a product of human conception is biologically incapable of achieving "humanness" seems radical until we consider the many products of conception lost by early miscarriage or stillbirth because of gross abnormalities. Although this approach makes organ procurement simple by denying the anencephalic baby the legal rights of personhood, there are compelling reasons for avoiding this stance. First, it is difficult to reach a consensus about personhood and what constitutes humanness. Secondly, denying personhood denigrates the pregnancy itself and may lead to a less respectful approach to the grieving family and to medical care of the fetus and newborn. Finally, there is the possibility of abuse; other fetuses or newborn babies, possibly with less severe handicaps, might be denied personhood.

Another attitude is that the anencephalic fetus is a dying person and that death is inevitable at or shortly after birth because of brain absence. The first point in favour of this attitude is that brain absence can be clearly defined and limited only to anencephalics, so individuals with less severe anomalies or injuries cannot be classed with anencephalic babies as exceptions for brain-death guidelines. Another point in favour of this attitude is that the anencephalic fetus is considered a person, albeit one doomed to death at birth. To consider the anencephalic baby as a person who is brain absent is to recognise his devastating anatomical and functional deficiency without demeaning his existence. He has rights and deserves respect, so removal of organs must not cause suffering, detract from the dignity of dying, or abridge the right to die. This is best done in the operating theatre as is currently being done for brain-dead subjects. This approach also provides a sound ethical rationale for the present practice of allowing the family to choose termination of an anencephalic pregnancy at any gestational age, and would eliminate potential incongruities, such as insisting on care of aborted anencephalic subjects.

Current laws seem to forbid removal of organs from an anencephalic subject until vital functions cease, by which time the organs and tissues are irreparably damaged. This is because anencephalic babies are not brain dead by the widely accepted whole-brain definition of death which requires "irreversible cessation of all functions of the entire brain, including the brain stem";[34] anencephalics may have lower-brain-stem activity capable of maintaining vital functions, although precariously, for hours after birth.

The whole-brain definition of death was drafted to protect the comatose patient whose injured brain might recover function. However, failure of the brain to develop is clearly different from injury to a functioning brain, and it was simply not considered when the brain-death definition was formulated. The extreme caution and safeguards needed in pronouncing brain death after brain injury should not apply to anencephaly, in which the physical structure necessary for recovery is absent. If failure of brain development, or brain absence, is recognised as the only exception to present brain-death statutes, society and the courts can then concentrate on the legal implications of regarding the anencephalic subject as being brain absent. I believe that brain absence will come to have the same medicolegal implications as brain death, but this will have to be recognised by society and confirmed by the courts.

If the anencephalic fetus is considered to be equivalent to brain-dead subjects for legal purposes, the family should be able to allow organ donation after delivery and to arrange the timing and place of delivery to facilitate transplantation.[35] Obstetrical decisions about how and when to end the pregnancy must be independent of plans to use the organs for transplantation. Members of the transplant team should not be involved in counselling or perinatal management, and the diagnosis of anencephaly should be confirmed by a panel independent of the transplant team and include a neurologist, a bioethicist, and a neonatologist. The family should also be able to decide before delivery whether they wish to see and hold the newborn.

Because many fetal disorders can now be diagnosed and even treated antenatally, we are learning to accept the fetus as an unborn patient.[30] We are also identifying fetuses so fatally damaged that survival outside the womb is impossible. The ability to transplant fetal organs may now give us the chance to recognise the contribution of this doomed fetus to mankind. If organs from prenatally diagnosed anencephalic fetuses can be obtained with safety for mother and respect for the fetus, the family should be allowed to salvage from their tragedy the consolation that their loss can provide life to another child.

I thank Dr John C. Fletcher, Dr Albert Jonsen, Professor John A. Robertson, Dr Mitchell Golbus, and colleagues at the Fetal Treatment Program, UCSF, for suggestions and review.

REFERENCES

1. Lum CT, Wassner SJ, Martin DE. Current thinking in transplantation in infants and children. *Ped Clins North Am* 1985; **32**: 1203-32.
2. Russell PS. Selective transplantation: An emerging concept. *Ann Surg* 1985; **201**: 255-62.
3. So SKS, Nevine TE, Chang PN, et al. Preliminary results of renal transplantation. *Transpl Proc* 1985; **17**: 182-83.
4. Eggers PW, Connerton R, McMullan M. The medicare experience with end-stage renal disease: Trends in incidence, prevalence, and survival. *Hlth Care Financing Rev* 1984; **5**: 69-88.
5. Lloyd-Still JD. Mortality from liver disease in children: Implications for hepatic transplantation program. *Am J Dise Child* 1985; **139**: 381-84.
6. Gartner JC, Zatelli, BJ, Starzl TE. Orthotopic liver transplantation. Two year experience with 47 patients. *Pediatrics* 1984; **74**: 140-45.
7. Baily LL, Jang J, Johnson W, Jolley WB. Orthotopic cardiac xenografting in the newborn goat. *J Thorac Cardiovasc Surg* 1985; **89**: 242-47.
8. Penkoske PA, Freidman RM, Rowe RD, Trusler GA. The future of heart and heart-lung transplantation in children. *Heart Transplant* 1984; **3**: 233-38.
9. Thomas ED. Marrow transplantation for nonmalignant disorders. *N Engl J Med* 1985; **312**: 46-47.
10. Barranger JA. Marrow transplantation in genetic disease. *N Engl J Med* 1984; **311**: 1629-30.
11. Simpson TJ, Golbus MS. In utero fetal hematopoietic stem cell transplantation. *Sem Perinatol* 1985; **9**: 68-74.
12. Prummer O, Raghavachar A, Werner C, et al. Fetal liver transplantation in the dog. *Transplantation* 1985; **39**: 349-55.
13. Brown J, Danilovs JA, Clark WR, Mullen YS. Fetal pancreas as a donor organ. *World J Surg* 1984; **8**: 152-57.
14. Tulipan NB, Zacar HA, Allen GS. Pituitary transplantation: Part I. Successful reconstitution of pituitary dependent hormone levels. *Neurosurgery* 1985; **16**: 331-35.

15. Chervenak FA, Farley MA, Walters LR, et al. When is termination of pregnancy during the third trimester morally justifiable? *N Engl J Med* 1983; **310**: 501-04.
16. Elwood JM, Elwood JH. Epidemiology of anencephalus and spina bifida. New York: Oxford University Press, 1980: 253-99.
17. Kinnaert P, Persign G, Cohen B, et al. Transplantation of kidneys from anenephalic donors, *Transplant Proc* 1984; **16**: 71-72.
18. Flake AW, Laberge JM, Adzick NS, et al. Auxiliary transplantation of the fetal liver I. Development of a sheep model, *J Pediatr Surg* 1986; **21**: 515-20.
19. Flake AW, Harrison MA, Sauer L, et al. Auxiliary transplantation of the fetal liver II. Functional evaluation of an intra-abdominal model. *J Pediatr Surg* (in press).
20. Bismuth H, Houssin D. Reduced-sized orthotopic liver graft in hepatic transplantation in children. *Surgery* 1984; **95**: 367-70.
21. Rudolph AM. Hepatic and ductus venosus blood flow during fetal life. *Hepatology* 1983; **3**: 245-58.
22. Barnard CN, Cooper DKC. Heterotopic versus orthotopic heart transplantation. *Transplant Proc* 1984; **16**: 886-92.
23. Thong YH, Robertson EF, Rischbieth GH, et al. Successful restoration of immunity in the DiGeorge Syndrome with fetal thymic epithelial transplat. *Arch Dis Child* 1978; **53**: 580-84.
24. Flake AW, Harrison MR, Adzick NS, Zanjani ED. Transplantation of fetal lamb hematopoietic stem cells *in utero*: The creation of hematopoietic chimeras, *Science* (in press).
25. Mandel TE. Transplantation of organ-cultured fetal pancreas: Experimental studies and potential clinical application in diabetes mellitus. *World J Surg* 1984; **8**: 158-68.
26. Bass BL, Schweitzer EJ, Harmon JW, et al. Anatomic and physiologic characteristics of transplanted fetal rat intestine. *Ann Surg* 1984; **200**: 734-41.
27. Fontan F, Choussat A, Deville C, et al. Aortic valve homografts in the surgical treatment of complex cardiac malformations. *J Thorac Cardiovasc Surg* 1984; **87**: 649-57.
28. Miller I. The immunity of the human foetus and newborn infant. Boston: Martinus Nijhoff, 1983.
29. Foglia RP, LaQuaglia M, DiPreta, J, et al. Can fetal and newborn allografts survive in an immunocompetent heart? *J Pediatr Surg* 1986; **21**: 608-12.
30. Harrison MR, Golbus, MS, Filly RA. The unborn patient. New York: Grune & Stratton, 1984.
31. Monoco AP. Clinical kidney transplantation in 1984. *Transplant Proc* 1985; **17**: 5-12.

32. Billingham RE, Brent L, Medawar PB. Actively acquired tolerance of foreign cells. *Nature* 1967; **214:** 179.

33. Lawson J. Delivery of the dead or malformed fetus. Intrauterine death during pregnancy with retention of fetus. *Clins Obs Gynecol* 1982; **9:** 745–56.

34. President's Commission for the Study of Ethical Problems in Medicine and Biomedical and Behavioral Research: Defining Death. US Government Printing Office, Washington DC. July 1981.

35. Harrison MR. Commentary. *Hastings Rep* 1986; **16:** 21–22.

NO

John D. Arras and Shlomo Shinnar

ANENCEPHALIC NEWBORNS AS ORGAN DONORS: A CRITIQUE

The debate over whether anencephalic newborns should be used as organ donors[1, 2] has entered a new phase with the recent announcements from West Germany[3] and California (*New York Times,* Oct 19, 1987, p A1) of kidney and heart transplants from anencephalic newborns. As we move from deliberation and debate to action, there is an urgent need to reflect on the ethical implications of this controversial procedure.

THE ISSUES

The case for taking hearts, paired kidneys, and other vital organs from anencephalic newborns is based on two distinct needs. First, there are many chronically ill infants, children, and adults who may benefit from organ transplant, and there is a relative scarcity of available donors. Second, there is the need of the parents of an anencephalic infant to salvage some good from a tragic situation. Allowing the infant to be used as an organ donor may help satisfy this need.[1, 3]

An important feature of anencephaly is the relative certitude of diagnosis and prognosis. Ultrasonography can now detect anencephaly in utero with relative certainty. The prognosis for these infants is death within hours, days, or weeks from birth, although there is some controversy over their exact life span. In view of the need for organs and the alleged uniqueness of anencephaly, it has been proposed that society consider such infants as persons who are born "brain absent." Anencephaly would be declared the *only* legitimate exception to our current insistence that all vital organ donors meet the criteria for whole-brain death.[1, 3] This would be useful in procuring neonatal organs, especially since the diagnosis of whole-brain death in the neonate is extremely difficult and fraught with uncertainty.[4, 7] The lack of established brain death criteria in the first week of life also poses additional problems for those who would use "brain dead" neonates as organ donors (*New York Times,* Oct 19, 1987, p A1).

From John D. Arras and Shlomo Shinnar, "Anencephalic Newborns as Organ Donors: A Critique," *Journal of the American Medical Association,* vol. 259, no. 15 (April 15, 1988), p. 2284. Copyright © 1988 by the American Medical Association. Reprinted by permission.

Advocates of the brain absent approach specifically decline to view anencephalic newborns as "nonpersons" and insist that these infants are "persons" deserving of respect. However, they state that since they are also brain absent, they should be functionally equivalent to brain dead insofar as vital organs might be harvested from them.[1, 3] Another approach for justifying the use of anencephalic newborns as organ donors would be to regard them as nonpersons—ie, as biologically human entities that nevertheless lack the prerequisites of "personal" life and thus lack full moral status.[8] This perspective provides the most direct route to salvaging their organs at the expense of redefining society's views of "personhood."

Despite the manifest importance of the "gift of life" to organ recipients and the laudable desire to help parents salvage some good from a tragedy, society must consider whether allowing anencephalic infants to be used as organ donors before they meet the traditional criteria for brain death is a morally acceptable and legitimate act. We believe it is not.

BRAIN ABSENT THEORY

Let us first address the issues posed by the brain absent theory. By insisting on the personhood of these infants, proponents of this scheme commit themselves to treat the anencephalic infant as a full member of the moral community, ie, one who has rights and is worthy of respect. The question is whether prolonging the infant's life by mechanical ventilation and then abruptly terminating it by harvesting vital organs is compatible with the minimum respect due to all persons. In Kantian philosophy, which is the source of many contemporary moral theories based on the concept of personhood, using one person merely as a means to benefit another constitutes a paradigmatic violation of moral law.[9] As "ends in themselves," persons have an intrinsic worth that cannot be reduced to their instrumental value to others. The investigators' claims notwithstanding, it is difficult to reconcile the treatment of anencephalic newborns outlined in the recent reports[3] (New York Times, Oct 19, 1987, p A1) with the notion of respect for personhood.

One response to this objection is to claim that if the anencephalic infant could (miraculously) reflect on his plight, he would consent to organ donation, since losing vital organs would not deprive him of anything he would desire. Similar arguments can be made using the social contract theory of Rawls,[10] in which the decision maker is unbiased because he does not know what role (parent, recipient, anencephalic infant, or physician) he would have in the societal drama and therefore tries to minimize the worst outcome, which may be a person in need of an organ with no available donor. However, these arguments are by no means unique to anencephalic newborns. They are equally applicable to other severely damaged infants as well as to adults in permanent vegetative states. We do not believe society is willing to harvest organs from living patients who have permanently lost the capacity for intelligent thought.

PERSONHOOD THEORY

Justifying the use of anencephalic newborns as organ donors by labeling them "nonpersons" creates the same uniqueness problem. In this philosophical theory, only beings capable of sapient life,

Sapient - having great wisdom or discernment.

Discern - Recognize or comprehend mentally

whatever that means, have the rights and privileges of "personhood."[7] If anencephalic newborns are nonpersons, one could perhaps justify using them as a mere means for the benefit of persons. Again, if the theory is carried out to its logical conclusion, other infants with conditions such as holoprosencephaly, hydranencephaly, and certain trisomies as well as adults in permanent vegetative states should be considered as potential organ donors.

Those who justify using anencephalic newborns as organ donors based on the fact that they will all die soon after birth[1,3] must deal with two objections. First, even a dying person is still a person and is entitled to a full measure of dignity and respect as discussed above. Second, there is nothing special in this respect about anencephaly. If the crucial issue is uniform early mortality, then a number of other conditions, such as Potter's syndrome and trisomy 13, would qualify.

The availability of reliable prenatal diagnosis has led some authors to conclude that abortion of anencephalic fetuses is justified even in the third trimester.[11] If we are willing to terminate a viable fetus just prior to term, why not terminate life just after delivery?[1,3] However, the moral justification for third-trimester abortion is based on the certitude of both diagnosis and prognosis and not on any inherently unique feature of anencephaly.[11] Many other conditions would meet the authors' criteria if reliable antenatal diagnosis were available.

BRAIN DEATH

Another fundamental objection to the proposals for amending the brain death statutes to define anencephalic infants as "dead" or "brain absent" is that this violates the spirit of our present brain death statutes regarding the definition of death.[4] Although anencephalic infants lack a cerebral cortex, they certainly have a brain stem that sustains and regulates a wide variety of vital bodily functions, including spontaneous respiration. Thus, it would be more accurate to describe them as "higher-brain absent" than as "brain absent." According to the present definition of brain death, ie, complete and irreversible cessation of all brain functions, including those of the brain stem, anencephalic infants are indisputably living human beings. Indeed, no one with spontaneous respirations meets the current criteria for brain death.[4, 5, 12] Permitting the use of anencephalic newborns as organ donors by defining them as legally dead requires a radical reformulation of our current definition of death.

One way to accomplish this would be to reinterpret the original intent of the whole-brain definition of death. One advocate of this approach has argued that the stringent safeguards built into the current brain death statutes were put there to protect comatose patients who might eventually recover some higher cortical functions. Since anencephalic infants lack the capacity ever to achieve such a level of existence, there is no need to protect them with such rigorous definitions of brain death.[1] Consequently, it is argued that taking organs from brain absent anencephalic newborns is ethically compatible with the spirit if not the letter of the laws governing brain death. Although the argument sounds plausible, it confuses a necessary condition for the definition of brain death with a sufficient condition. Of course, any adequate definition of brain death must preclude the possibility of meaningful recovery.

However, it is one thing to note that a person is incapable of recovery of higher cortical functions and/or is imminently dying but quite another to say that he or she is dead.

Why should irreversible cessation of activity of the entire brain be necessary for a definition of death? According to the President's Commission, the brain, including the brain stem, performs an irreplaceable function in sustaining and regulating the physiological systems that keep us alive. Once it ceases to perform these vital tasks, modern technology can continue to oxygenate other organs, for a time creating a simulacrum of life, but cannot substitute for the spontaneous integrative functions that the Commission identified as the sine qua non of human life. The Commission insisted on a rigorous definition of brain death not solely to protect comatose patients, but because it believed that anything short of whole-brain death was not equivalent to the death of the human being.[2, 4] The Commission also specifically insisted that organ donors be *dead*, not just irrevocably brain damaged or imminently dying. This position has been cogently reiterated recently by the former executive director of the Commission.[2] Thus, the attempt to reconcile the use of anencephalic newborns as organ donors with current principles of brain death founders on a flawed account of the rationale for accepting whole-brain death as death of the human being.

CONCLUSIONS

Current public policy and practice embody two fundamental principles: first, that vital organs may not be taken from the living for the benefit of others and, second, that for brain death to be considered the moral and legal equivalent of the death of the person, the strict criteria for whole-brain death must be satisfied. The second principle is accepted as sound public policy even by many, including one of us (J.D.A.), who do not fully agree with the President's Commission's philosophical rationale for choosing whole-brain death. The use of anencephalic newborns as organ donors is incompatible with both of these generally accepted principles. Advocates of using these infants as organ donors can invoke the more controversial "higher brain" definitions of either death or personhood to justify their proposal.[8, 13] However, to be consistent, infants with other severe brain malformations as well as adults in chronic vegetative states should then also be candidates for use as organ donors. We believe that the current principles of the strict definition of brain death are sound public policy and good ethics. We hope that, after careful scrutiny and debate, the use of anencephalic infants as organ donors is rejected. Admirable goals should not be advanced by improper means.

REFERENCES

1. Harrison MR: Organ procurement for children: The anenephalic fetus as donor. *Lancet* 1986;2:1383–1386.
2. Capron AM: Anencephalic donors: Separate the dead from the dying. *Hastings Cent Rep*, February 1987, pp 5–9.
3. Holzgreve W, Beller FK, Bucholz B, et al: Kidney transplantation from anencephalic donors. *N Engl J Med* 1987;316:1069–1070.
4. President's Commission for the Study of Ethical Problems in Medicine and Biomedical and Behavioral Research: *Defining Death*. US Government Printing Office, 1981.
5. Guidelines for the determination of brain death in children: Report of the task force. *Pediatrics* 1987;80:298–300.
6. Coulter D: Neurologic uncertainty in newborn intensive care. *N Engl J Med* 1987; 316:870–874.

7. Volpe JJ: Brain death determination in the newborn. *Pediatrics* 1987;80:293–297.

8. Engelhardt HT Jr: *The Foundations of Bioethics.* New York, Oxford University Press Inc, 1986.

9. Kant I: *Groundwork of the Metaphysics of Morals,* Paton HJ (trans). New York, Harper & Row Publishers Inc. 1964.

10. Rawls J: *A Theory of Justice.* Cambridge, Mass, Harvard University Press, 1971.

11. Chervenak FA, Farley MA, Walters L, et al: When is termination of pregnancy during the third trimester justifiable? *N Engl J Med* 1984;310:501–504.

12. Ad Hoc Committee of the Harvard Medical School to Examine the Definition of Death: A definition of irreversible coma. *JAMA* 1968;205:337–340.

13. Green MB, Wikler D: Brain death and personal identity. *Philos Public Affairs* 1980;9:105–133.

POSTSCRIPT

Should Newborns Without Brains Be Used as Organ Donors?

In October 1987 physicians at Loma Linda University Medical Center in California—the same institution that operated on Baby Fae (see Issue 14)—transplanted the heart of Baby Gabrielle, a Canadian anencephalic baby, into the chest of another Canadian baby, known as Baby Paul. Baby Paul survived and is reported to be doing well.

Loma Linda then established a research program to transplant organs from anencephalic babies. The protocol called for a determination of brain death before the organs could be retrieved. In September 1988 the program was suspended. Dr. Leonard C. Bailey announced that not a single procedure had been performed, even though a dozen anencephalic babies had been flown to Loma Linda from around the country.

The medical team encountered several problems. Only two of the twelve infants turned out to be possible donors; the rest were unsuitable because their organs deteriorated before brain death occurred. The heart of one of the two babies who were suitable donors went unused because there was no appropriate recipient at the time; in the other case a possible heart recipient was available, but the blood type was incompatible.

All the babies in the program died within one or two days after they were removed from the respirator; however, one baby survived for two months after removal. Physicians involved in the program experienced considerable stress. They also reported that babies with less severe defects than anencephaly had been offered to them as potential donors. Dr. Joyce Peabody, the hospital's chief of neonatology, declared, "The slippery slope is real."

"The Anencephalic Newborn as Organ Donor," a case study in *Hastings Center Report* (April 1986), offers two views of the question. Also see Larry R. Churchill and Rosa Lynn B. Pinkus, "The Use of Anencephalic Organs: Historical and Ethical Dimensions," *Milbank Q* (1990). Three articles opposing the practice are: "Anencephalic Donors: Separate the Dead from the Dying," by Alexander Morgan Capron, *Hastings Center Report* (February 1987); "From Canada with Love: Anencephalic Newborns as Organ Donors?" by George J. Annas, *Hastings Center Report* (December 1987); and "The Use of Anencephalic Infants as Organ Sources: A Critique," by D. Alan Shewmon et al., *Journal of the American Medical Association* (March 24/31, 1990).

ISSUE 18

Should There Be a Market in Body Parts?

YES: Lori B. Andrews, from "My Body, My Property," *Hastings Center Report* (October 1986)

NO: Thomas H. Murray, from "Gifts of the Body and the Needs of Strangers," *Hastings Center Report* (April 1987)

ISSUE SUMMARY

YES: Attorney Lori B. Andrews believes that donors, recipients, and society will benefit from a market in body parts so long as owners—and no one else—retain control over their bodies.

NO: Ethicist Thomas H. Murray argues that the gift relationship should govern transfer of body parts because it honors important human values, which are diminished by market relationships.

In 1976 John Moore was treated for hairy-cell leukemia at the University of California at Los Angeles. His enlarged spleen was removed; Moore's condition improved. In the course of seven years of follow-up, Moore was asked by his physicians to return frequently to UCLA from his home in Seattle to have his blood tested. When he became concerned about the frequency of the visits and the amount of blood drawn, he learned that, as a by-product of his treatment, scientists had been able to use his cells to grow a potentially commercially valuable patented cell line, which they named Mo. (Cell line means cells that continuously reproduce in a culture without differentiating.) Moore sued, claiming that he had not given consent for this use of his body parts, and asked for a share of any profits. The physicians claimed that Moore had waived his interest in his body parts when he authorized the removal of his spleen on a routine consent form.

In a similar case, Hideaki Hagiwara, a postdoctoral biology student at the University of California at San Diego, suggested to a colleague, Dr. Ivor Royston, that cancer cells from Hagiwara's mother could be used to create a human monoclonal antibody—that is, an antibody that reacts specifically with a certain kind of cancerous cell. After the new cell line was completed, Hagiwara claimed that he had an economic interest in the procedure since he had suggested the idea and the cells had come from his mother.

These cases are unusual only because they resulted in lawsuits. The practice of using patients' body parts or tissues for research with potential commercial applications is widespread. According to a survey conducted by a subcommittee of the U.S. House of Representatives, about half of 81 medical schools responding to the questionnaire use patients' fluids or tissues for research. About one-fifth of the patent applications filed by these schools in the five years previous to the survey had used materials derived from patients. Three times as many patents had originated in patients' body parts from 1980 to 1984 as had occurred between 1975 and 1979.

Should patients have the right to consent to the use of their body parts and to share in any profits that might accrue? Or does the value mainly derive from the scientists' labors? The following selections approach this problem from different viewpoints. Lori B. Andrews believes that it is time to acknowledge that body parts are personal property and that individuals must have the ability to transfer and sell them, and thus to participate in any economic rewards. Thomas H. Murray, on the other hand, warns that treating body parts as property will diminish their symbolic and human value. He argues for a continuation of the gift relationship, which strengthens the bonds between strangers.

YES

Lori B. Andrews

MY BODY, MY PROPERTY

Tangible items are generally considered to be property. As new potentials for body parts unfold in research, diagnostics, and therapy, the question arises—should they be considered property as well? Current policy allows people to donate solid organs, but not to sell them. A federal law forbids sales of organs for transplant in interstate commerce[1] and certain state laws ban payment for specified organs as well.[2] This perspective—that bodily parts and products are gifts, not compensable items of property—underlies researchers' use of a patient's tissue to produce potentially marketable products.

THE PROPERTY APPROACH AND INDIVIDUAL CONTROL

Throughout the legal lore, judges have reacted with horror to the idea that body parts may be property. Nevertheless, many legal decisions treat the body as a type of property. The law allows me to make gifts of certain body parts and even to destroy my body entirely. Not only do I have a property-like interest in my own body, I may have rights that could be considered property rights in other people's bodies. Tort law allows me to recover for harm to my child, such as it allows me recovery for damage to my car. In most instances, I can collect damages if an autopsy is performed on my next of kin without my consent.

Since the legal treatment of bodies and body parts sounds suspiciously like property treatment, why is there such a reluctance to label it as such? One major fear is that bodily property could be transferred to others (the legal term is alienable) and we could become slaves, not in a market for our bodies, but in a market for body parts. However, characterizing body parts as property does not mean that they must be completely transferable. As Susan Rose-Ackerman points out, many forms of property have restrictions on alienability.[3] There may be restrictions on who holds them, what actions are required or forbidden, and what kinds of transfers are permitted. Some types of properties can be given as gifts, but not sold (items made of the fur

From Lori B. Andrews, "My Body, My Property," *Hastings Center Report* (October 1986). Copyright © 1986 by The Hastings Center. Reprinted by permission.

or feathers of endangered species, for example). Other types of properties (such as the holdings of a person who is bankrupt) can be sold, but not given as gifts.

Even under current policy, the body can be considered property, the kind of property that can be transferred without payment, but not sold. However, restraints on payment need strong moral and legal justification. The Ontario Law Reform Commission recently faced the issue of paying for body parts in the context of artificial reproduction. After deciding that donating sperm, eggs, or embryos was ethically, morally, and socially acceptable, the Commission noted that any restriction on available services (for example, by prohibiting commercial banks for gametes and embryos) "must be scrutinized very carefully; it would be futile and frustrating to give with one hand, only to take with the other."[4]

The property approach recognizes people's interest in controlling what happens to their body parts. It provides a legal basis for a remedy as theories of privacy, autonomy, or assault do not when inappropriate actions are taken with respect to extracorporeal bodily materials. The presumption that the authority belongs to the individual who provided the body parts would be a starting point, which would at least assure that the regulatory and institutional policies developed be measured against some standard. . . .

Some lawyers and researchers argue that there is no need to inform people that body parts removed in the course of treatment may be used for research or commercial purposes, so long as the patient is not exposed to any additional physical risk due to the research. Currently, under federal regulations covering federally funded research, consent is not required to do research on such pathological or diagnostic specimens, so long as the subjects cannot be identified.[5] In such cases, consent is given under the general hospital admission form, which states that the part may be used for teaching or research before it is destroyed. But the hospital consent form does not say that the patient may refuse to allow bodily materials to be used and still retain the patient/physician relationship and be treated. Only when the human material is taken primarily for research purposes is consent required. Even then, if the research poses "no more than minimal risk" and involves only collection of some body excretions, including blood, placenta or amniotic fluid, it may be given an expedited review by an Institutional Review Board; while consent is not specifically required, presumably the IRB can seek consent if the subjects are identifiable.[6] The failure to extend consent to all categories of research on human body parts and the failure even to raise the issue of compensation puts patients at a distinct psychological and economic disadvantage. . . .

There is support for informing patients about the potential uses of the body parts, even among groups that now gain commercially from using those parts. The Licensing Executive Society Biotechnology Committee recently surveyed its members, who generally represent organizations that use human tissues, fluids, or cells for research or development purposes. Of those responding, twenty-two believed that research or commercialization should occur *only* with the patient's prior consent; two felt consent was unnecessary. Thirteen felt that a person has a right to receive compensation for the use of his or her fluid, tissues, or cells, while eight did not.

THE MARKET'S EFFECT ON DONORS

The property approach requires the individual's consent before her body parts can be used by others. But in some instances, body parts—such as kidneys or corneas—may be in such short supply or a particular patient may have such a rare tissue or fluid type that the issue of payment to donors will arise, as it did in the Moore and Hagiwara cases. . . .

Naturally, the need for money is not a justification for any action (we would not want the person to become a contract killer for a fee). But it is difficult to justify a prohibition on payment for what otherwise would be a legal and ethical act—giving up body parts for someone else's valid use. Similarly, the analogy to slavery is inapposite. We do not want people to sell themselves into slavery *nor* do we want them to "give" themselves into slavery without pay. In contrast, with respect to organ donation or the development of a diagnostic or therapeutic product from bodily materials, the underlying activity is one we want to encourage. . . .

GUARDING AGAINST COERCION

Just as we would not condone a labor system that did not allow people to choose their own employers, we should insist that paid donations from living people be voluntary: that is, made by the person himself or herself. It is one thing for people to have the right to treat their own bodies as property, quite another to allow others to treat a person as property. A hospital should not be allowed to take, sell, and use blood or eggs from a comatose woman to help pay her costs of hospitalization. People should be prohibited from selling their relative's body parts when the relative dies (unless the deceased left orders to that effect). Nor should judges be allowed to sentence offenders to pay their fines in body product donations (once the property approach has established a market value for them). If this seems farfetched, consider that there already have been instances in which judges sentenced defendants to give blood transfusions. Similarly, an eighteenth-century British statute allowed judges to order anatomical dissection of hanged murderers.[7] It is possible to maintain that people are priceless by not allowing others to treat a person's body commercially either before or after death and by giving people the power to refuse to sell their body parts.

A decision to sell certain types of body parts—nonregenerative ones (such as a kidney) or parts that could give rise to offspring (sperm, eggs, and embryos)—has lifelong implications. With respect to other decisions of long-lasting consequences (such as marriage), society has sometimes adopted added protections to assure that the decision has been carefully made. A similar approach might be used with regard to body parts. In this area, only competent adults should be allowed to decide to sell. There should be a short waiting period (like the cooling-off period that protects consumers from door-to-door salesmen) between the agreement to sell an organ and its removal, and the donor should be required to observe certain formalities (such as signing a witnessed consent form).

Only the person who owns the body part should be allowed to sell it. This approach has two goals. The first is to assure that others do not treat one's body as property. For example, it will prevent the harms associated with holding the body as security until funeral costs are paid.[8] The second is to attempt to assure that the individual is adequately compensated for the body part by limiting the amount any middleman receives. If the middleman cannot "sell" the part, but can only be compensated for bringing together the donor and recipient, the donor may more likely receive adequate compensation and the transaction will less likely be viewed as excessively commercial. There might even be limitations on what the middleman (physician or entrepreneur) receives, similar to the statutory limitation in some states of "reasonableness" in the amount of money an attorney receives in connection with arranging a private adoption. . . .

Giving an individual sole rights over his or her body parts is in keeping with attitudes toward the body held in other areas of law. Attempted suicide and suicide are no longer considered crimes.[9] However, aiding and abetting a suicide is a crime. Competent individuals can refuse a readily available lifesaving treatment, but their physicians cannot withhold it. Thus, people are allowed to control what is done to their bodies (even to the point of physical damage) in ways that other individuals are not.

Ironically, our current policy is just the reverse. Other people seem to have property rights in our body parts, but we do not. In a British case, an accused man who poured his urine sample down the sink was found guilty of stealing it from the police department.[10] And although an individual has no property interest in his or her cell lines, scientists are quick to claim a property interest in those cell lines. Such a claim was the basis of a six-year conflict between microbiologist Leonard Hayflick and the National Institutes of Health. The conflict was over which side owned a cell line that Hayflick had developed with embryonic living tissue under NIH funding and then sold to scientists around the world.[11] . . .

THE MARKET'S EFFECT ON RECIPIENTS

We can protect potential donors from the market's effect by attempting to assure that donations are voluntary and by limiting donations to body parts that do not unreasonably affect the person's ability to function. But how does a market affect potential recipients? The policy of prohibiting payment for body parts and products has been justified as protecting potential recipients by raising the quality of donations and preventing a situation in which body parts are affordable only by the rich.

The work of Richard Titmuss on policies governing blood donation raised serious questions of quality control when blood is sold.[12] Among other things, he argued that paid donors have an incentive not to disclose illnesses or characteristics that might make their blood of dubious quality. Subsequent work by Harvey Sapolsky and Stan Finkelstein[13] challenged Titmuss's conclusions. They pointed to a Government Accounting Office study in which some voluntary groups in the United States reported hepatitis rates as high as the worst paid groups; and some commercially collected blood was nearly as good as the best of the volunteer blood.

Even if paid donors are more likely to misrepresent their condition than are volunteer donors, payment need not be banned on quality control grounds since tests are available to assess the fitness of the donor. In this country we allow payment for blood and sperm, although it is easy to lie about their quality; yet we do not allow payment for body organs such as kidneys, although organ transplantation offers more independent checks on quality. Nor is banning payment the only mechanism to enhance quality, since if known risks are not disclosed, liability may follow. While this may not offer sufficient protection to the recipients of blood (since donors may not be solvent), organ donors would be better paid and a portion of that money could be used to buy insurance. When a person sells organs contingent on death, payment to an estate could be withheld if it was clear that he failed to disclose a known harmful condition. Already, the Ontario Law Reform Commission has recommended enacting a criminal law prohibiting people selling their gametes from knowingly concealing infectious and genetic disorders.

A market in solid organs is also thought harmful to potential recipients because of the possibility that only the rich will be able to afford organs. On the issue of the poor selling and the rich buying body parts, Thomas Murray says, "Our consciences can tolerate considerable injustice, but such naked, undisguised profiteering in life would be too much for us."[14] Yet other equally troublesome but less visible inequities are already occurring in allocating other kinds of medical care. When a drug company prices a medication necessary for someone's life beyond a person's reach or a physician with unique skills refuses to accept patients who receive Medicare, that is also profiteering in life, but the injustice may be overlooked. Currently at least fifty different types of artificial body parts (such as artificial blood vessels and joints) have been designed to substitute for human ones.[15] It is as important ethically to address discrimination between rich and poor recipients with respect to those products as it is with respect to human body parts. A visible market in body parts may lull people out of complacency to address more general issues of allocation in health care. . . .

THE MARKET'S EFFECT ON SOCIETY

Will a market in body parts harm society by creating an attitude that people are commodities? The body is a symbol of the whole person and degrading it can be viewed as an assault to the whole person. Our distaste with viewing the body as property is, in part, a reaction to our belief that human beings should have no price.

Certainly people are more than the sum of their parts.[16] But treating the body as property does not mean it is a person's only property. Cognitive functions can be included within the property characterization. Indeed, they already are, for example, under the legal doctrine of copyright, patent, and other so-called "intellectual property" rights. I view my uniqueness as a person as more related to my intellectual products than my bodily products. (Definitions of personhood, for example, rarely revolve around the possession of body parts, but rather focus on sentience or other cognitive traits.) Arguably it commercializes me less as a person to sell my bone marrow than to sell my intellectual products. Thus, I do not view payment of body parts as commercializing people. The danger I see in the sale of a physical (as opposed to a mental) bodily product comes from the potential for physical harm in removing the bodily material or living without it. This danger can be handled by limiting the types of body parts that can be sold and the circumstances under which they can be sold.

Selling body parts has also been criticized as harmful to society because it could diminish altruism. But in our society, the basics of life—food, shelter, health care—are already sold. Nevertheless, many people continue to act altruistically, devoting time, money, or goods to provide needy people with those basics. The possibility of selling tissue or organs seems only a modest further step toward a market, unlikely to change vastly the impulse toward altruism. Even people who take advantage of the market may engage in altruistic behavior. One patient, Ted Slavin, received up to $10.00 per milliliter from commercial enterprises for his blood, which was used in manufacturing diagnostic kits for hepatitis B virus. At the same time, he provided additional blood—at no charge—to a research project at the Fox Chase Cancer Center, which used it to develop a vaccine against hepatitis B.[17] . . .

To guard against the appearance that people are commodities, we must not let other people treat one's body parts as property. Body parts will thus not be salable in the sense of cars, farm animals, or baseball cards. There will be no means for a tax man or physician to put a lien against a person's body parts. Nor can relatives choose to sell a person's parts after his or her death. However, it differs from previous notions of quasi-property by recognizing the right of an individual to compensation for certain types of body parts. Under this approach, human beings have the right to treat certain physical parts of their bodies as objects for possession, gift, and trade, but they do not become objects so long as others cannot treat them as property.

THE MARKET'S EFFECT ON THE DOCTOR/PATIENT RELATIONSHIP

The treatment of body parts as property will help curtail activities by physicians, researchers, and their attorneys that deny individuals information about or control over body parts that will be removed.

Implicit in many arguments made by physician/researchers is that the removed body part belongs to the doctor, not the patient. Why do physicians feel that way? I can only speculate that it is because society allows medical practitioners to do things to a patient's body (for example, cut it up) that no one else (other than the patient) is allowed to do. Perhaps this gives physicians the feeling that the patient's body belongs in some sense to them.

Physicians argue that getting patients' permission to use their body parts and products would change the relationship between patients and physicians or researchers. Some argue that discussing the research with the patient may imply that a patient has a right to direct the scope or direction of the study. But that is absurd. Just because IBM is required to make certain disclosures to me when I buy a share of stock does not mean that I can set policy for the operation of the company.

Related to this is an argument that paying for the patient's cells, tissue, fluids, or organs would tie up physicians in endless negotiation with their patients. But when payment for human biological material is required, it is no more disastrous to the research enterprise than payment for pipettes, microscopes, animals, or laboratory equipment. It may represent a modest increase in the cost of doing business (just as an increase in fuel prices would raise the costs of lighting the laboratory). But the money paid would go to a good cause, slightly enhancing the resources of medical patients at a time when they need money to pay for medical care. If the patient is unwilling to sell rights to the biological materials, the physician need not barter; she can simply avoid using that specimen and approach other patients. Moreover, we allow the patient to pay the physician for services without being concerned that it will lead to endless negotiations.

Just as physicians raise the price for their services to cover rising malpractice insurance rates, so they will charge slightly more for the right to use the specimens of some patients for research. If it strikes you as unfair (it does me) to force patients to pay for the research by increasing medical costs, consider that under the current system the "cost" of the human specimens is borne entirely by the patients who own them and who do not even get in return a right to refuse to participate.

Another reason has been advanced against disclosure: it would decrease patient-physician trust if the patient were aware that the physician might develop a commercial product from the patient's body parts. Yet this begs the question of whether the information is relevant. It might diminish the patient's trust to know the success rate and unnecessary surgery rates of a practitioner or health care facility; yet this information is clearly relevant to patient decision making.

There is a similar concern that disclosing the commercial potential of human body parts may tarnish the image of the researchers by making it appear that profit rather than scientific knowledge is their goal. However, the media is already informing the public about the relationship between researchers and the corporate sector. "The public cannot help but see that the goals of some scientists—clinical or basic—are different than in the past," says Leon Rosenberg, dean of the Yale University School of Medicine. "The biotechnology revolution has moved us, literally or figuratively, from the classroom to the boardroom and from the *New England Journal* to the *Wall Street Journal*."[18]

Finally people point to the difficulty of assigning values to body parts as an implicit barrier to the property approach. But the value of many items that are currently bought and sold (such as paintings or jewels) is difficult to assess. This is no reason to prohibit the market from developing a particular price. . . .

In a variation on the value argument, physician/researchers seem to imply that the patient has already been paid for the body part by receiving the benefits of the surgery. John Moore, for example, was allegedly helped by his treatment at UCLA. (This argument is harder to make when the patient dies or otherwise does not recover.) But patients may feel they have already paid for their health benefits in the price of the surgery. The patient has a right to know about the research so that she can choose the "price" she is willing to pay for the surgery. Perhaps she would rather choose a surgeon whose price is set solely in terms of dollars and insurance coverage rather than one who commercially exploits, say, her ovaries.

THE FUTURE OF THE BODY AS PROPERTY

Some of the finest advances in society have resulted from a refusal to characterize human beings (blacks, women, children) as property. Why, then, am I arguing for a property approach here?

Let me emphasize that I am advocating not that people be treated by others as property, but only that they have the autonomy to treat their own parts as property, particularly their regenerative parts. Such an approach is helpful, rather than harmful, to people's well-being. It offers potential psychological, physical, and economic benefits to individuals and provides a framework for handling evolving issues regarding the control of extracorporeal biological materials.

It is time to start acknowledging that people's body parts are their personal property. This is distinguishable from the past characterizations of people as property, which were immoral because they failed to take into account the nonbodily aspects of the individual (blacks and women were deemed incapable of rational thought) and they created the rights of ownership by others (masters, husbands, parents). Allowing people to transfer and sell their own body parts, while protecting them from coercion, does not present those dangers.

REFERENCES

1. 42 U.S.C. 274(e) (1984).

2. Cal. Penal Code § 367f (West 1986) (exception for sale by patient); D.C. Code Ann. § 6–2601 (Supp. 1985); Fla. Stat. Ann. § 873.01 (West Suppl. 1986); La. Rev. Stat. Ann. § 17.2280 (West 1982); Md. Health General Code Ann. § 5.408 (Supp. 1985); Mich. Comp. Laws Ann. § 333.10204 (West Supp. 1986); N.Y. Pub. Health Law § 4307 (McKinney 1985); Va. Code § 32.1–289.1 (1985). Additionally, in Arkansas there is a specific prohibition on the sale of eyes after death. Ark. Stat. Ann. § 82–410.2; § 82–410.13 (1976).

3. Susan Rose-Ackerman, "Inalienability and the Theory of Property Rights," *Columbia Law Review* 931 (1985), 85.

4. Ontario Law Reform Commission, *Report on Human Artificial Reproduction and Related Matters* (Ontario: Ministry of the Attorney General, 1985).

5. 45 C.F.R. 46.101(b)(5) (1985).

6. 45 C.F.R. 46.110(b) (1985).

7. Matthews, p. 205.

8. Such practices are described in *Jefferson County Burial Soc. v. Scott*, 218 Ala. 354, 118, S. 644 (1928).

9. A 1975 law review article, "Criminal Aspects of Suicide in the United States," 7 *North Carolina Central Law Journal* 156, 158 n. 19–21 (1975) listed only three states (Oklahoma, Texas, and Washington) which still had laws against attempted suicide. Those statutes have since been repealed.

10. *R. v. Welsh*, (1974) R.T.R. 478, reported in Matthews, pp. 223–24.

11. Constance Holden, "Hayflick Case Settled," *Science* 215 (1982), 271.

12. Richard Titmuss, *The Gift Relationship: From Human Blood to Special Policy* (New York: Vintage, 1972).

13. Harvey M. Sapolsky and Stan N. Finkelstein, "Blood Policy Revisited—A New Look at 'The Gift Relationship,'" *Public Interest*, 46 (1977), 15.

14. Thomas H. Murray, "The Gift of Life Must Always Remain a Gift," *Discover* 7:3 (March 1986), 90.

15. See, e.g., L. L. Hench, "Biomaterials," *Science* 208 (1980), 826.

16. See Leon R. Kass, "Thinking About the Body," *Hastings Center Report*, 15:1 (February 1985), 20.

17. Baruch S. Blumberg, Irving Millman, W. Thomas London, et al., "Ted Slavin's Blood and the Development of HBV Vaccine," *New England Journal of Medicine* 312 (1985), 189 (letter).

18. Leon E. Rosenberg, "Using Patient Materials for Production Development: A Dean's Perspective," *Clinical Research* 33:4 (October 1985), 452–54.

NO

Thomas H. Murray

GIFTS OF THE BODY
AND THE NEEDS OF STRANGERS

Human bodies have value, and not just to the persons whose bodies they are. Organs can be transplanted; tissues used for research and product development. One way of looking at these body parts is as property, to be bought and sold.[1] Another way—the approach I want to examine—is to see them as gifts. This may seem at first a simpler concept, but it is far from that. The idea of "gift" has deep and sometimes contradictory cultural meanings, which can illuminate the appropriate stance we should take toward modern biotechnology.

There are two modern conceptions of gifts. On the one hand, William Blackstone, the great legal commentator, wrote in 1767 that "gifts are always gratuitous"—that is, requiring "no consideration or equivalent." A gift in this sense is, as the *Oxford English Dictionary* defines it, "the transference of property in a thing by one person to another, voluntarily and without any valuable consideration." Givers are free to give or not; recipients are free to accept or not, and after acceptance, free to do whatever they like with the gift.

But if gifts are so bereft of obligations of any kind, why is there a second strain of sentiment about them? Ralph Waldo Emerson, in his essay on "Gifts," illustrated the power of gifts to bind one person to another. He wrote: "It is not the office of a man to receive gifts. How dare you give them? We wish to be self-sustained. We do not quite forgive a giver."[2] In a more modern context and with a hint of irony, the historian Michael Ignatieff echoes a similar sentiment: "The bureaucratized transfer of income among strangers has freed each of us from the enslavement of gift relations."[3]

How can the notion of gifts as gratuitous and completely voluntary be reconciled with the idea that gifts are the cause of degradation, dependence, and enslavement? Neither idea captures the full significance of the gift in human relations. The first perspective sees only that gifts carry no formal *legal* obligations. This is correct, but not very important. In this sense, gifts are opposed to contracts—forms of social exchange specifying in sometimes numbing detail precisely what is being exchanged for what. Of course, the obverse is also true: anything *not* explicitly required in the contract is permitted, and no other new obligations arise outside the limited sphere of relationship created by the contract. The second perspective sees correctly that gifts may entangle people in relationships that will impose great but vague moral obligations.

The first view assumes that only legal obligations matter. The second view understands that gifts create moral obligations, but focuses only on their ugly, manipulative potential. It fails to see that relationships based on gifts can and do play positive roles in regulating family and social life, in promoting solidarity in the face of powerful forces of alienation, and in serving essential social values that are not well served by markets, commerce, and contract. . . .

GIFTS, PRUDENCE, AND MORAL OBLIGATIONS

The notion that either donors or recipients could have obligations in gift relations seems foreign to the modern mind. The concept of "obligation," at least as it is used by moral philosophers, does not seem to fit gift relationships. Perhaps one should speak of an etiquette rather than an ethic of gifts. But such a weak term would belie the powerful ties that can be created by gifts, the strong indebtedness a recipient may feel, and the grave harm an ignorant, inconsiderate, or malicious giver may do.

There is certainly a heavy dose of prudence in many gift exchanges. Using gifts to establish personal relationships need not entail any heavy moral obligations. If you desire the relationship, then respond appropriately to the gift; if you do not, refuse the gift.

There are, however, occasions when an individual may feel obliged, morally, to make certain gifts. Suppose a member of your family was suddenly in dire need of food or shelter—or bone marrow. Perhaps not everyone will feel an obligation to give in response to this need, but many will. Some might describe it as charity or supererogation, something noble but not obligatory. But many would think they had failed more fundamentally if they did not offer some gift, however modest, that addressed the need. Another example: in a relationship of long duration characterized by great caring, one party abruptly ceases to show gratitude or to reciprocate. The harm done the other, as well as the devaluation of the relationship and of both parties, is substantial enough to count as a moral harm. Such relationships contain a set of implied promises, which were broken by the sudden, uncaring way in which they were sundered. Remember that a common way of expressing gratitude is to say "much obliged." The language of obligation may discomfit some philosophers, but it seems to reflect more accurately the importance of at least certain gift relationships.

Here are three interrelated suggestions—too informal to be called "claims" or hypotheses—that may be helpful in clarifying our thinking about gifts in general and gifts of the body in particular:

1. Significant gifts are commonly given in response to the needs of individuals and societies. I mean *need* here as opposed to mere *desire*; but human needs in a wide sense, encompassing not merely basic survival—food, clothing, and shelter—but also the requirements for flourishing in a particular society—art, beauty,

preparation for participation in adult life (including, in industrialized nations, literacy and education) and, not least, peace among groups, a measure of community, and intimate relationships.

2. The degree of *moral* (and not merely prudential) obligation one feels (and should feel) to make a gift is greatest when the recipient's need is greatest. The more universal the need (such as for adequate food) the more likely people are to feel a sense of obligation to give to those more distant.

3. Mass bureaucratic societies need to affirm what it is citizens share with their neighbors. Gifts, especially gifts to assuage needs, and most especially gifts of the body, are one of the most significant means we have to affirm that solidarity. Thomas Merton, writing of the Buddhist's begging bowl, says it "represents the ultimate theological root of the belief, not just in a right to beg, but in openness to the gifts of all beings as an expression of the interdependence of all beings. . . ."[4] Gifts of the body, ministering to the need for health, are in this sense affirmations of interdependence. . . .

MORAL OBLIGATIONS, GRATITUDE, AND GRACIOUSNESS

In a study of related kidney donors, Roberta Simmons and her colleagues found that when recipients did not express what the donors considered a reasonable amount of gratitude, the donor felt angry and used—a "sucker." One donor reported: "I would say for three months [the recipient] tried to avoid me. I was never so crushed. I would call him up and he would be as cold as ice. I was destroyed. To this day I don't mention

the kidney in front of him. Whenever I do, it turns him off. He has never come out and said 'Thank you.' "[5]

Reciprocating the gift, in an appropriate form, at an appropriate time, is also important. Alvin Gouldner, a sociologist, argues for a "norm of reciprocity" that is "no less universal and important an element of culture than the incest taboo." He says it is "a dimension to be found in all value systems and, in particular, as one among a number of 'Principal Components' universally present in moral codes."[6] Just what constitutes appropriate reciprocation depends on particular cultural norms and the specifics of the relationship. It need not be "tit-for-tat" if, for example, the donor is a parent and the recipient a ten-year-old child, whose means are not adequate to return full economic value of the parent's gift. Similar cultural and relationship factors determine what is an appropriate time for reciprocation. Seneca's warning is correct for some situations, but not all. (Not exchanging Christmas presents simultaneously could be insulting to the person who gave the present.)

A third recipient obligation is what Camenisch calls "grateful use." He argues that "grateful acceptance of the gift indicates the concurrence of the recipient's will with the donor's and/or implies consent to comply with that will." He suggests that the moral language of "stewardship" often applies to the use of gifts. Searching for more precise criteria for grateful use, he offers two: "the nature of the gift itself and what we can discover of the donor's intention for its use." It would be wrong to treat something dear to the donor in an undignified manner, as merely a commodity; likewise it would be wrong to use it in a way the donor would disapprove of.

All three obligations—grateful use, grateful conduct, and reciprocation—stem from the purpose of gift exchange—building moral relationships, and perhaps as well from the nature of at least certain significant gifts. Mauss says that among the Maori "to give something is to give a part of oneself. . . . while to receive something is to receive a part of someone's spiritual essence." It is not necessary to accept the Maori's animistic beliefs to grasp that in some gifts, the giver offers symbolically a part of himself or herself. Simply recall an occasion when someone treated with indifference a gift that you had regarded as special and important. In some way, the rejection of the gift was a personal rejection. (This is true more than metaphorically in gifts of the body.) . . .

GIFTS TO STRANGERS

Perhaps Arrow's most striking criticism of Titmuss is his claim that Titmuss wishes to promote "impersonal altruism." He does not wish to encourage the "richness of family relationships or the close ties of a small community" but rather a "diffuse expression of confidence in the workings of society as a whole." But Arrow says, "Such an expression of impersonal altruism is as far removed from the feelings of personal interaction as any marketplace."

Arrow is certainly correct. It cannot be the rewards of immediate personal relationships that prompt impersonal altruism. But when he goes on to describe British blood donors as "an aristocracy of saints" and to express doubt that a voluntary system could work elsewhere, he is wrong—factually wrong—as the movement to an almost entirely voluntary system of whole blood procurement in the

U.S. shows. This cannot be ascribed to the British tradition of Fabian socialism with which Arrow tries to explain the British experience.

Something more than a vague sentiment is at work in the instance of blood donation, something powerful that escapes any simple explanation in terms of pure self-interest—or pure altruism. Ignatieff grasps the problem when he notes: "We think of belonging in moral terms as direct impingement on the lives of others: fraternity implies the closeness of brothers. Yet the moral relations that exist between my income and the needs of strangers at my door pass through the arteries of the state." This would pose no problem if the needs of strangers exerted no moral pull on us; if we felt no relationship with them. But, as Ignatieff notes, "We need justice, we need liberty, and we need as much solidarity as can be reconciled with justice and liberty."

Relationships governed by markets keep moral and social dimensions to a bare minimum. Gifts, by their open-endedness, defy such minimization. Impersonal gifts such as blood or body parts or charity may not regulate relationships between specific individuals, but they serve other functions by regulating larger relationships and honoring important human values, precisely those threatened by massive and impersonal bureaucracies.

For one thing, impersonal gifts acknowledge an entire realm of moral relationships and moral obligations wider than intimate, family ones, and wider still than legal, contractual ones. Further, these obligations are often *unchosen*.

Gifts to strangers affirm the solidarity of the community over and above the depersonalizing, alienating forces of mass society and market relations. They signal that self-interest is not the only significant human motivation. And they express the moral belief that it is good to minister to fundamental human needs, needs for food, health care, and shelter, but also needs for beauty and knowledge. These universal needs irrevocably tie us together in a community of needs, with a shared desire to satisfy them, and see them satisfied in others.

Finally, these gifts remind us that wealth is merely a means to an end, and that not all valuable things can be purchased, among them love, friendship, fellow-feeling, and trust. These "moral" assets of individuals and of societies are "noneconomic" in still another way. They are not "scarce resources" that are consumed as they are offered. Arrow cautions us not "to use up recklessly the scarce resources of altruistic motivation." The truth is more likely the opposite: To a considerable extent, employing "moral assets" generously increases rather than decreases the supply.

GIFTS, SOLIDARITY, AND SOCIAL INSTITUTIONS

It may well be that the way a society structures the exchange of such "moral assets" affects their supply just as the structure of markets affects the supply of ordinary commodities. Titmuss's survey of blood donors in Great Britain revealed that the overwhelming majority, when asked why they were giving, cited non-self-interested reasons. Among them (with spelling and punctuation preserved):

Knowing I mite be saving somebody life;
You cant get blood from supermarkets and chaine stores. People themselves must come forward;

I thought it just a small way to help people—as a blind person other opportunities are limited.

Gratitude for good health appears in some:

Briefly because I have enjoyed good health all my life and in a small way it is a way of saying 'Thank you' and a small donation to the less fortunate.

Others write of reciprocating a gift:

To try and repay in some small way some unknown person whose blood helped me recover from two operations. . . . ;
Some unknown person gave blood to save my wifes life.

Other reasons offered included a general sense of social duty and the perception that there was a need for blood.

A more recent study of blood procurement inspired by skepticism of Titmuss's account focused primarily on the U.S. In that work Alvin Drake, Stan N. Finkelstein, and Harvey Sapolsky found that the bleak portrait of motivation for giving and quality of blood in the U.S. painted by Titmuss was unwarranted a decade later, and may even have been an unfair picture at the time Titmuss's book was published.[7] The details of their differences are not important here. Much more significant is the authors' carefully documented research on the beliefs, values, and practices of potential blood donors in the U.S. By 1982, about 70 percent of all whole blood was being provided on a purely voluntary basis. Roughly a quarter was being given through "blood credit" or "blood insurance" programs, which could be seen as quasi-voluntary. Paid donors constituted no more than 3 to 4 percent, and that proportion was declining.

Drake, Finkelstein, and Sapolsky found that the principal impediment to fulfilling the need for whole blood was lack of coordination and competence in the regional procurement agencies. Where efforts were well organized, as they had been for years in Connecticut and in upstate New York, local needs could be met with purely voluntary programs. The researchers found a strong and consistent opposition to the use of paid donors. Americans overwhelmingly preferred to have their community's need for whole blood met with volunteer donors.

When they examined the reasons American blood donors gave for their generosity, they found it was "simply a general awareness of the continuing need for blood." "All our own experiences lead us to believe that participation in the whole-blood supply is the natural, unforced response of a great many people once they are exposed to a mild degree of personal solicitation and some convenient donation opportunities."

The saga of the transformation of the American whole-blood supply from a largely paid to a virtually all-volunteer system is not a simple one. Much of it concerns rivalries among organizations. But one important fact is clear: the voluntary agencies could not have emerged victorious unless the American people were willing to donate adequate amounts of whole blood. This willingness in turn rests, I believe, on deeply held convictions about the obligation to give to those in need, and about the ethical inappropriateness of commercializing whole blood.

It is a massive effort at giving to strangers. Roughly eight million Americans donate each year. In its scale, its lack of monetary rewards, and its distance between donor and recipient, the whole-blood procurement system in the U.S. is a remarkable example of impersonal gifts. It suggests something very important that a society would be so generous in this realm and would reject so clearly a market approach to the supply and distribution of a good.

The gift of blood is doubly expressive. It affirms solidarity in a gift that is quintessentially human. Blood represents individual life and vitality, and at the same time it signifies the oldest, most primitive tie that affirms solidarity and binds people to one another. Perhaps one of the oldest and most persistent human problems has been to reconcile the loyalties and attachments defined by blood—the ties of family—with the need for, at a minimum, peace but, better, solidarity, with strangers—those with whom we do not share blood. From these roots comes the political importance of marriage between groups in potential conflict, and perhaps as well the symbolic value of "blood brotherhood."

Blood is life, but also kinship. Giving blood to strangers is not just any gift, but a vital one that expresses and affirms our bonds with those strangers. If, on the other hand, we would rather deny our brotherhood, then mixing blood could be a serious threat. Titmuss reports that in South Africa a set of regulations issued in 1962 required that "European" and "non-European" donors be kept separate, and that the records of their donations also be kept apart. Furthermore, "[a]ll containers of blood and blood products have to be labelled by 'racial origin.' " Although South Africa has relied primarily on voluntary donations, authorities at gold mines in the Transvaal region purchased blood from mining company employees. The rates in 1967 were four Rands per pint for whites; one

Rand per pint for "Bantus, Colored and Asians."

Profiting from others' blood is sometimes seen as a particularly heinous form of exploitation. A plasmapheresis center opened in Managua, Nicaragua, in 1973 that purchased plasma and exported it. The center was owned in part by the dictator Somoza. At the funeral of a popular newspaper editor who had criticized Somoza for "inhuman trade in the blood of Nicaraguans" and who had been murdered, a large crowd burned several buildings, among them the plasmapheresis center.[8]

Blood can connect people, or it can divide them. Contemporary inhabitants in the U.S., no less than the Trobrianders or Maori or other traditional societies, seem to believe that some things are *sacra*—"sacred" in the nondenominational sense of dignified human "property"—and that it is morally preferable to procure and distribute certain kinds of property, including *sacra*, but other things as well, outside the otherwise dominant system of market and contract. . . .

GIFTS, THE BODY, AND BIOMEDICAL RESEARCH

What has been said until now does not settle the question of what should happen to human tissues in contemporary biomedicine. It does, however, demonstrate that certain body parts are and ought to be treated as gifts and not as personal property.

Even if certain parts or products of the body are *sacra* and hence fit for gift but not commerce, it does not follow that all are equally so.[9] If I could find a buyer for my urine, it is doubtful that any great moral outcry would arise, no more than accompanies the sale of hair or finger-nails. But then these products are less central to what characterizes living human persons, members of the human community, than kidneys, for example, or blood. In any case, the nature of the gift, its meaning and significance within the community, will determine whether it belongs to the realm of commodities or the circle of gifts.

A second issue concerns the relationship between the giver—the patient or research subject in the case of biomedicine—and the recipient—the physician or researcher. The patient-physician relationship has long been described with apparently inconsistent images. On the one hand, physicians earn their money by seeing patients, and in that sense it is clearly a commercial relationship, a trade of money for service. At the same time the noncommercial aspects of the relationship are stressed. The very words used to describe what physicians do—they "take care of" patients—come from the language of personal, moral, nonmarket relationships. Physicians are expected to act in the patient's best interest, and not to try to cut the best deal for themselves; they are in a "fiduciary" relationship with their patients.

To the extent that people see their relationship with physicians as not strictly a market one, then an ethic of personal gifts may apply. (People quite commonly make gifts to their medical and nursing caretakers after an episode of illness.) With the increasing commercialization of medicine, people's expectations may be changing, and the nature of the physician-patient relationship, always an ideal only partially realized, may change accordingly. At some future time, the gift may become irrelevant to the clinic.

The emergence of the physician-researcher-entrepreneur complicates things immensely. It is one thing to have someone offer to buy something. It is quite another to give it to someone with whom we believe there is a more or less personal, noncommercial relationship, and to learn only later that what was given as a gift, especially if it was a "sacred" gift, has been diverted to commerce. The mixed roles of biomedical researchers who may also be clinicians, who may also be entrepreneurs, make it difficult to know what set of moral expectations apply. By blurring the distinctions, we jeopardize the future of physician-patient relationships. One could say cynically that such relationships always were commercial, and that it is better to be explicit about it. But if important social values were served by stressing the noncommercial dimensions of those relationships, then the threat is a serious one.

Lastly, consider the problem of how to think about impersonal gifts. Normally there is a distinction drawn between eleemosynary and civil corporations. The former are "organized for charitable purposes"; the latter, according to the Oxford English Dictionary, for "business purposes." Universities and most medical research centers, along with charities, learned societies, and the like, are eleemosynary organizations. When people are asked to make gifts of money—or of their tissues—to university-based medical research, whether or not they actually give, they see this as a reasonable request. Pleas for gifts by a profit-seeking firm, in contrast, would be perceived as ludicrous.

One of the ways to express solidarity with "strangers" is by contributing to the satisfaction of basic human needs and desires, especially those not well served by the system of trade and markets. These two systems have long existed side by side, an implicit acknowledgment that neither one alone is adequate for human flourishing and for sustaining community. In place now is an informal system of gifts of human biological materials to noncommercial organizations. Relying on this system fulfills many of the social values mentioned earlier as the justifications for gift exchanges. They include expressing solidarity in the face of illness and suffering, and declaring respect and support for biomedical research and teaching.

PURSUIT OF THE GOOD

Gifts help to create and sustain intimate personal relationships. In the face of impersonal bureaucracies, gifts to "strangers" affirm a number of vital social values including our solidarity with others in our community, and our vision of human flourishing, individual and social, that require more than the thin relationships established by markets and contracts.

Individuals in market societies, especially intellectuals, may delude themselves into believing that needs are indistinguishable from desires, that the body is merely a commodity like any other, and that we have no moral bonds with the members of our communities other than those we have freely chosen. But the evidence of charitable practices in general and gifts of the body in particular affirm the belief that there *are* human needs—biological and cultural; that the body, especially in its health-giving and life-saving manifestations, should not be treated as a mere commodity; and that we are bound together by our often needy bodies (and by our other, non-physiological needs) into a community of needs. In this community—really multiple communities, sometimes overlapping, some like ripples extending wider and wider around a core—we can recognize the needs of others through our shared embodiment. And we can minister to those needs by sharing the fruits, the very living tissues of the body.

How we choose to handle the transfers of human biological materials from patients and research subjects to teachers and researchers will declare how we regard the human body. If certain human parts are "dignified," then our social traditions suggest they may be given, but not sold, and ownership of them is only of a special, limited kind.

Moreover, like the choice of obtaining blood for transfusions, the system chosen for obtaining human biological materials will carry whatever symbolic weight attaches to the relationship to the "strangers at our door," as Ignatieff calls our fellow inhabitants of mass society. These gifts of the body, ministering to the needs of strangers, connect us in our mutual quest to relieve suffering and to pursue our good, separately and together.

ACKNOWLEDGMENTS

I am grateful to many people whose gifts of time and thought enabled me to clarify further my own thinking on the issues discussed in this paper. Here I can mention only a few: William Winslade, Ronald Carson, and Harold Vanderpool critiqued versions of this article. I want to thank also Gladys White and the U.S. Congress Office of Technology Assessment. I did much of the research on which this paper is based for their project, "New Developments in Biotechnology: Ownership of Human Tissues and Cells."

REFERENCES

1. Lori B. Andrews, "My Body, My Property," *Hastings Center Report* 16:5 (October 1986), 28–38.

2. Ralph Waldo Emerson, "Gifts," *Essays of Ralph Waldo Emerson* (Norwalk, CT: Easton Press, 1979), pp. 212–13.

3. Michael Ingatieff, *The Needs of Strangers: An Essay on Privacy, Solidarity, and the Politics of Being Human* (New York: Viking, 1984), pp. 18–141.

4. Thomas Merton, *The Asian Journals*, eds. Naomi Burton et al. (New York: New Directions, 1973), pp. 341–42.

5. Roberta G. Simmons, Susan D. Klein, and Richard L. Simmons, *Gift of Life: The Social and Psychological Impact of Organ Transplantation* (New York: Wiley, 1977), p. 325.

6. Alvin W. Gouldner, "The Norm of Reciprocity: A Preliminary Statement," *American Sociological Review* 25:2 (1960), 171.

7. Richard M. Titmuss, *The Gift Relationship* (New York: Pantheon, 1971).

8. Piet J. Hagen, *Blood: Gift or Merchandise* (New York: Alan R. Liss, 1982), pp. 168–69.

9. Thomas H. Murray, "On the Ethics of Commercializing the Human Body." Paper prepared for U.S. Congress Office of Technology Assessment, April 1986.

POSTSCRIPT

Should There Be a Market in Body Parts?

John Moore's case was dismissed three times by state courts in California, but in August 1988 the 2nd District Court of Appeals in Houston ruled that he had the right to sue UCLA. The court said, "A patient must have the ultimate power to control what becomes of his or her tissue. To hold otherwise would open the door to a massive invasion of human privacy and dignity in the name of medical progress." However, in July 1990 the California Supreme Court ruled that a patient does not have property rights over body tissue and that letting patients sue for rights in research resulting from their tissue would threaten "to destroy the economic incentive to conduct important medical research." The court also stated that the physician has a "fiduciary duty" to tell the patient if there is interest in studying his tissue. Two articles written on this subject are George J. Annas, "Whose Waste is it Anyway? The Case of John Moore," *Hastings Center Report* (October/November 1988), and John J. Howard, "Biotechnology, Patients' Rights and the *Moore* Case," *Food Drug Cosmetic Law Journal* (July 1989).

The Hagiwara case was settled by an agreement in which the University of California was given the patent and the Hagiwara family received an exclusive license to market the cell line in Japan and Asia. For the researcher's view of this case, see Ivor Royston, "Cell Lines from Human Patients: Who Owns Them?" *Clinical Research*, vol. 33 (1985).

The Congressional Office of Technology Assessment has issued a comprehensive report called *New Developments in Biotechnology: Ownership of Human Tissue* (Government Printing Office, 1987). In an article called "Research that Could Yield Marketable Products from Human Materials: The Problem of Informed Consent," *IRB: A Review of Human Subjects Research* (January/February 1986), Robert J. Levine argues that it is unlikely that research designed to develop marketable products from human materials will present any problems to the research-subject relationship that cannot be resolved within the framework of existing informed consent regulations. See also Emanuel D. Thorne, "Tissue Transplants: The Dilemma of the Body's Growing Value," *Public Interest* (Winter 1990); Nancy E. Field, "Evolving Conceptualizations of Property: A Proposal to De-Commercialize the Value of Fetal Tissue," *Yale Law Journal* (October 1989); and Margaret S. Swain and Randy W. Marusyk, "An Alternative to Property Rights in Human Tissue," *Hastings Center Report* (September/October 1990).

ISSUE 19

Should Health Care for the Elderly Be Limited?

YES: Daniel Callahan, from "Limiting Health Care for the Old?" *The Nation* (August 15/22, 1987)

NO: Amitai Etzioni, from "Spare the Old, Save the Young," *The Nation* (June 11, 1988)

ISSUE SUMMARY

YES: Philosopher Daniel Callahan believes that since health care resources are scarce, people who have lived a full natural life span should be offered care that relieves suffering but not expensive life-prolonging technologies.
NO: Sociologist Amitai Etzioni argues that rationing health care for the elderly would encourage conflict between generations and would invite restrictions on health care for other groups.

America is aging. In 1965 the 18.5 million people over the age of 65 accounted for only 9.5 percent of the population. By 1987 the number had climbed to 29 million, or 12 percent of the population. The number of people over 85—the "old old"—is the fastest-growing age group in the United States. By the year 2040 the elderly will represent 21 percent of the population.

Older people are more likely to need health care than the young. In 1980 people over 65 accounted for 29 percent of the total American health care expenditures of $219.4 billion. By 1986 the bill had risen to $450 billion, and the share devoted to the elderly to 31 percent. The costs of Medicare—the federal program that supports the health care of people over 65—are projected to increase from $75 billion in 1986 to $114 billion in the year 2000, measured in current, not inflated dollars.

While Medicare coverage of nursing homes and home care remains inadequate to meet the need, organ transplants are now covered. The typical cost of such an operation is $200,000.

Many (but not all) elderly people do not want to have their lives prolonged through the use of expensive technology such as kidney dialysis, respirators, and intensive care. They fear losing control of their medical care and dying "hooked up to tubes."

There are many competing interests vying for the increasingly scarce health care dollar. Groups representing patients suffering from particular diseases—cancer, AIDS, diabetes, heart disease, to name just a few—advocate increased spending on research and care. Those who speak for the poor, especially poor children, point out that they often do not have access to the most basic medical care, such as immunizations. The costs of treating premature, low-birth-weight infants are extremely high; yet programs that provide prenatal care and adequate nutrition to mothers at risk, which might prevent many such births, are inadequately funded.

In such a complex web of competing claims, when not all interests can be met, how should decisions to ration care be determined? Should age be one criterion? In Great Britain, which has a National Health Service and centralized planning, patients over the age of 55 have been routinely denied kidney dialysis ostensibly on "medical" grounds, even though the procedure is performed in the United States on very old patients.

Should we begin to follow this pattern in the United States? The following selections present the contrasting views. Daniel Callahan says we must confront realities: in the interest of ensuring adequate health care to the younger generation, we must limit the kinds of care that will be available to those who have lived a full natural life span. Amitai Etzioni objects to this call to ration health care to the elderly on the grounds that it will lead to denying care to people of younger ages and other groups deemed less productive to society.

YES

Daniel Callahan

LIMITING HEALTH CARE FOR THE OLD

Is it sensible, in the face of the rapidly increasing burden of health care costs for the elderly, to press forward with new and expensive ways of extending their lives? Is it possible even to hope to control costs while simultaneously supporting innovative research, which generates new ways to spend money? Those are now unavoidable questions. . . .

Anyone who works closely with the elderly recognizes that the present Medicare and Medicaid programs are grossly inadequate in meeting their real and full needs. The system fails most notably in providing decent long-term care and medical care that does not constitute a heavy out-of-pocket drain. Members of minority groups and single or widowed women are particularly disadvantaged. How will it be possible, then, to provide the growing number of elderly with even present levels of care, much less to rid the system of its inadequacies and inequities, and at the same time add expensive new technologies?

The straight answer is that it will be impossible to do all those things and, worse still, it may be harmful even to try. It may be so because of the economic burdens that would impose on younger age groups, and because of the requisite skewing of national social priorities too heavily toward health care. But that suggests to both young and old that the key to a happy old age is good health care, which may not be true.

In the past few years three additional concerns about health care for the aged have surfaced. First, an increasingly large share of health care is going to the elderly rather than to youth. The Federal government, for instance, spends six times as much providing health benefits and other social services to those over 65 as it does to those under 18. And, as the demographer Samuel Preston observed in a provocative address to the Population Association of America in 1984, "Transfers from the working-age population to the elderly are also transfers away from children, since the working ages bear far more responsibility for childrearing than do the elderly."

Preston's address had an immediate impact. The mainline senior-citizen advocacy groups accused Preston of fomenting a war between the genera-

From Daniel Callahan, "Limiting Health Care for the Old?" *The Nation* (August 15, 1987). Adapted from Daniel Callahan, *Setting Limits* (Simon & Schuster, 1987). Copyright © 1987 by Daniel Callahan. Reprinted by permission of Simon & Schuster, Inc.

tions. But the speech also stimulated Minnesota Senator David Durenberger and others to found Americans for Generational Equity (AGE) to promote debate about the burden on future generations, particularly the Baby Boom cohort, of "our major social insurance programs." Preston's speech and the founding of AGE signaled the outbreak of a struggle over what has come to be called "intergenerational equity," which is now gaining momentum.

The second concern is that the elderly, in dying, consume a disproportionate share of health care costs. "At present," notes Stanford University economist Victor Fuchs, "the United States spends about 1 percent of the gross national product on health care for elderly persons who are in their last year of life. . . . One of the biggest challenges facing policy makers for the rest of this century will be how to strike an appropriate balance between care for the [elderly] dying and health services for the rest of the population."

The third issue is summed up in an observation by Dr. Jerome Avorn of the Harvard Medical School, who wrote in *Daedalus*, "With the exception of the birth-control pill, [most] of the medical-technology interventions developed since the 1950s have their most widespread impact on people who are past their fifties—the further past their fifties, the greater the impact." Many of the techniques in question were not intended for use on the elderly. Kidney dialysis, for example, was developed for those between the ages of 15 and 45. Now some 30 percent of its recipients are over 65.

The validity of those concerns has been vigorously challenged, as has the more general assertion that some form of rationing of health care for the elderly

might become necessary. To the charge that old people receive a disproportionate share of resources, the response has been that assistance to them helps every age group: It relieves the young of the burden of care they would otherwise have to bear for elderly parents and, since those young will eventually become old, promises them similar care when they need it. There is no guarantee, moreover, that any cutback in health care for the elderly would result in a transfer of the savings directly to the young. And, some ask, Why should we contemplate restricting care for the elderly when we wastefully spend hundreds of millions on an inflated defense budget?

The assertion that too large a share of funds goes to extending the lives of elderly people who are terminally ill hardly proves that it is an unjust or unreasonable amount. They are, after all, the most in need. As some important studies have shown, it is exceedingly difficult to know that someone is dying; the most expensive patients, it turns out, are those who were expected to live but died. That most new technologies benefit the old more than the young is logical; most of the killer diseases of the young have now been conquered.

There is little incentive for politicians to think about, much less talk about, limits on health care for the aged. As John Rother, director of legislation for the American Association of Retired Persons, has observed, "I think anyone who wasn't a champion of the aged is no longer in Congress." Perhaps also, as Guido Calabresi, dean of the Yale Law School, and his colleague Philip Bobbitt observed in their thoughtful 1978 book *Tragic Choices*, when we are forced to make painful allocation choices, "Evasion, disguise, temporizing . . . [and] averting our eyes enables us to save some lives even when we will not save all."

I believe that we must face this highly troubling issue. Rationing of health care under Medicare is already a fact of life, though rarely labeled as such. The requirement that Medicare recipients pay the first $520 of hospital care costs, the cutoff of reimbursement for care after 60 days and the failure to cover long-term care are nothing other than allocation and cost-saving devices. As sensitive as it is to the senior-citizen vote, the Reagan Administration agreed only grudgingly to support catastrophic health care coverage for the elderly (a benefit that will not help very many of them), and it has already expressed its opposition to the recently passed House version of the bill. It is bound to be far more resistant to long-term health care coverage, as will any administration.

But there are reasons other than the economics to think about health care for the elderly. The coming economic crisis provides a much-needed opportunity to ask some deeper questions. Just what is it that we want medicine to do for us as we age? Other cultures have believed that aging should be accepted, and that it should be in part a time of preparation for death. Our culture seems increasingly to dispute that view, preferring instead, it often seems, to think of aging as hardly more than another disease, to be fought and rejected. Which view is correct?

Let me interject my own opinion. The future goal of medical science should be to improve the quality of old people's lives, not to lengthen them. In its longstanding ambition to forestall death, medicine has reached its last frontier in the care of the aged. Of course children and young adults still die of maladies that are open to potential cure; but the highest proportion of the dying (70 percent) are over 65. If death is ever to be humbled, that is where endless work remains to be done. But however tempting the challenge of that last frontier, medicine should restrain itself. To do otherwise would mean neglecting the needs of other age groups and of the old themselves.

Our culture has worked hard to redefine old age as a time of liberation, not decline, a time of travel, of new ventures in education and self-discovery, of the ever-accessible tennis court or golf course and of delightfully periodic but thankfully brief visits from well-behaved grandchildren. That is, to be sure, an idealized picture, but it arouses hopes that spur medicine to wage an aggressive war against the infirmities of old age. As we have seen, the costs of such a war would be prohibitive. No matter how much is spent the ultimate problem will still remain: people will grow old and die. Worse still, by pretending that old age can be turned into a kind of endless middle age, we rob it of meaning and significance for the elderly.

There is a plausible alternative: a fresh vision of what it means to live a decently long and adequate life, what might be called a "natural life span." Earlier generations accepted the idea that there was a natural life span—the biblical norm of three score and ten captures that notion (even though in fact that was a much longer life span than was typical in ancient times). It is an idea well worth reconsidering and would provide us with a meaningful and realizable goal. Modern medicine and biology have done much, however, to wean us from that kind of thinking. They have insinuated the belief that the average life span is not a natural fact at all, but instead one that is strictly dependent on the state of medical knowledge and skill. And there is much to that belief as a statistical fact: The average life expectancy continues to increase with no end in sight.

But that is not what I think we ought to mean by a natural life span. We need a notion of a full life that is based on some deeper understanding of human needs and possibilities, not on the state of medical technology or its potential. We should think of a natural life span as the achievement of a life that is sufficiently long to take advantage of those opportunities life typically offers and that we ordinarily regard as its prime benefits—loving and "living," raising a family, engaging in work that is satisfying, reading, thinking, cherishing our friends and families. People differ on what might be a full natural life span; my view is that it can be achieved by the late 70s or early 80s.

A longer life does not guarantee a better life. No matter how long medicine enables people to live, death at any time—at age 90 or 100 or 110—would frustrate some possibility, some as-yet-unrealized goal. The easily preventable death of a young child is an outrage. Death from an incurable disease of someone in the prime of young adulthood is a tragedy. But death at an old age, after a long and full life, is simply sad, a part of life itself.

As it confronts aging, medicine should have as its specific goals the averting of premature death, that is, death prior to the completion of a natural life span, and thereafter, the relief of suffering. It should pursue those goals so that the elderly can finish out their years with as little needless pain as possible—and with as much vitality as can be generated in contributing to the welfare of younger age groups and to the community of which they are a part. Above all, the elderly need to have a sense of the meaning and significance of their stage in life, one that is not dependent on economic productivity or physical vigor.

What would medicine oriented toward the relief of suffering rather than the deliberate extension of life be like? We do not have a clear answer to that question, so longstanding, central and persistent has been medicine's preoccupation with the struggle against death. But the hospice movement is providing us with much guidance. It has learned how to distinguish between the relief of suffering and the lengthening of life. Greater control by elderly persons over their own dying—and particularly an enforceable right to refuse aggressive life-extending treatment—is a minimal goal.

What does this have to do with the rising cost of health care for the elderly? Everything. The indefinite extension of life combined with an insatiable ambition to improve the health of the elderly is a recipe for monomania and bottomless spending. It fails to put health in its proper place as only one among many human goods. It fails to accept aging and death as part of the human condition. It fails to present to younger generations a model of wise stewardship.

How might we devise a plan to limit the costs of health care for the aged under public entitlement programs that is fair, humane and sensitive to their special requirements and dignity? Let me suggest three principles to undergird a quest for limits. First, government has a duty, based on our collective social obligations, to help people live out a natural life span but not to help medically extend life beyond that point. Second, government is obliged to develop under its research subsidies, and to pay for under its entitlement programs, only the kind and degree of life-extending technology necessary for medicine to achieve and serve the aim of a natural life span. Third, beyond the point of a natural life span, government should provide only the means necessary for the relief of suffering, not those for life-extending technology.

A system based on those principles would not immediately bring down the cost of care of the elderly; it would add cost. But it would set in place the beginning of a new understanding of old age, one that would admit of eventual stabilization and limits. The elderly will not be served by a belief that only a lack of resources, better financing mechanisms or political power stands between them and the limitations of their bodies. The good of younger age groups will not be served by inspiring in them a desire to live to an old age that maintains the vitality of youth indefinitely, as if old age were nothing but a sign that medicine has failed in its mission. The future of our society will not be served by allowing expenditures on health care for the elderly to escalate endlessly and uncontrollably, fueled by the false altruistic belief that anything less is to deny the elderly their dignity. Nor will it be aided by the pervasive kind of self-serving argument that urges the young to support such a crusade because they will eventually benefit from it also.

We require instead an understanding of the process of aging and death that looks to our obligation to the young and to the future, that recognizes the necessity of limits and the acceptance of decline and death, and that values the old for their age and not for their continuing youthful vitality. In the name of accepting the elderly and repudiating discrimination against them, we have succeeded mainly in pretending that, with enough will and money, the unpleasant part of old age can be abolished. In the name of medical progress we have carried out a relentless war against death and decline, failing to ask in any probing way if that will give us a better society for all.

NO

Amitai Etzioni

SPARE THE OLD, SAVE THE YOUNG

In the coming years, Daniel Callahan's call to ration health care for the elderly, put forth in his book *Setting Limits*, is likely to have a growing appeal. Practically all economic observers expect the United States to go through a difficult time as it attempts to work its way out of its domestic (budgetary) and international (trade) deficits. Practically every serious analyst realizes that such an endeavor will initially entail slower growth, if not an outright cut in our standard of living, in order to release resources to these priorities. When the national economic "pie" grows more slowly, let alone contracts, the fight over how to divide it up intensifies. The elderly make an especially inviting target because they have been taking a growing slice of the resources (at least those dedicated to health care) and are expected to take even more in the future. Old people are widely held to be "nonproductive" and to constitute a growing "burden" on an ever smaller proportion of society that is young and working. Also, the elderly are viewed as politically well-organized and powerful; hence "their" programs, especially Social Security and Medicare, have largely escaped the Reagan attempts to scale back social expenditures, while those aimed at other groups—especially the young, but even more so future generations—have been generally curtailed. There are now some signs that a backlash may be forming.

If a war between the generations, like that between the races and between the genders, does break out, historians may accord former Governor Richard Lamm of Colorado the dubious honor of having fired the opening shot in his statement that the elderly ill have "got a duty to die and get out of the way." Phillip Longman, in his book *Born to Pay*, sounded an early alarm. However, the historians may well say, it was left to Daniel Callahan, a social philosopher and ethicist, to provide a detailed rationale and blueprint for limiting the care to the elderly, explicitly in order to free resources for the young. Callahan's thesis deserves close examination because he attempts to deal with the numerous objections his approach raises. If his thesis does not hold, the champions of limiting funds available to the old may have a long wait before they will find a new set of arguments on their behalf.

In order to free up economic resources for the young, Callahan offers the older generation a deal: Trade quantity for quality; the elderly should not be given life-*extending* services but better years while alive. Instead of the relentless attempt to push death to an older age, Callahan would stop all development of life-extending technologies and prohibit the use of ones at hand for those who outlive their "natural" life span, say, the age of 75. At the same time, the old would be granted more palliative medicine (e.g., pain killers) and more nursing-home and home-health care, to make their natural years more comfortable.

Callahan's call to break an existing ethical taboo and replace it with another raises the problem known among ethicists and sociologists as the "slippery slope." Once the precept that one should do "all one can" to avert death is given up, and attempts are made to fix a specific age for a full life, why stop there? If, for instance, the American economy experiences hard times in the 1990s, should the "maximum" age be reduced to 72, 65—or lower? And should the care for other so-called unproductive groups be cut off, even if they are even younger? Should countries that are economically worse off than the United States set their limit, say, at 55?

This is not an idle thought, because the idea of limiting the care the elderly receive in itself represents a partial slide down such a slope. Originally, Callahan, the Hastings Center (which he directs) and other think tanks played an important role in redefining the concept of death. Death used to be seen by the public at large as occurring when the lungs stopped functioning and, above all, the heart stopped beating. In numerous old movies and novels, those attending the dying would hold a mirror to their faces to see if it fogged over, or put an ear to their chests to see if the heart had stopped. However, high technology made these criteria obsolete by mechanically ventilating people and keeping their hearts pumping. Hastings et al. led the way to provide a new technological definition of death: brain death. Increasingly this has been accepted, both in the medical community and by the public at large, as the point of demise, the point at which care should stop even if it means turning off life-extending machines, because people who are brain dead do not regain consciousness. At the same time, most doctors and a majority of the public as well continue strongly to oppose terminating care to people who are conscious, even if there is little prospect for recovery, despite considerable debate about certain special cases.

Callahan now suggests turning off life-extending technology for all those above a certain age, even if they could recover their full human capacity if treated. It is instructive to look at the list of technologies he would withhold: mechanical ventilation, artificial resuscitation, antibiotics and artificial nutrition and hydration. Note that while several of these are used to maintain brain-dead bodies, they are also used for individuals who are temporarily incapacitated but able to recover fully; indeed, they are used to save young lives, say, after a car accident. But there is no way to stop the development of such new technologies and the improvement of existing ones without depriving the young of benefit as well. (Antibiotics are on the list because of an imminent "high cost" technological advance—administering them with a pump implanted in the body, which makes their introduction more reliable and better distributes dosages.)

One may say that this is Callahan's particular list; other lists may well be drawn. But any of them would start us down the slope, because the savings that are achieved by turning off the machines that keep brain-dead people alive are minimal compared with those that would result from the measures sought by the people calling for new equity between the generations. And any significant foray into deliberately withholding medical care for those who can recover does raise the question, Once society has embarked on such a slope, where will it stop?

Those opposed to Callahan, Lamm and the other advocates of limiting care to the old, but who also favor extending the frontier of life, must answer the question, Where will the resources come from? One answer is found in the realization that defining people as old at the age of 65 is obsolescent. That age limit was set generations ago, before changes in life styles and medicines much extended not only life but also the number and quality of productive years. One might recognize that many of the "elderly" can contribute to society not merely by providing love, companionship and wisdom to the young but also by continuing to work, in the traditional sense of the term. Indeed, many already work in the underground economy because of the large penalty—a cut in Social Security benefits—exacted from them if they hold a job "on the books."

Allowing elderly people to retain their Social Security benefits while working, typically part-time, would immediately raise significant tax revenues, dramatically change the much-feared dependency-to-dependent ratio, provide a much-needed source of child-care workers and increase contributions to Social Security (under the assumption that anybody who will continue to work will continue to contribute to the program). There is also evidence that people who continue to have meaningful work will live longer and healthier lives, without requiring more health care, because psychic well-being in our society is so deeply associated with meaningful work. Other policy changes, such as deferring retirement, modifying Social Security benefits by a small, gradual stretching out of the age of full-benefit entitlement, plus some other shifts under way, could be used readily to gain more resources. Such changes might be justified prima facie because as we extend life and its quality, the payouts to the old may also be stretched out.

Beyond the question of whether to cut care or stretch out Social Security payouts, policies that seek to promote intergenerational equity must be assessed as to how they deal with another matter of equity: that between the poor and the rich. A policy that would stop Federal support for certain kinds of care, as Callahan and others propose, would halt treatment for the aged, poor, the near-poor and even the less-well-off segment of the middle class (although for the latter at a later point), while the rich would continue to buy all the care they wished to. Callahan's suggestion that a consensus of doctors would stop certain kinds of care for all elderly people is quite impractical; for it to work, most if not all doctors would have to agree to participate. Even if this somehow happened, the rich would buy their services overseas either by going there or by importing the services. There is little enough we can do to significantly enhance economic equality.

Do we want to exacerbate the inequalities that already exist by completely eliminating access to major categories of health care services for those who cannot afford to pay for them?

In addition to concern about slipping down the slope of less (and less) care, the *way* the limitations are to be introduced raises a serious question. The advocates of changing the intergenerational allocation of resources favor rationing health care for the elderly but nothing else. This is a major intellectual weakness of their argument. There are other major targets to consider within health care, as well as other areas, which seem, at least by some criteria, much more inviting than terminating care to those above a certain age. Within the medical sector, for example, why not stop all interventions for which there is no hard evidence that they are beneficial? Say, public financing of psychotherapy and coronary bypass operations? Why not take the $2 billion or so from plastic surgery dedicated to face lifts, reducing behinds and the like? Or require that all burials be done by low-cost cremations rather than using high-cost coffins?

Once we extend our reach beyond medical care to health care, if we cannot stop people from blowing $25 billion per year on cigarettes and convince them to use the money to serve the young, shouldn't we at least cut out public subsidies to tobacco growers before we save funds by denying antibiotics to old people? And there is the matter of profits. The high-technology medicine Callahan targets for savings is actually a minor cause of the increase in health care costs for the elderly or for anyone—about 4 percent. A major factor is the very high standard of living American doctors have, compared to those of many other nations. Indeed, many doctors tell interviewers that they love their work and would do it for half their current income as long as the incomes of their fellow practitioners were also cut. Another important area of saving is the exorbitant profits made by the nondoctor owners of dialysis units and nursing homes. If we dare ask how many years of life are enough, should we not also be able to ask how much profit is "enough"? This profit, by the way, is largely set not by the market but by public policy.

Last but not least, as the United States enters a time of economic constraints, should we draw new lines of conflict or should we focus on matters that sustain our societal fabric? During the 1960s numerous groups gained in political consciousness and actively sought to address injustices done to them. The result has been some redress and an increase in the level of societal stress (witness the deeply troubled relationships between the genders). But these conflicts occurred in an affluent society and redressed deeply felt grievances. Are the young like blacks and women, except that they have not yet discovered their oppressors—a group whose consciousness should be raised, so it will rally and gain its due share?

The answer is in the eye of the beholder. There are no objective criteria that can be used here the way they can be used between the races or between the genders. While women and minorities have the same rights to the same jobs at the same pay as white males, the needs of the young and the aged are so different that no simple criteria of equity come to mind. Thus, no one would argue that the teen-agers and those above 75 have the same need for schooling or nursing homes.

At the same time, it is easy to see that those who try to mobilize the young—led by a new Washington research group, Americans for Generational Equity (AGE), formed to fight for the needs of the younger generation—offer many arguments that do not hold. For instance, they often argue that today's young, age 35 or less, will pay for old people's Social Security, but by the time that they come of age they will not be able to collect, because Social Security will be bankrupt. However, this argument is based on extremely farfetched assumptions about the future. In effect, Social Security is now and for the foreseeable future overprovided, and its surplus is used to reduce deficits caused by other expenditures, such as Star Wars, in what is still an integrated budget. And, if Social Security runs into the red again somewhere after the year 2020, relatively small adjustments in premiums and payouts would restore it to financial health.

Above all, it is a dubious sociological achievement to foment conflict between the generations, because, unlike the minorities and the white majority, or men and women, many millions of Americans are neither young nor old but of intermediate ages. We should not avoid issues just because we face stressing times in an already strained society; but maybe we should declare a moratorium on raising new conflicts until more compelling arguments can be found in their favor, and more evidence that this particular line of divisiveness is called for.

POSTSCRIPT

Should Health Care for the Elderly Be Limited?

In 1988 Congress passed the Medicare Catastrophic Coverage Act, which protects Medicare recipients from liabilities for hospital care, doctors' services, and prescription drugs over specified amounts. It also provides modest additional coverage for care in skilled nursing facilities, hospices, and at home.

A study of patients' and families' preferences for medical intensive care reported in the *Journal of the American Medical Association* (August 12, 1988) concluded that personal preferences may conflict with any health policy that limits the allocation of intensive care based on age, function, or quality of life.

Daniel Callahan's views are amplified in his book *Setting Limits: Medical Goals in an Aging Society* (Simon & Schuster, 1987). See Paul Homer and Martha Holstein, eds., *A Good Old Age: The Paradox of Setting Limits* (Touchstone, 1990), for responses to Callahan's arguments. For contrasting views on age as a criterion for medical care, see Mark Siegler, "Should Age Be a Criterion for Health Care?" and James F. Childress, "Ensuring Care, Respect, and Fairness for the Elderly," both in the *Hastings Center Report* (October 1984). Other articles on the subject include Harry R. Moody, "Age-Based Entitlements to Health Care: What are the Limits?" *Mount Sinai Journal of Medicine* (May 1989), and Nancy S. Jecker and Robert A. Pearlman, "Ethical Constraints on Rationing Medical Care by Age," *Journal of the American Geriatrics Society* (November 1989). Marshall B. Kapp opposes Callahan's view in "Rationing Health Care: Will it Be Necessary? Can it Be Done Without Age or Disability Discrimination?" *Issues in Law & Medicine* (Winter 1989). Pat Milmoe McCarrick's "The Aged and the Allocation of Health Care Resources" (Scope Note #13, Kennedy Institute of Ethics, 1990) offers a good bibliography.

A plan currently under review in Oregon would eliminate Medicaid coverage for operations considered to be too costly, ineffective, or rare, and would ration health care based on a list that gives priority to preventive measures.

For discussions of the general problems of allocating scarce resources, see Henry J. Aaron and William B. Schwartz, *The Painful Prescription: Rationing Hospital Care* (Brookings Institution, 1984); Ronald Bayer, Arthur L. Caplan, and Norman Daniels, eds., *In Search of Equity: Health Needs and the Health Care*

System (Plenum Press, 1983); Larry R. Churchill, *Rationing Health Care in America: Perceptions and Principles of Justice* (University of Notre Dame Press, 1987); Victor R. Fuchs, *The Health Economy* (Harvard University Press, 1986); Paul T. Menzel, *Strong Medicine: The Ethical Rationing of Health Care* (Oxford University Press, 1990); David Mechanic, *Painful Choices: Research Essays on Health Care* (Transaction Publishers, 1989); Daniel Callahan's *What Kind of Life: The Limits of Medical Progress* (Simon & Schuster, 1990); and the report of the President's Commission for the Study of Ethical Problems in Medicine and Biomedical and Behavioral Research, *Securing Access to Health Care* (Government Printing Office, 1983). See Edward L. Schneider and Jack M. Guralnik, "The Aging of America: Impact on Health Care Costs," *Journal of the American Medical Association* (May 2, 1990) for a discussion of how the rapid increase in the elderly population will affect health care costs.

ISSUE 20

Should Dying Patients Have Greater Access to Experimental Drugs?

YES: Nathaniel Pier, from "The Emperor Has No Clothes: Notes on AIDS Drug Testing and Access," *AIDS Treatment News* (August 12, 1988)

NO: Douglas D. Richman, from "Public Access to Experimental Drug Therapy: AIDS Raises Yet Another Conflict Between Freedom of the Individual and Welfare of the Individual and Public," *Journal of Infectious Diseases* (March 1989)

ISSUE SUMMARY

YES: Physician Nathaniel Pier argues that the current, cautious system of drug approval consigns large numbers of people with AIDS to death without giving them the chance to fight back by taking experimental medications.
NO: Physician Douglas D. Richman believes that unproven therapies are unlikely to prolong life or improve its quality and instead have significant potential for harm.

When is it ethically justifiable for scientists to involve human beings in biomedical and behavioral research? This question has been high on the agenda of biomedical ethics for 50 years. And just when the answers seemed to be at least tentatively in place, the new disease of acquired immunodeficiency syndrome (AIDS) challenged many of the assumptions, rules, and practices that evolved during the post–World War II era. The process of review, analysis, and change is still underway.

Most of the ethical issues that have arisen around epidemiological and behavioral studies have concerned the traditional research review questions of protecting subjects from risk (in this case, social or psychological risk) through breaches of confidentiality. The context of a highly stigmatized, new, and still ultimately fatal infectious disease has made these issues more compelling. In the case of clinical trials and other mechanisms of access to investigational drugs, however, the traditional protectionist stance has been challenged, and it is here that the ethics of research and the processes of drug development are changing most profoundly.

The current federal drug approval process emphasizes protecting consumers from unsafe and ineffective drugs; the Food and Drug Administration (FDA) is the government agency charged with that responsibility. In

1962, as a result of the birth in Europe and Australia of thousands of newborns with severe birth defects caused by the drug thalidomide, U.S. laws were strengthened. The drug was never approved for marketing in the United States because a cautious FDA official asked for more data. Before 1962 a drug company sponsor could market a new drug unless the FDA, after reviewing safety data, disapproved. After 1962 a sponsor could market a drug only if the FDA specifically approved. The process of drug approval was thus lengthened and, in the view of many, made too cumbersome.

Although the FDA's own rules do not require it, approval of new drugs relies heavily on data obtained in randomized controlled trials (RCTs). The RCT is considered more reliable than other research designs because random allocation to one or another drug, therapy, dosage, or placebo (an inert substance) counteracts potential bias in assignment if the investigator were to make the choice. Furthermore, variables such as patient characteristics that might affect the outcome tend to be evenly distributed if patients are randomized. An RCT must have a control group; that is, a group of patients who do not receive the test drug or therapy but are in all other respects as similar as possible to the patients who do receive the drug or therapy.

Although the RCT's reliability makes it especially valuable, it is limited in two ways: first, the study population is typically restricted to people who fit a specific medical profile and thus many patients are not eligible to receive the study drug; and second, the results may not be applicable to types of patients other than those in the study.

Before the advent of AIDS, there were some patients, mainly cancer patients and patients suffering from rare diseases, who opposed restricted access to experimental drugs. AIDS activists have vastly increased pressure on regulatory agencies and drug sponsors. The changes they propose, and in some cases have effected, would increase the early availability of drugs for many diseases in addition to AIDS.

Much of the controversy over access to experimental drugs derives from conflicting views of the purpose of clinical trials. Investigators see them as *research* (an activity designed to produce generalizable knowledge). Patients (and some clinicians) see them as *therapy* (medical practice designed to benefit individuals). Patients want to believe that all aspects of a clinical trial are designed to benefit him or her directly, and surely investigators hope that patients will benefit; but this is not the purpose of the trial.

In the following selections, Nathaniel Pier asserts that AIDS patients and physicians need more and better treatment options and that "the emperor" (the government) "has no clothes" (is failing to provide these options despite its proclamations to the contrary), while Douglas D. Richman maintains that properly designed clinical studies of experimental drugs will relieve the most suffering and do the most good, certainly in the long run and almost certainly in the short run.

YES

THE EMPEROR HAS NO CLOTHES: NOTES ON AIDS DRUG TESTING AND ACCESS

There has been something lost in the struggle to find therapies for AIDS. The individual patient with the counsel and guidance of his or her physician must have the right to make choices, to have options. People with AIDS and at risk for AIDS have abdicated their responsibility far too much to the medical establishment and the research establishment to make these decisions for them.

The primary role of a clinician is to synthesize with a patient a course of action that makes sense. This means every patient is offered the opportunity of choosing from the options that are available, under the careful guidance of their clinician. This should not be a major issue. Yet in treating AIDS, these options are limited by restricted access to experimental drugs.

The current system of doing drug studies has failed. It has been bureaucratized to the point where it takes two to three years to test a drug that should be tested in two to four months. There is no proof that this system works. Let us go back to the system where individual clinicians are given the opportunity of synthesizing a course of action appropriate to each patient's situation. This implies freer access to experimental drugs.

Under supervised protocols from a national group, we should get access to drugs that are in Phase II trials, including drugs that have not had efficacy demonstrated. Clinicians should be allowed to authorize the use of these drugs with patients' consent. [Editor's note: drugs in "Phase II" testing have already passed the "Phase I" test for dosage, toxicity, and safety.] It should be up to the patient with the clinician's guidance to make such decisions. The fact that we have to wait two to four years for a drug like lentinan or dideoxycytidine to come down as a potentially useful drug is not fair to the patients who have no other options, who are simply going to die.

The present system is essentially telling patients with immune deficiency disease, "We don't care about you, go home and die. We will cure this

This article was reprinted by permission from *AIDS Treatment News*, a semimonthly newsletter. *AIDS Treatment News* provides the most accurate, up-to-date treatment information available while also examining public policy issues. Available by subscription only; to request more information write to P.O. Box 411256, San Francisco, CA 94141 or call either 800-TREAT-1-2 (800-873-2812) or 415-255-0588.

disease in our own time with our designer drugs." Every patient should demand to have access to a number of experimental options through their clinician, and these options should be offered to them as supervised protocols.

A good example of an equitable drug testing system is the multidrug protocols for cancer. If you are diagnosed as having colorectal cancer, for example, your oncologist ties in to a national computer where your statistics are kept confidentially and analyzed. Out the other end comes a protocol. Not only are you allowed to participate in a potentially life-saving drug regimen, but the data collected from you goes back to a center that very quickly will collect information as to whether this particular combination of drugs works.

We should be doing this in AIDS. . . .

We would not need to do complex virological or immunological tests on everyone. The studies requiring such tests should be done in smaller protocols at major medical centers. For example, in my proposed system, once a month the physician would do the routine blood work specified in the protocol and send the data to the NIH, and the physician will also fill in clinical data. Probably within three or four months we could find out which treatment combinations are best. People with AIDS should be demanding that the system be reformed to allow anybody at risk access to these drugs under supervised protocols. I hope that groups advocating for people with AIDS will adopt this as a primary goal. It should be the *patient's* option to use experimental drugs under guidance, supervision, and monitoring.

The system now in place for developing, testing, and distributing AIDS drugs is not working; it is not producing new therapeutic options. It is also discriminatory. Only 4000 people out of an estimated 1.5 million HIV seropositives in this country have been enrolled in trials. The vast majority are white males. It is clear that the people designing this system do not understand AIDS and who is affected by it. AIDS advocates need to start saying that the emperor has no clothes. Let us start a system that is going to work—one where people with AIDS-related problems get rapid access to experimental drugs in protocol, on a routine basis through their clinicians, whether private physicians or at a clinic.

Let us stop wasting time. I have done my rounds of researchers and AIDS drug testing centers. There is nothing new—there are no new drugs close to approval. It is a scandal that our system with its funding still is not producing. It is completely unreasonable that nearly two years after AZT was first released there has been no new drug made available and combination therapies using antivirals and immunomodulators are not being tested. It is unreasonable that Frank Young of the FDA says that very few drugs are likely to be approved between now and 1991, when we are losing 48 people a day to this disease.

We must stop this idea that testing drugs on a small number of patients, then on a slightly larger number of patients is a reasonable approach when people are dying. We want to make experimental therapies available to people as a matter of course, as a matter of therapy, so that clinicians caring for AIDS patients can get access to these drugs under supervised protocols. Not only would patients have more options, but we would also learn quickly what works.

The system is not working, so let us come up with a new system. Let us use experimental treatments as potential therapy for ailing patients, and do it in a manner that is going to provide useful information. We must set up a national registry, check out protocols of combination therapies, and let people use them. . . .

As a result of the lack of access to drugs, a high underground drug network has arisen. A problem with the treatment underground is that for the last two-and-a-half years we have tried naltrexone, AL 721, antabuse, dextran sulfate. Something has come along every few months that has offered people hope and access to therapy that they could not get other places. That is very important. But I, as a clinician, am tired of my patients not knowing which of these therapies is the best to choose, tired of patients being bamboozled by people into taking this or that or the other thing, tired of not being able to assess whether an approach or combination therapy is really benefiting the patients. We need a working system able to rapidly test new therapies so that when a therapy comes along, we can evaluate the efficacy very quickly.

What I am proposing is very clear. We need a national registry of treatment protocols. If a patient has an AIDS-related problem at any stage of the illness, and if that patient elects to try to intervene, there should be protocols available to that patient's clinician. There should be multiple protocols for every stage of the disease, so that we can quickly assess which intervention might make a difference.

These protocols should be available not just through a few selected centers or just in the major cities, not just to the lucky few who can afford to go to doctors who can get them into these studies. They should be available to every physician who treats AIDS patients. We know enough about this disease to develop a logical approach involving antiviral, immunomodulatory, prophylactic, and anti-inflammatory therapies.

There are enough drugs to be tried so that we could develop these protocols in a few weeks and make them available to clinicians through a national computer. The data from these combination trials could start pouring in, and we would know within a few months which of the available combinations are working best, rather than the years and years that it is currently taking.

This approach will give patients hope and access to humane, well-supervised medical treatments, instead of allowing them to live in fear or desperation or in search of the few trials available. It will allow them to participate in a larger effort, to find which therapies work best for everybody, making their situation meaningful not only for themselves but for the world.

Clinicians want to participate, to know what is happening with the research and what the future plans are. We want to reduce the secrecy, the sense that scientific data are proprietary or exclusive in the face of this epidemic. The current system simply has not produced the goods. And if Dr. Frank Young's prediction of few new drugs approved by 1991 is any indication, it will not produce the goods for a long time to come. This consigns large numbers of people to death without giving them the dignity of the chance to fight back. This is not an acceptable human or reasonable approach to conducting research in this epidemic.

After five years of being on the front lines, my heartfelt feeling is that the top priority for people with AIDS and people who care about AIDS is to demand access to experimental therapies. I appeal to people to organize this effort immediately, to bring it forward in their local groups, then present the case to their politicians, and to the people who supervise the present medical system of testing drugs. It is time we told them that the emperor has no clothes. It is time to insist on wider access to promising therapies, and rapid testing of existing drugs to develop better treatment options.

NO

Douglas D. Richman

PUBLIC ACCESS TO EXPERIMENTAL DRUG THERAPY: AIDS RAISES YET ANOTHER CONFLICT BETWEEN FREEDOM OF THE INDIVIDUAL AND WELFARE OF THE INDIVIDUAL AND PUBLIC

With tens of thousands of human immunodeficiency virus (HIV)-infected persons facing the prospect of a relentlessly fatal illness, there is understandable impatience with any apparent delay or restrictions in making effective therapeutic measures available quickly and widely. However, it is critical to understand how important the word "effective" is in this formulation. Urgency and hope have prompted patients and physicians to pursue treatments with alternative therapies and unproven experimental drugs. These include megavitamins, psychospiritual exercises, and pharmaceuticals of all levels of sophistication.

Many who do this say, "I already have a fatal illness and you purists have no cure to offer. What have I got to lose?" While the pressure to administer experimental drugs in poorly controlled circumstances is understandable, the net result is the opposite of that desired. These unproven therapies are unlikely to prolong life or improve its quality. More important, they have significant potential for harm, and may make a difficult situation worse. An analogy may help make the point. If my 1979 Volvo conks out on the freeway, I may raise the hood and see that motor is not running. Given my rudimentary understanding of the internal combustion engine, I may decide to fix it by bashing it once with a sledge hammer. While this may fix the problem, the odds are that it will not, and, in fact, it will actually be harmful. We are more complicated than my Volvo's engine and our knowledge of the pathophysiology of AIDS is even less than my understanding of the engine. Thus a random unproved attempt at therapy is unlikely to be effective and more likely to do harm than to be merely neutral. The dream of the winning lottery ticket for AIDS therapy seems to be especially prevalent.

From Douglas D. Richman, "Public Access to Experimental Drug Therapy: AIDS Raises Yet Another Conflict Between Freedom of the Individual and Welfare of the Individual and Public," *Journal of Infectious Diseases*, vol. 159, no. 3 (March 1989). Copyright © 1989 by the University of Chicago Press. Reprinted by permission.

Fortunately, drugs that to date have undergone the most extensive uncontrolled use in the community are relatively nontoxic, for example, ribavirin, AL721, and dextran sulfate. Only survivors can give live testimonials. Whether these compounds have any true benefit cannot be ascertained by uncontrolled use. Had one of these drugs been effective, then a promptly performed controlled study would have permitted thousands of needy patients access to the drug years earlier. The ineffectual or toxic drugs will continue to waste the valuable financial resources, energies, and hopes of thousands of patients.

People raise the question, "why is it necessary to employ complex placebo-controlled studies to prove the efficacy of a new form of therapy? The open administration of penicillin to patients with bacterial meningitis or endocarditis in the 1940s was sufficient to document efficacy." The answer, I think, is quite clear. HIV infection and AIDS are not identical to pneumococcal meningitis or endocarditis. The latter infections are uniformly fatal in days to weeks and any survivors are clear successes of therapy. The natural history of AIDS and other HIV infections is complex and unpredictable in any individual and is not the direct and immediate consequence of the multiplication of the organism. It is unrealistic to expect a cure for a chronic disease caused by a pathogen that integrates its genome into the host's genome. Suppression of infection is a more realistic objective at present.

While uncontrolled studies in patients with AIDS could reveal a completely curative drug, they would miss drugs like zidovudine (Retrovir, 3'-azido, 3'-deoxythymidine; AZT) that help but don't cure, and they would not unmask drugs that look good on paper but have more toxicity than efficacy (do more harm than good). This is not just academic theory. In the field of antiviral therapy alone, numerous anecdotal claims were made for the benefits of corticosteroids for chronic hepatitis B, of iododeoxyuridine for herpes simplex encephalitis, and cytosine arabinoside for disseminated herpes zoster. These clinical observations made by concerned physicians were proved to be erroneous in randomized, double-blind, placebo-controlled studies [1-6]. In fact, the study drug in each case did more harm than the placebo. Were it not for controlled studies, thousands of patients would still be receiving harmful treatment.

It took only two years after AZT was shown to inhibit the replication of HIV in vitro to prove its clinical efficacy and obtain licensure. Accomplishing this in two years represents unprecedented speed in drug development. While two years is a lifetime for someone with a progressive fatal disease, it takes some time to demonstrate clinical efficacy and prevent the widespread use of harmful forms of therapy. For the first four years that AIDS and its related diseases were recognized, physicians had little to offer but treatment of opportunistic infections and malignancies and general support.

Had AZT been available for open use in 1986, it would likely have been discarded as toxic and ineffective. In the placebo-controlled study, no impact on opportunistic infections was discerned for at least six weeks; an impact on survival required even longer [7]. Toxicity, especially anemia requiring transfusion and granulocytopenia, occurs within two months of starting AZT therapy [8]. AIDS in many respects resembles cancer or leukemia. Although we would like a penicillin for AIDS, we have to think more like oncologists than like infectious disease doctors. For the present, therapy will probably require the prolonged use of toxic drugs aimed at suppression rather than cure and regimens with cycles and combinations of drugs.

Physicians and patients alike would like to believe that when the patient's condition improves it is because of what the physician did, and when the patient's condition fails to improve, it is despite what the physician did. With a little experience in medicine, we learn that some conditions improve regardless of what the physician did and some do poorly because of what the physician did.

Both patients and health care providers are frustrated by the suffering and the relentless progression that characterize the course of AIDS. The reflex wish by all is for a simple solution—a relief of the suffering and an escape from the relentless progression. Thus, the obvious response to this reflex is to offer any treatment with even a glimmer of hope. The idea of experimentation or research in the midst of this desperation may seem to lack compassion. On the contrary, I propose that properly designed clinical studies of experimental drugs will relieve the most suffering and do the most good, certainly in the long run and almost certainly in the short run.

The purpose of experimental drug therapy is to determine which drugs work and which drugs do not work. Once an effective drug is identified, further studies determine how best to use it; for example, what regimens to use and which patient groups will benefit from therapy.

The major goals of experimental drug therapy are to increase the quantity and quality of life; in other words, to delay mortality and to reduce morbidity. The reduction of morbidity includes reducing the suffering from disease and minimizing the toxicity of therapy. These goals should be practical. They should be obtained as expeditiously as possible. The ideal drug for a chronic disease should be orally administered. The price of therapy should be low.

The proper clinical evaluation of a promising antiretroviral compound requires an expeditious dose-escalating study to assess safety, tolerance, pharmacokinetics, and possible virological and immunologic endpoints. If these results are encouraging, the prompt documentation of safety and efficacy requires a randomized double-blind study. The control should be placebo if no effective therapy is known; it should be a regimen proved to be effective, for example AZT, in populations for whom benefit is accepted. Conduct of proper studies is a great responsibility that clinical investigators, government representatives, and the pharmaceutical industry must accept with the maximal efficiency and cooperation. . . .

It has been argued that this "establishment" has no monopoly on the capability of conducting proper drug evaluation and that useful drug evaluation can be conducted in the private community. Any mechanism that will provide better or faster information is to be encouraged. Any study, however, must appreciate that the value of its conclusion is no better than the study design and the quality of the data. Thus any study including community research initiatives must consider informed consent; controlled study design including subject numbers, subject characteristics, endpoint criteria, well-characterized study compounds, patient and physician compliance with dosing regimens, and other protocol components; accurate and retrievable data collection; and proper study monitoring and analysis.

The information network, especially in the gay community, is extensive. Within days of the hint of a new hope, newsletters and gossip spread information, misinformation, recipes and rumors. This search for cures results in individuals trying home remedies and nonprofit purchasing cooperatives. Also, businessess have sprung up, many of which misrepresent facts to exploit the hope and desperation of the sick and of the worried well. Proponents of the open availability of experimental drugs will argue, "It's my own body, I can do with it as I wish. Moreover, I have a life-threatening disease." In our society individuals should and do have rights of free choice. We are free to do many things that may be unsafe and self-destructive. Hand guns, tobacco, alcohol, junk food, and not wearing set belts come to mind. The problem is to set the proper limits on individual freedoms when those freedoms have impacts on society and, for those of us interested in trying to control the epidemic and to relieve suffering, to purse the most effective course possible.

The open distribution of unproved drugs is not compassionate, and this approach in fact often delays access of needy patients and health care workers to the critical information that will prolong life and reduce suffering. Such distribution may: (1) give false hope to a desperate patient; (2) waste patient or medical care resources; (3) subject patients to unappreciated toxicity or toxicity that is not compensated by benefit; (4) delay or prevent documentation of benefit or proper use of a drug; and (5) delay licensure and general availability of a useful drug.

Although the most important consequence of experimental drugs is that they may delay or prevent the determination of whether or not drugs work, there are probably other consequences as well. AIDS has become an economic catastrophe, both to many persons suffering from the disease and for a society that must assume most of the costs of care. The individual choice to experiment with a drug may result in serious toxicity, untoward interactions with standard therapies, delay or avoidance of proven therapies, and delay of documentation of new effective drugs. With the cost of each case of AIDS in the tens of thousands of dollars, these decisions have financial consequences for which society must pay, and they remove resources from an arena that offers both short- and long-term benefit.

An additional consequence of the availability and promotion of unproved drugs is the interference with the controlled studies that offer the best (only) hope of identifying effective agents. Moreover, when patients enroll in studies, some continue to use such drugs, often without the knowledge of the investigators. Thus, they destroy the validity of the study and create false data about toxicity that could prompt us to discard as too toxic a useful drug. For example, ribavirin might add to the hematologic toxicity of AZT and it does interfere with the activity of AZT in cell culture [9].

Many who support uncontrolled experimentation seem to presume that the establishment is withholding secret cures because of greed, glory, disinterest, or malice towards groups considered socially undesirable. Denials by the accused are of no value; nevertheless, it is worth pointing out that ethical investigators make no claims or promises and they charge no fees or expenses for the investigational component of their work.

Both the purpose of experimental drug therapy and the limitations of open administration of unproved drugs can be summarized in a simple paradigm. Numerous drugs have been proposed to treat serious HIV infection. For every 10 candidates perhaps one is effective, one is toxic, and most are relatively safe and useless. A patient seeks help from a doctor. The doctor has 10 bottles of pills from which to choose. One will prolong and improve the quality of the patient's life. One will cause extreme sickness. Eight are highly touted placebos. Even if there were no regulatory agency like the FDA, only a well-conducted clinical investigation in experimental drug therapy would permit a caring, thoughtful physician to choose the correct bottle of pills for a hopeful patient.

REFERENCES

1. Stevens DA, Jordan GW, Waddell TF, Merigan TC. Adverse effect of cytosine arabinoside on disseminated zoster in a controlled trial. N Engl J Med 1973; 289:873-8

2. Boston Interhospital Virus Study Group and the NIAID-Sponsored Cooperative Antiviral Clinical Study. Failure of high dose 5-Iodo-2'-deoxyuridine in the therapy of herpes simplex virus encephalitis. N Engl J Med 1975; 292:600-3

3. Sagnelli E, Maio G, Felaco FM, Izzo CM, Manzillo G, Pasquale G, Filippini P, Piccinino F. Serum levels of hepatitis B surface and core antigens during immunosuppressive treatment of HBsAg-positive chronic active hepatitis. Lancet 1980; 2:395-7

4. Lam KC, Lai CL, Ng RP, Trepo C, Wu PC. Deleterious effect of prednisolone in HBsAg-positive chronic active hepatitis. N Engl J Med 1981; 304:380-6

5. European Association for the Study of the Liver. A multicenter randomized clinical trial of low-dose steroid treatment in chronic active HBsAg positive liver disease (abstract). Gastroenterology 1984; 86:1317

6. Hoofnagle JH, Davis GL, Pappas SC, Hanson RG, Peters M, Avigan MI, Waggoner JG, Jones EA, Seeff LB. A short course of prednisolone in chronic type B hepatitis. Ann Intern Med 1986; 104:12-7

7. Fischl MA, Richman DD, Grieco MH, Gottlieb MS, Volberding PA, Laskin OL, Leedom JM, Groopman JE, Mildvan D, Schooley RT, Jackson GG, Durak DT, King D, AZT Collaborative Working Group. The efficacy of azidothymidine (AZT) in the treatment of patients with AIDS and AIDS-related complex: a double-blind, placebo-controlled trial. N Engl J Med 1987; 317:185-91

8. Richman DD, Fischl MA, Grieco MH, Gottlieb MS, Volberding PA, Laskin OL, Leedom JM, Groopman JE, Mildvan D, Hirsch MS, Jackson GG, Durack DT, Nusinoff-Lehrman S, AZT Collaborative Working Group. The toxicity of azidothymidine (AZT) in the treatment of patients with AIDS and AIDS-related complex: a double-blind, placebo-controlled trial. N Engl J Med 1987; 317:192-7

9. Vogt MW, Hartshorn KL, Furman PA, Chou TC, Fyfe JA, Coleman LA, Crumpacker C, Schooley RT, Hirsch MS. Ribavirin antagonizes the effect of azidothymidine on HIV replication. Science 1987; 235:1376-9

POSTSCRIPT

Should Dying Patients Have Greater Access to Experimental Drugs?

There are several new mechanisms through which people with AIDS and other life-threatening illnesses can obtain access to promising but still unproven drugs. A drug company may obtain from the FDA a "Treatment IND" (Investigational New Drug), that is, permission to distribute to eligible patients a drug that is nearing approval but has not completed the process. As of March 1990, 18 Treatment INDs had been approved, six of them for AIDS/HIV drugs.

A process called "parallel track" makes it possible for patients to receive some AIDS/HIV drugs much earlier in the approval process. Promising drugs are made available, at about the same time, both to subjects enrolled in clinical trials and to patients who might benefit from the drug but are not eligible for the trials because of their medical profile or because they live too far from the trial site. Two drugs have been approved for distribution under parallel track conditions.

In addition to the more traditional academic research institutions, research studies are also being conducted in community-based settings. In this way more patients can be enrolled in drug trials, and promising alternative therapies that might not engage the interest of major drug companies can be studied.

In August 1990 the National Committee to Review Current Procedures for Approval of New Drugs for Cancer and AIDS, appointed in 1988 by former vice president George Bush, recommended sweeping changes to speed the delivery of new drugs. For a strong defense of the traditional clinical trial system, see Sheila C. Mitchell and Jay Steingrub, "The Changing Clinical Trials Scene: The Role of the IRB," *IRB: A Review of Human Subjects Research* (July/August 1988). In "Faith (Healing), Hope, and Charity at the FDA: The Politics of AIDS Drug Trials," George J. Annas argues against transforming the FDA "from a consumer protection agency into a drug promotion agency" (in Lawrence O. Gostin, ed., *AIDS and the Health Care System*, Yale University Press, 1990). Frank E. Young, the former FDA commissioner, and his colleagues report on changes in agency policy in "The FDA's New Procedures for the Use of Investigational Drugs in Treatment," *Journal of the American Medical Association* (April 15, 1988). Harold Edgar and David J. Rothman provide a helpful analysis of the background of drug regulation in "New Rules for New Drugs: The Challenge of AIDS to the Regulatory Process," *Milbank Quarterly* (Supplement 1, 1990). Also see Benjamin Freedman and the McGill/Boston Research Group, "Nonvalidated Therapies and HIV Disease," *Hastings Center Report* (May/June 1989) and the *Final Report of the National Committee to Review Current Procedures for Approval of New Drugs for Cancer and AIDS* (August 1990).

ISSUE 21

Should the United States Follow the Canadian Model of a National Health Program?

YES: Steffie Woolhandler and David U. Himmelstein, from "A National Health Program: Northern Light at the End of the Tunnel," *Journal of the American Medical Association* (October 20, 1989)

NO: Ronald Bronow, from "A National Health Program: Abyss at the End of the Tunnel—The Position of Physicians Who Care," *Journal of the American Medical Association* (May 9, 1990)

ISSUE SUMMARY

YES: Physicians Steffie Woolhandler and David U. Himmelstein propose a sweeping reform of health care financing, following the Canadian model of a single-source system of payment, to ensure equity of access and efficiency.
NO: Physician Ronald Bronow, on behalf of an organization called Physicians Who Care, believes that problems of underfinancing and rationing in the Canadian system would be magnified in the American setting.

The American health care system is the most expensive in the world. No other country spends as much—11.5 percent of the Gross National Product—on health care. The American health care system is also among the most technologically advanced in the world. On the negative side, however, the American health care system is among the least equitable in the world. Approximately 37 million people have no medical insurance; some have employers who do not provide health insurance as a benefit, others are unemployed, and still others are uninsurable because of current or prior health problems such as cancer, heart disease, or AIDS. Many more millions have medical insurance that does not pay for expensive items like prescription drugs, outpatient care, or nursing home care. Publicly funded programs such as Medicare (for the elderly and those with end-stage kidney disease) and Medicaid (for the very poor) spend more and more each year to provide less and less coverage. Those who are hardest hit by the lack of financial support for health care are the poorest populations, especially children.

The United States is the only industrialized country other than South Africa that does not have some form of national health insurance. In some countries, such as the United Kingdom, health care is provided through a National Health Service, which employs physicians and other health care workers. In other countries, such as West Germany, a national health insurance plan covers all citizens. In the United States the traditional form of payment for health care is "fee for service," that is, a patient pays a doctor for an office visit, procedure, or other service, the free market sets the rates, and the costs are paid by private insurance, largely obtained as an employment benefit. There are about 1,500 private insurance companies providing health insurance, and each state regulates insurance according to its own laws. Each state also sets its own Medicaid eligibility and reimbursement standards.

Industry is trying to lower medical costs through a number of mechanisms: shifting the costs to employees; reducing hospital utilization by requiring second opinions and by limiting lengths of stay; and limiting choices of the provider. Although these cost-containment measures reduce the physician's discretion in recommending treatment, they may also reduce unnecessary surgery and other unnecessary forms of treatment. In June 1985 the U.S. Supreme Court upheld a Massachusetts statute requiring that certain health care benefits be provided to residents who are insured under employee health care plans.

No one—doctors, patients, hospital administrators, or government officials—is happy with the present system. It is generally accepted that it is too costly, inequitable, irrational, and enmeshed in red tape. However, there is no agreement as to the solution. Patient choice and physician autonomy are long-standing values in American health care, and any system that appears to limit these values is suspect. Recently economists and physicians have looked to Canada for guidance. The following two selections present differing views on whether the Canadian experience is applicable to the United States. On behalf of a group called Physicians for a National Health Program, Steffie Woolhandler and David U. Himmelstein argue that the Canadian model of a single payer would provide a rational, pragmatic, and ethical framework for reform. Ronald Bronow, a representative of another group, Physicians Who Care, acknowledges the difficulties in the United States but warns that the Canadian solution will only bring rationing and fewer resources.

YES

Steffie Woolhandler and David U. Himmelstein

A NATIONAL HEALTH PROGRAM: NORTHERN LIGHT AT THE END OF THE TUNNEL

Few would dispute that our health care system is deeply troubled. Thirty-seven million Americans are uninsured, health care costs continue their exuberant growth, and bureaucracy increasingly intrudes in the examining room. Opinion on solutions is more divided.

We and many colleagues have proposed a sweeping reform of health care financing[1] because we are convinced that lesser measures will fail, as they have for the past quarter century. Expanding Medicaid,[2] mandating that employers provide health benefits,[3] setting up state risk pools, and similar piece-meal attempts to expand access either fuel inflation or install intrusive cost-management bureaucracies—usually both.[4] Providing more care to those currently uninsured must raise costs if resources are not diverted from elsewhere in the system. Unless bureaucracy is trimmed, these resources will be siphoned from existing clinical care, a process invariably overseen by yet another layer of bureaucrats.

Medicare epitomizes the problem. It improved access for the elderly, but costs soared and diagnosis related groups resulted.[5] Moreover, cost-management bureaucracies are not only intrusive but expensive, leading to a steady fall in the care-bureaucracy ratio, which is now little better than 3:1.[6] For each dollar spent for the clinical components of care, 30 cents is spent for administrators and their tools.[6] Resources seep silently but inexorably from the clinic to the administrative suite. The shortage of bedside nurses coexists with a proliferation of Registered Nurse utilization reviewers and preadmission screeners. Few physicians now escape the pleasure of their scrutiny.

Such an enormous bureaucratic burden is a peculiarly American phenomenon. Our insurance companies take 12% of their premiums for overhead[7]; Canada's program runs for less than 3% overhead.[6] We devote more than 18% of hospital spending to administration and billing; Canada devotes

From Steffie Woolhandler and David U. Himmelstein, "A National Health Program: Northern Light at the End of the Tunnel," *Journal of the American Medical Association*, vol. 262, no. 15 (October 20, 1989), pp. 2136-2137. Copyright © 1989 by the American Medical Association. Reprinted by permission.

8%.[6,8] United States physicians spend 45% of gross income for professional expenses, much of it for billing; our Canadian colleagues spend 36%.[9,10] Overall, we spend 2.6% of our gross national product for health care bureaucracy, while Canada spends 1.1%.[6] Reducing our health administrative apparatus to the Canadian level would have saved about $2 billion this year.

Unfortunately, piecemeal tinkering cannot reverse bureaucratic hypertrophy. The key to administrative simplicity in Canada is the single-source system of payment[11]: in each province, virtually all bills are paid by the provincial insurance plan. Hospitals do little or no billing and need not keep track of the charges for individual patients.[12] They are paid a global annual budget to cover all costs, much as a fire department is funded in the United States. Physicians bill by checking a box on a simple insurance form and submitting it to the provincial plan. Fee schedules are negotiated annually between the provincial medical associations and governments.[12,13] All patients have the same (complete) coverage.

The fragmentation of insurance coverage in the United States (with > 1500 different plans) requires the current herculean administrative efforts. Hospitals must determine eligibility, keep track of charges, and bill for each patient individually; coverage and regulations vary widely. Each insurer employs legions (6000 people work for Blue Cross of Massachusetts alone) to market their plans and minimize their costs, often by simply shifting those costs onto patients, other insurers, the government, or hospital red ink. Physicians must deal with an increasingly complex tangle of insurance forms and requirements. Our group

practice pays about 10% of gross revenues to a billing service, a typical figure.[6]

The national health program (NHP) we propose would create a single tax-funded comprehensive insurer in each state, federally mandated but locally controlled.[1] Everyone would be fully insured for all medically necessary services and private insurance duplicating the NHP coverage would be proscribed, as would patient copayments and deductibles. The current byzantine insurance bureaucracy with its tangle of regulations and wasteful duplication would be dismantled. Instead, the NHP in each state would disburse all funds, and central administrative costs would be limited by law to 3% of total health spending. Cost-shifting efforts would be pointless—there would be nowhere to shift costs to. Marketing of insurance plans, health maintenance organizations, and hospitals would also be eliminated, saving billions of dollars annually.

We expect that initially the NHP would cause little change in the total costs of care, with savings on administration and billing approximately offsetting the costs of expanded care.[14] The Canadian experience suggests the increase in use of care would be modest after an initial surge,[15] with most of the rise occurring among the poor and those with serious symptoms.[16,17]

Demonstration projects in one or more states might precede nationwide implementation. In these demonstrations, and during the phasing in of a nationwide system, funding would mimic existing patterns to minimize economic disruption—but all payment would be funneled through the NHP. Thus, Medicare and Medicaid monies would go to the NHP; employers would pay an NHP tax equivalent to the average now spent for health benefits; and individuals would pay a tax equivalent to the current average out-of-pocket expenditure.

The NHP would pay each hospital and nursing home a global budget to cover all operating expenses. This operating budget would be negotiated annually based on past expenditures, previous financial and clinical performance, projected changes in costs and use, and proposed new and innovative programs. Capital projects would be funded through separate appropriations from the NHP, and the use of operating funds for capital purchases or profits would be prohibited to minimize incentives for hospitals to skimp on care. Under this payment scheme, many administrative tasks would disappear. There would be no hospital bills to keep track of, no eligibility determination, and no need to attribute costs and charges to individual patients.

Physicians would enjoy a free choice of practice settings and styles. They could elect to be paid on a fee-for-service basis or receive salaries from health maintenance organizations, hospitals, or other institutional providers. The representative of the fee-for-service practitioners (perhaps the state medical society) and the state's NHP board would negotiate a simplified binding-fee schedule. Practitioners who accepted payment from the NHP could bill patients directly only for uncovered services (as is done for cosmetic surgery in Canada). The effort and expense of billing would be trivial: stamp the patient's NHP card on a billing form, check a box, send in all the bills once a week, and receive full payment for virtually all services—with an extra payment for any bill not paid within 30 days. Health maintenance organizations and group practices could elect to be paid a capitation fee to cover all services except inpatient hospitalization, which would be funded through hospitals' global budgets. Regulations on capital funding and profits would be similar to those for hospitals. Financial incentives for physicians based on the health maintenance organization's financial performance would be prohibited.

A similar system has worked well in Canada for nearly 20 years.[4,12,18] There are virtually no financial barriers to care and fewer nonfinancial barriers than in our country.[19] Health spending per capita, though 30% below the US figure, is the second highest in the world.[20] It remained stable as a proportion of gross national product largely because bureaucracy has not hypertrophied and because the NHP, as the sole source of funds for health care, is able to set and enforce overall budgetary limits.[11] Despite disputes about the adequacy of funding for high-technology care,[21] most observers agree that quality of care has remained on a par with the United States and health status is at least as good as in our country.

Regulation of practice in Canada consists mainly of setting ceilings on aggregate physician reimbursement, hospital budgets, and capital spending and monitoring for outlandish abuses (e.g., a single family physician who billed for $250,000 for urinalyses in 1 year).[11,13] Detailed oversight of the clinical encounter has proved unnecessary and clinical freedom is better preserved than in our country.[22,23] Although Canadian physicians have battled government over adequate funding, physician incomes are high and have more than kept pace with inflation.[13] Overall, 69% of Canadian physicians rate their NHP good or excellent, 61% believe it has improved health status, and the same proportion express satisfaction with their own practices.[24] Medicine remains a much sought after career, attracting nearly three times as many applicants per medical school place (and per capita) as in the United States.[25-27]

The Canadian system enjoys overwhelming support among patients.[19] Indeed, only 3% of Canadians would go back to the US-style system that predated their NHP.[19] In contrast, 61% of Americans favor a Canadian-style reform,[19] more than twice as many as support patchwork approaches like extending Medicaid.[28] United States corporations are also increasingly interested in fundamental health policy reform. Thus, Chrysler's health insurance costs ($700 per car in the United States vs $223 in Canada) have spurred Lee Iacocca to consider supporting an NHP (*Baltimore Sun.* April 16, 1989:2D).

Despite such popular and powerful support, the NHP we propose faces important political obstacles. The virtual elimination of private health insurance will meet stiff opposition from the insurance industry and necessitate a large-scale retraining program for employees of insurance companies (many might be employed as support personnel to free nurses for clinical tasks). Although business as a whole would see no rise in its health care costs, firms not now providing health benefits would face increased taxes without the offset provided by the elimination of health insurance premiums.

The long-term financial viability of the system we propose is critically dependent on achieving and maintaining administrative simplicity. The Canadian macromanagement approach to cost control—setting overall budgetary limits—is inherently less intensive administratively than the current US micromanagement approach that depends on case-by-case scrutiny of billions of individual expenditures and encounters. However, even in a Canadian-style system, vigilance and statutory limits on administrative spending will likely be needed to curb the tendency of bureaucracy to reproduce and amplify itself.

An NHP would solve the cost-vs-access conflict by slashing bureaucratic waste and improving health planning. It would reorient the way we pay for care and eliminate financial barriers to access, but preserve the physician-patient relationship. An NHP would offer patients a free choice of physicians and hospitals, and physicians a free choice of practice style and hospital affiliation. How many failed patchwork reforms, how many patients turned away from care they can't afford, how many dollars spent on bureaucracy, before we arrive at the only viable solution—a universal, comprehensive, publicly administered national health program?

REFERENCES

1. Himmelstein DU, Woolhandler S, the Writing Committee of the Working Group on Program Design. A national health program for the United States: a physicians' proposal. *N Engl J Med.* 1989; 320:102–108.

2. Thorpe KE, Siegel JE, Dailey T. Including the poor: the fiscal impacts of Medicaid expansion. *JAMA*, 1989; 261:1003–1007.

3. The National Leadership Commission on Health. *For the Health of a Nation: A Shared Responsibility.* Ann Arbor, Mich: Health Administration Press; 1989.

4. Evans RG. Finding the levers, finding the courage: lessons from cost containment in North America. *J Health Polit Policy Law.* 1986; 11:585–615.

5. Aiken LH, Bays KD. The Medicare debate: round 1. *N Engl J Med.* 1984; 311:1196–1200.

6. Himmelstein DU, Woolhandler S. Cost without benefit: administrative waste in U.S. health care. *N Engl J Med.* 1986; 314:441–445.

7. Levit KR, Freeland MS. National Medical care spending. *Health Aff.* 1988; 7(5):124–136.

8. *Administrative and Supportive Services.* Ottawa, Canada: Health Information Division, Dept of Health and Welfare; 1981.

9. Reynolds RA, Ohsfeldt RL, eds. *Socioeconomic Characteristics of Medical Practice.* Chicago, Ill: American Medical Association; 1984.

10. *Estimates of Physicians' Earnings, 1973–1982.* Ottawa, Canada: Health Information Division, Dept of National Health and Welfare; 1983.

11. Evans RG, Lomas J., Barer ML, et al. Controlling health expenditures: the Canadian reality. *N Engl J Med.* 1989; 320:571–577.

12. Iglehart JK. Canada's health care system. *N Engl J Med.* 1986; 315:202–208, 778–784.

13. Barer ML, Evans RG, Labelle RJ. Fee controls as cost control: tales from the frozen north. *Milbank Q.* 1988; 66:1–64.

14. Himmelstein DU, Woolhandler S. Free care: a quantitative analysis of the health and cost effects of a national health program. *Int J Health Serv.* 1988; 18:393–399.

15. LeClair M. The Canadian health care system. In: Andreopoulos S, ed. *National Health Insurance: Can We Learn From Canada?* New York, NY: John Wiley & Sons Inc; 1975:11–92.

16. Enterline PE, Salter V, McDonald AD, McDonald JC. The distribution of medical services before and after 'free' medical care: the Quebec experience. *N Engl J Med.* 1973; 289:1174–1178.

17. Siemiatycki J, Richardson L, Pless IB. Equality in medical care under national health insurance in Montreal. *N Engl J Med.* 1980; 303:10–15.

18. Taylor MG. *Health Insurance and Canadian Public Policy: The Seven Decisions That Created the Canadian Health Insurance System and Their Outcomes.* Montreal, Canada: McGill-Queens University Press; 1987.

19. Blendon RJ. Three systems: a comparative survey. *Health Manage Q.* 1989; 11:1–10.

20. Scheiber GJ, Poullier J-P. Recent trends in international health care spending. *Health Aff.* 1987; 6(3):105–112.

21. Task Force on the Allocation of Health Care Resources. *Health: A need for Redirection.* Ottawa: Canadian Medical Association; 1984.

22. Hoffenberg R. *Clinical Freedom.* London, England: Nuffield Provincial Hospitals Trust; 1987.

23. Relman AS. American medicine at the crossroads: signs from Canada. *N Engl J Med.* 1989; 320:590–591.

24. Stevenson HM, Williams AP, Vayda E. Medical politics and Canadian Medicare: professional response to the Canada Health Act. *Milbank Q.* 1988; 66:65.

25. Jonas HS, Etzel SI. Undergraduate medical education. *JAMA.* 1988; 260:1063–1071.

26. Ryten E. Medical schools in Canada. *JAMA.* 1988; 260:1157–1161.

27. US Bureau of the Census. *Statistical Abstract of the United States: 1989.* Washington, DC: Government Printing Office; 1989.

28. Seaver DJ, Huske MS. *Health Care Attitude Survey Shows Surprising Results.* Cambridge, Mass: Arthur D Little; 1988.

NO

Ronald Bronow

A NATIONAL HEALTH PROGRAM: ABYSS AT THE END OF THE TUNNEL—THE POSITION OF PHYSICIANS WHO CARE

Doctors Woolhandler and Himmelstein,[1] in their Commentary in the October 29, 1989, issue of THE JOURNAL, argue that a national health program based on the Canadian system is the best solution to the crisis in American health care financing. The authors, however, fail to recognize the negative repercussions of such a system, the consequences of which are now being fully realized in Canada.

The province of Saskatchewan started compulsory universal health insurance in 1961. The same province was among the first to announce it had run out of money for medical care services for 1987 and would be unable to pay for them for the rest of the year. Following a funding freeze imposed by Premier Grant Devine's Conservative government, Saskatchewan's hospitals faced a critical shortage of beds, with 1870 patients waiting for surgery at Saskatoon's University Hospital alone (*Macleans.* February 13, 1989:32). At the present time, health care in most provinces consumes more than one third of the total provincial budget, and the costs continue to rise. The province of Ontario shows projected expenditures for 1989 and 1990 of close to $14 billion, on total government revenues of $40 billion (W. Goodman, MD, oral communication, January 1990). Canadian provincial health and finance ministers recently issued a report arguing that the future quality of the system is threatened because the rate of growth in federal transfer payments to the provinces has averaged 9%, while health care expenditures are rising at an average rate of 11.3%—a familiar scenario. But, despite this, Prime Minister Mulroney has proposed a 2-year freeze on federal payments to the 10 provinces, moneys needed to help finance health care programs (*New York Times,* January 28, 1990:F13). A heated debate is raging over whether Canada can continue to afford the 20-year-old publicly funded universal system. The Canadian Medical Association and Canadian Hospital Association have

From Ronald Bronow, "A National Health Program: Abyss at the End of the Tunnel—The Position of Physicians Who Care," *Journal of the American Medical Association*, vol. 263, no. 18 (May 9, 1990), pp. 2488-2489. Copyright © 1989 by the American Medical Association. Reprinted by permission.

warned that underfinancing and rationing have created a two-tiered health care system in which those with money go to private clinics or the United States, while those without political connections and/or financial resources wait in "long queues." Moore[2] has warned that "unless a financing system creates incentives to dampen consumer demand, expenditure caps will only result in more rationing, reductions in the use of new technologies, and the further subjection of health care budgets to special interest group politics." Canada is faced with a system in which the funding is finite and limited, while the demands of the patients are not. The mounting strains on the system of medical care have raised the prospect that so-called user fees may eventually be needed to discourage Canadians from making needless medical visits (*Globe and Mail*. November 17, 1989:A12).

The politicians, to cope with the crisis, are restricting access to medical care. Hospitals across the country are taking beds out of service, limiting the number of operations they perform, and cutting back on other services, as provincial governments battle to keep down health care costs. There is a shortage of critical care and neonatal beds in Ontario. The Ontario Medical Association confirms that there has been a net decrease of about 2000 beds in the province during the past 1 to 2 years.[3] In Toronto an estimated 1000 people are facing waits of as long as a year for bypass operations at three hospitals. In Ontario the normal wait for cataract surgery is 5 to 6 months (*Financial Post*. January 20, 1989:11). During the past 2 years, most of the provinces have sought to curb costs by telling hospitals they will no longer pay for operating deficits (*Macleans*. February 13, 1989:32). Emergency departments in large hospitals in major Canadian cities have been shut down because of lack of beds. Important teaching hospitals have been unable to purchase new equipment without cutting back on traditional services.[4] More and more Canadian hospital beds are being occupied by elderly patients who stay there longer than 60 days, and whose costs are well below average. This prevents physicians from using the beds to treat short-term, acutely ill patients, exactly the opposite of the US system.[5]

Canadian politicians have blamed physicians for the mounting crisis. The Canadian government is arguing that physicians are refusing to advise their patients to use medical procedures that are the best value, but insist on advising patients on the best possible treatment. Certainly, physicians in Ontario have freely admitted this. Dr Henry Gassman, speaking on behalf of Ontario doctors, was quoted in the *Toronto Sun* on February 4, 1989: "Your doctor will not enter into any agreement which will sacrifice the accessibility or quality of care in favor of the government's agenda of cost reduction." The conflict arises because the government wants the physicians to serve as the "gatekeeper" who controls the rationing of medical services, and the physicians do not want the job.[6] Also in Ontario, the Health Ministry has told two hospital administrations that for them to receive desperately needed funding, the physicians on the staff must accept "alternative payment methods." The alternatives being considered include fixed salary for physicians and capitation. Ontario Health Minister Elinor Caplan stated, "We have said for quite some time that, as we look at alternative approaches to delivery of services, that there should be options available for both providers and consumers." She said, "We've been encouraging communities to look at innovative and creative proposals for the delivery of those kinds of services" (*Globe and Mail*. January 18, 1989:A8).[7] In Quebec, the government has put a ceiling on certain categories of income. Any fees earned by a general practitioner in excess of $164, 108 (Canadian) a year are reimbursed at a rate of 25%.[8] In 1987, the Manitoba government disposed of the system of binding arbitration for fee negotiations with the Manitoba Medical Association after physicians had been awarded a 5.7% fee increase. British Columbia has capped growth of physicians' payments at 3% per year.[5]

It has been argued that the above stories are merely anecdotal. If so, their sheer number demands attention. Our primary concern is that health care decisions are being made by the state, not the individual.

Considering the many Canadian problems and the rescinding here of the Medicare Catastrophic Coverage Act, it is unlikely that Congress will pass any major health care financing legislation in the immediate future. Our government, in struggling with its own budget deficits, will not be willing to transfer a very large segment of private financing to the tax rolls.[9] It would then have to finance health care for large poverty populations, a nonexistent situation in Canada. And, the price tag for a Canadian-style health care system? At least $339 billion in additional taxes, according to a study prepared for the National Center for Policy Analysis (*Business Insurance*. March 5, 1990:B8). Despite this, I see two quite different scenarios as to where American medicine will be by the turn of the century.

SCENARIO 1

There will be increased funding for health care for the poor. This will come from either state, county, or federal funds and will be funded by a direct tax increase, either federal or state. Other possibilities include a value-added tax, sales tax, or taxes on alcohol and tobacco consumption. There will be basic levels of health care coverage for the indigent. This coverage will be determined by guidelines worked out from treatment outcomes analysis, funds available, and value to society.

(During the early 1990s, the costs of American technology continued to overwhelm the short-term saving from managing of health care.[10] The following system of financing evolved, following extensive public debate.)

Every working American will be covered by a basic employer-funded program. Policies will be based on a $250 (or higher) yearly deductible payment. This will create less third-party interference and make insurance costs more predictable. If the employee decides to buy his or her own policy, the employer will contribute the same amount as for the employer-funded plan. Premiums, deductibles, and copayments will be tax deductible by the person paying the bill. But, the employer-funded premiums will be treated as taxable income to the employee (*New York Times*, February 21, 1990:A5). State pools and tax credits will help to ease the burden on small businesses. Health care decisions, again, will be made by the physician and the patient rather than the third party. The increased deductible will discourage overutilization, both by the patient and by the physician.[11] The costs of managing care will be dramatically decreased as insurance companies pay health benefits according to scientific guidelines used in medicine. The results of scientific outcomes analysis will be disseminated to the practicing physician. The insurance companies will use these guidelines to determine payment rather than questioning the physician's decision step-by-step, creating paperwork and increased bureaucratic costs. This shift in policy will have been initiated by the 1989 study from the National Academy of Science, which showed that utilization review, by managing site and duration of treatment rather than the need for services, did not alter the pattern of continued high rates of increase in health care costs. All savings had been largely offset by administrative costs and increased use of outpatient services.[12,13]

Health maintenance organizations will be limited to Kaiser-style staff-model plans. Independent practice associations based in physicians' offices will disappear as the health maintenance organizations find it impossible to make a profit in such groups without excessively rationing care.

The malpractice system will be reorganized into a workers' compensation-style commission. Claims will be heard, fault determined, and money awarded based on injuries and loss of further earning potential. Billions of dollars in unnecessary tests and procedures will be saved by taking malpractice out of the tort system.

Medicine will devise effective systems to punish bad physicians, while Congress will pass legislation to protect those who sit on peer review panels from charges of anticompetitiveness.

Outcomes and practice-pattern analysis of individual physicians will identify cost-effective, quality providers who will be rewarded by the payers. Physicians who overcharge and overutilize will also be identified. They will be advised to change their practice patterns or not continue on insurance company panels.

SCENARIO 2

Frustrations from the failure of managed care to slow medical inflation, along with the push of Congress to blame physicians for the health care crisis, will create a government one-payer system. Patients will believe they will be entitled to complete, free medical care. This will create a credit-card mentality among the American public. As in Canada, there will be unlimited demand for services with finite resources.[12] This will create delays in diagnostic testing and therapy, particularly surgical. As the money runs out of the "global budget," physicians will be blamed for overutilizing resources to increase their personal income. Punitive measures will then be instituted, such as salary caps and decreased future payments based on the budget deficit.

The overall quality of care in the United States will decrease as costs skyrocket and physicians lose their autonomy and their decision-making power. Patients who can afford it will seek private care, although most people will accept the system because it's free, and, as in Canada and England, public expectations will be significantly diminished.[14]

As was noted in the late 1980s, the quality of incoming medical students will continue to decrease. As doctors lose their decision-making power, they will also lose the joy of practicing medicine. Congress and the news media will answer by stating that physicians are basically greedy and will on to other fields when they realize they cannot make as much money in medicine.

Who could tip the balance between the two scenarios? American physicians. Will they lead, or watch from the sidelines? We will see what happens.

REFERENCES

1. Woolhandler S, Himmelstein DU. A national health program: northern light at the end of the tunnel. *JAMA*, 1989; 262:2136–2137.

2. Moore S. America's current love affair with the Canadian health system. *Health Care Trends Rep.* February 1989:1, 15, 16.

3. Nesdoly D. Guest editorial. *Fam Pract.* November 25, 1989:4.

4. Reece R. The Canadian health care system model. *Reece Rep.* April 1989:6.

5. Six tough questions. *Calif Phys.* October 1989:32n49.

6. Slemon C. *Health Care in Ontario: Ontario Libertarian Party Position Paper,* Toronto, Canada: Ontario Libertarian Party:1989.

7. Berube B, McAllister J. Blackmailed: Ontario doctors held to ransom over hospital. *Med Post.* January 14, 1989:1.

8. Lemieux P. Socialized medicine: the Canadian experience. *Freeman.* March 1989:97.

9. Kirshner E. Insider interview with Bernard S. Tresnwki. *Healthweek.* December 4, 1989:12–15.

10. Iglehart J. A conversation with William B. Schwartz. *Health Aff.* Fall 1989:71–73.

11. Manning W, Newhouse J, Duan N, et al. Health insurance and the demand for medical care: evidence from a randomized experiment. *RAND Health Insurance Experiments Series.* Santa Monica, Calif: RAND Corp: February 1988:24.

12. Moore S. The future of utilization management. *Health Care Trends Rep.* November 1989:1, 15, 16.

13. *Controlling Costs and Changing Patient Care? The Role of Utilization Management.* Washington, DC: National Academy Press: October 1989.

14. Iglehart J. A conversation with William B. Schwartz. *Health Aff.* Fall 1989:64–67.

POSTSCRIPT

Should the United States Follow the Canadian Model of a National Health Program?

The Bipartisan Commission on Health Care, appointed by former president Reagan and chaired by Senator John D. Rockefeller 4th (D.-W. Va.), proposed in March 1990 that employers be required either to provide their employees with insurance that covered hospital and doctor bills and preventive care or to contribute to a fund that would provide such coverage. Minnesota is one of the few states to experiment with state-subsidized health insurance; after two years of operation, nearly half of the eligible population has enrolled and participants have made greater use of preventive services. Several states, including New York, are implementing step-by-step changes. In January 1991, New York State began covering primary and preventive care for children under 13 whose families have incomes below a certain level. The plan does not cover costs of hospitalization of specialized dental, vision, or speech treatment. In addition, the New York State Department of Health has developed a proposal for universal health insurance. For a discussion of this proposal, see Dan E. Beauchamp and Ronald L. Rouse, "Universal New York Health Care: A Single-Payer Strategy Linking Cost Control and Universal Access," *The New England Journal of Medicine* (September 6, 1990).

For more detail on the Canadian system, see John K. Iglehart's three-part report "Canada's Health Care System," *The New England Journal of Medicine* (July 17, September 18, and December 18, 1986). A longer version of the proposal by Physicians for a National Health Program was published in *The New England Journal of Medicine* (January 12, 1989). A two-part series that emphasizes incremental, not radical, change is Alain Enthoven and Richard Kronick, "A Consumer-Choice Health Plan for the 1990s: Universal Health Insurance in a System Designed to Promote Quality and Economy," *The New*

England Journal of Medicine (January 5 and 12, 1989). Joseph A. Califano, Jr., a former secretary of Health, Education and Welfare (now the Department of Health and Human Services), advocates in *America's Health Care Revolution: Who Lives? Who Dies? Who Pays?* (Random House, 1986) a sweeping program of change: altering American health habits, reducing by half the number of hospital beds, and curbing excessive fees and profits. Also see Nicholas E. Davies and Louis H. Felder, "Applying Brakes to the Runaway American Health Care System: A Proposed Agenda," *Journal of the American Medical Association* (January 5, 1990).

CONTRIBUTORS
TO THIS VOLUME

EDITOR

CAROL LEVINE is the executive director of the Citizens Commission on AIDS for New York City and Northern New Jersey. She is managing editor of *IRB: A Review of Human Subjects Research* and was formerly editor of the *Hastings Center Report*, periodicals published by the Hastings Center in Briarcliff Manor, New York. Ms. Levine received her B.A. in history from Cornell and an M.A. in public law and government from Columbia University. She was codirector of the Hastings Center project on "AIDS and the Ethics of Public Health," and she writes and lectures widely on AIDS and other issues in bioethics.

STAFF

Marguerite L. Egan   Program Manager
Brenda S. Filley   Production Manager
Whit Vye   Designer
Libra Ann Cusack   Typesetting Supervisor
Juliana Arbo   Typesetter
David Brackley   Copy Editor
David Dean   Administrative Assistant
Diane Barker   Editorial Assistant
James and David Filley   Graphics

AUTHORS

LORI B. ANDREWS is a research fellow with the American Bar Foundation and a senior scholar at the Center for Clinical Medical Ethics at the University of Chicago. She is the principal author of *Feminist Perspectives on Reproductive Technologies* (American Bar Foundation, 1987) and the author of *Between Strangers: Surrogate Mothers, Expectant Fathers, and Brave New Babies* (Harper & Row, 1989).

MARCIA ANGELL is a physician and an executive editor of *The New England Journal of Medicine*.

GEORGE J. ANNAS is the Edward R. Utley Professor of Law and Medicine in the Schools of Medicine and Public Health at Boston University. He is the author of *The Rights of Doctors, Nurses, and Allied Health Professionals* (Avon, 1983).

JOHN D. ARRAS is the philosopher-in-residence in the Department of Epidemiology and Social Medicine at Albert Einstein College of Medicine/Montefióre Medical Center in New York City.

AMERICAN MEDICAL ASSOCIATION is a society of physicians, which was organized in 1847 to promote the science and art of medicine and the betterment of public health. Its main activities include evaluating drugs, foods, and medical equipment; coordinating research; and improving medical education standards.

MICHELE BARRY is a physician and a researcher with the Tropical Medicine and International Health Program in the School of Medicine at Yale University.

DIANA BAUMRIND is a research psychologist and the principal investigator for the Family Socialization and Developmental Competence Project of the University of California's Institute for Human Development in Berkeley, California. She has contributed numerous articles to professional journals and books and is on the editorial board for *Developmental Psychology*.

SISSELA BOK is an associate professor in the Department of Philosophy at Brandeis University in Waltham, Massachusetts, where she has taught since 1985. Her publications include *Lying: Moral Choice in Public and Private Life* (Random House, 1979) and *A Strategy for Peace: Human Values and the Threat of War* (Pantheon Books, 1989).

RONALD BRONOW is a physician and a member of the National Organization of Physicians Who Care in San Antonio, Texas.

DANIEL CALLAHAN, a philosopher, is the founder and director of The Hastings Center's Institute of Society, Ethics, and the Life Sciences and a member of the editorial advisory boards for *Technology in Society* and the *Journal of Bioethics*.

SIDNEY CALLAHAN is an associate professor in the Department of

Psychology at Mercy College in Dobbs Ferry, New York. Her publications include *The Illusion of Eve: Modern Women's Quest for Identity* (Sheed, 1965) and *Parenting: Principles and Politics of Parenthood* (Doubleday, 1973).

ARTHUR L. CAPLAN received his Ph.D. from Columbia University in 1979. He is the director of the Center for Biomedical Ethics at the University of Minnesota in Minneapolis. He is the coeditor of *Scientific Controversies: Case Studies in the Resolution and Closure of Disputes in Science and Technology* (Cambridge University Press, 1985), with H. Tristram Engelhardt, Jr.

FRANK A. CHERVENAK is a physician in the Department of Obstetrics and Gynecology in the New York Hospital of Cornell Medical Center.

JAMES F. CHILDRESS is a professor of medical education and a professor and chairman of religious studies at the University of Virginia at Charlottesville. He is a fellow of The Hastings Center's Institute of Society, Ethics, and the Life Sciences; a member of the Society of Christian Ethics; and a member of the American Theological Society. His publications include *Moral Responsibility in Conflicts: Essays on Nonviolence, War and Conscience* (Louisiana University Press, 1982) and *Who Should Decide: Paternalism in Health Care* (Oxford University Press, 1982).

PAUL CHODOFF is a physician and a clinical professor of psychiatry in the School of Medicine at George Washington University. He is the coeditor, with Sidney Bloch, of *Psychiatric Ethics* (Oxford University Press, 1981).

DOUGLAS CONDIT is the senior physician assistant in the Department of Cardiothoracic Surgery at Albert Einstein College of Medicine/Montefióre Medical Center in New York City.

CHARLES J. DOUGHERTY is a professor of philosophy and chairman of the Department of Philosophy at Creighton University in Omaha, Nebraska. He is the author of *Ideal, Fact, and Medicine: A Philosophy for Health Care* (University Press of America, 1985).

AMITAI ETZIONI is a professor in the Department of Sociology at George Washington University, where he has taught since 1968. He is a member of the board of Canadian Peace Research Institute and a member of the National Alliance for Safer Cities. His publications include *Capital Corruption: The New Attack on American Democracy* (Transaction Books, 1984) and *Moral Dimension: Toward a New Economics* (Free Press, 1988).

ROBERT W. M. FRATER is a professor and chairman of the Division of Cardiothoracic Surgery at Albert Einstein College of Medicine/Montefióre Medical Center in New York

City. He is a member of the editorial board for *Cardiac Chronicle: Journal of Cardiac Surgery*, a fellow of the Royal College of Surgeons, and a fellow of the American College of Cardiology.

BEVERLY WILDUNG HARRISON is a professor of Christian ethics at the Union Theological Seminary in New York. She is the author of *Our Right to Choose: Toward a New Ethic of Abortion* (Beacon Press, 1984) and *Making the Connections: Essays in Feminist Social Ethics* (Beacon Press, 1986).

MICHAEL R. HARRISON is the director of the Fetal Treatment Program at the University of California's San Francisco Medical Center.

WILLIAM R. HENDEE is the vice president of science and technology for the American Medical Association in Chicago, Illinois. He received his Ph.D. in physics from the University of Texas in 1962.

DAVID U. HIMMELSTEIN is a physician and a member of Physicians for a National Health Program at Cambridge, Massachusetts.

ALBERT R. JONSEN, a philosopher, is a professor and the chairman of the Department of Medical Ethics at the University of Washington's School of Medicine. He is on the board of directors for the Foundation of Critical Care Medicine and the Sierra Foundation, and is the author of *Clinical Ethics: A Prac-*

tical Approach to Ethical Decisions in Clinical Medicine (Macmillan, 1986).

MICHAEL H. KOTTOW is a physician at Olga Children's Hospital in Stuttgart, Federal Republic of Germany.

HERBERT T. KRIMMEL is a professor of law in the School of Law at Southwestern University in Los Angeles, California.

JEROD M. LOEB is a member of the American Medical Association's Group on Science and Technology.

JOANNE LYNN is an associate professor of health care services and medicine in the School of Medicine at George Washington University. She is the editor of *By No Extraordinary Means: The Choice to Forgo Life-Sustaining Food and Water* (Indiana University Press, 1986).

LAURENCE B. McCULLOUGH is a philosopher at the Center for Ethics, Medicine, and Public Issues at Baylor College of Medicine.

GILBERT MEILAENDER is a professor in the Department of Religion at Oberlin College. He is the author of *Friendship: A Study in Theological Ethics* (University of North Dakota Press, 1981); *The Theory and Practice of Virtue* (University of North Dakota Press, 1984); and *The Limits of Love: Some Theological Explorations* (Pennsylvania State University Press, 1987).

BERNARD C. MEYER is in the private practice of psychiatry in New York. He is a clinical professor of psychiatry at Mount Sinai Hospital School of Medicine.

The late **STANLEY MILGRAM** was a professor of psychology at the Graduate School and University Center of the City University of New York. He is the author of *Obedience to Authority: An Experimental View* (Harper & Row, 1975).

NANCY MILLIKEN is a physician in the Department of Obstetrics, Gynecology, and Reproductive Services at the University of California at San Francisco.

THOMAS H. MURRAY is the director of the Center for Biomedical Ethics in the School of Medicine at Case Western Reserve University in Cleveland, Ohio. He is the coeditor of *Feeling Good, Doing Better* (Humana, 1984) and *Which Babies Shall Live?* (Humana, 1985), with Arthur L. Caplan.

LAWRENCE J. NELSON is a philosopher in the Department of Medicine, Clinical Faculty Program in Medical Ethics, at the University of California at San Francisco.

DAVID ORENTLICHER is a physician and a lawyer with the Ethics and Health Policy Counsel and the Council on Ethical and Judicial Affairs for the American Medical Association.

DAVID T. OZAR is an associate professor and a director of graduate studies in health care ethics in the Department of Philosophy at Loyola University in Chicago, Illinois. He is also an adjunct associate professor at Loyola University's School of Medicine.

LYNN M. PETERSON is an assistant professor of medical ethics in the Department of Social Medicine and an assistant professor of surgery in the Department of Surgery at Harvard University.

The late **NATHANIEL PIER** was a New York City physician, AIDS researcher, and member of the Institutional Review Board of the Community Research Initiative.

TOM REGAN is an animal rights activist and a professor of philosophy at North Carolina State University. His publications include *All That Dwell Therein: Animal Rights and Environmental Ethics* (University of California Press, 1982) and *The Case for Animal Rights* (University of California Press, 1983).

DOUGLAS D. RICHMAN is a professor in the Department of Pathology and Medicine at the University of California at San Diego and a professor in the San Diego Veterans Administration Medical Center. He is also a member of the San Diego AIDS Clinical Treatment Group.

JOHN A. ROBERTSON is a professor of law in the School of Law at the University of Texas in Austin.

ALFRED M. SADLER, JR., practices internal medicine in Monterey, California. He served as a chief consultant to the Commissioners on Uniform State Laws in drafting the Uniform Anatomical Gift Act.

BLAIR L. SADLER is the president of the Children's Hospital of San Diego. She served as a chief consultant to the Commissioners on Uniform State Laws in drafting the Uniform Anatomical Gift Act.

M. ROY SCHWARZ is the senior vice president of medical education and science for the American Medical Association in Chicago, Illinois. He received his M.D. from the University of Washington's School of Medicine in 1963.

SHLOMO SHINNAR is on the staff of the Department of Neurology and the Department of Pediatrics at Albert Einstein College of Medicine/Montefióre Medical Center in New York City.

MARK SIEGLER is a professor of medicine and the director of the Center for Clinical Medical Ethics in the Pritzker School of Medicine at the University of Chicago. He is the coauthor of *Medical Innovation and Bad Outcomes: Legal, Social, and Ethical Responses* (Health Administration Press, 1987).

STEVEN J. SMITH, Ph.D., is a senior scientist in the Division of Drugs and Toxicology for the American Medical Association.

THOMAS S. SZASZ is a psychiatrist, a psychoanalyst, and a professor in the Department of Psychiatry at State University of New York's Upstate Medical Center at Syracuse, New York, where he has taught since 1956. He is the senior and visiting scholar for the Faculty Improvement Program of the Eli Lilly Foundation and a member of the Board of Governors of the International Academy of Forensic Psychology.

JAMES W. TEGTMEIER is a student in the School of Law at Boston University.

SIDNEY H. WANZER is a physician with Emerson Hospital in Concord, Massachusetts.

STEFFIE WOOLHANDLER is a physician in the Division of Social and Community Medicine at the Cambridge Hospital of Harvard Medical School.

INDEX